# Performing Arts Medicine

# Performing Arts Medicine

LAUREN E. ELSON, MD
Director of Dance Medicine
Physical Medicine and Rehabilitation
Sports Medicine
Harvard Medical School
Boston, MA, United States

Spaulding Rehabilitation
Charlestown, MA, United States

ELSEVIER

# ELSEVIER

3251 Riverport Lane
St. Louis, Missouri 63043

Performing Arts Medicine

ISBN: 978-0-323-66212-3

*Publisher:* Cathleen Sether
*Content Strategist:* Kayla Wolfe
*Editorial Project Manager:* Sandra Harron
*Production Project Manager:* Kiruthika Govindaraju
*Cover Designer:* Alan Studholme

Typeset by TNQ Technologies

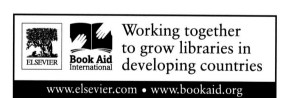

# List of Contributors

**Kathryn E. Ackerman, MD, MPH**
Assistant Professor
Medicine
Harvard Medical School
Boston, MA, United States

Director — Female Athlete Program
Divisions of Sports Medicine and Endocrinology
Boston Children's Hospital
Boston, MA, United States

Associate Director — Sports Endocrine Research Lab
Neuroendocrine Unit
Boston Children's Hospital
Boston, MA, United States

**Marshall Chasin, MSc, AuD**
Director of Audiology
Audiology
Musicians' Clinics of Canada
Toronto, ON, Canada

**John P. Chong, MD, FRCPC**
Medical Director
Artists' Psychophysiology and Ergonomics
Musicians' Clinics of Canada
Hamilton, ON, Canada

**Kathleen L. Davenport, MD, CAQSM**
Physical Medicine and Rehabilitation
Sports Medicine
Memorial Rehabilitation Institute
Hollywood, FL, United States

Company Physician Miami City Ballet
Miami, FL, United States

**Randall W. Dick, MS, FACSM**
American College of Sports Medicine
Indianapolis, IN, United States

**Jayme Rose Dowdall, MD**
Assistant Professor
University of Nebraska Medical Center
Nebraska Medicine
Omaha, NE , United States

**Lauren E. Elson, MD**
Director of Dance Medicine
Physical Medicine and Rehabilitation
Sports Medicine
Harvard Medical School
Boston, MA, United States

Spaulding Rehabilitation
Charlestown, MA, United States

**Joana L. Fraser, MD, RYT**
Clinical Instructor
Sports Medicine
Boston Children's Hospital
Boston, MA, United States

**Marina Gearhart, BA**
Research Coordinator
Division of Sports Medicine
Boston Children's Hospital
Boston, MA, United States

**Matthew Grierson, MD**
Physical Medicine and Rehabilitation
Sports Medicine
Seattle Spine and Sports Medicine
Seattle, WA, United States

**Scott Homer, MD, BM Jazz Studies**
Instructor
Physical Medicine and Rehabilitation
Harvard Medical School
Boston, MA, United States

Spaulding Rehabilitation
Charlestown, MA, United States

Associate Physiatrist Orthopedic Surgery, Hand Division
Brigham and Women's Hospital
Boston, MA, United States

**Melody Hrubes, MD**
Assistant Professor
Physical Medicine and Rehabilitation
Sports Medicine
University of Illinois at Chicago Hospital
Chicago, IL, United States

**Nancy Kadel, MD**
Orthopaedic Surgeon
Group Health Physicians
Seattle, WA, United States

**Lynda Mainwaring, PhD, C. PSYCH**
Associate Professor
Faculty of Kinesiology and Physical Education
University of Toronto
Toronto, ON, Canada

**Shulamit Mor, PhD, C. PSYCH**
Mor Centre for Performance Psychology
York University
Toronto, ON, Canada

**Steven Rock, MD**
Primary Care Sports Medicine
Musculoskeletal Center
Medical Associates Clinic
Dubuque, IA, United States

**Selina Shah, MD, FACP**
Sports and Dance Medicine
Walnut Creek, CA, United States

**Heather Southwick, PT, MSPT**
Director of Physical Therapy
Boston Ballet
Boston, MA, United States

**Andrea Stracciolini, MD, FAAP, FACSM**
Sports Medicine
Boston Children's Hospital
Boston, MA, United States

Waltham, MA, United States

**Serena Weren, DMA**
Assistant Professor of Music
College of Music and Fine Arts
Loyola University New Orleans
New Orleans, LA, United States

**Matthew Wyon, PhD, MSc**
Professor Dance Science
Institute of Sport and Health Sciences
University of Wolverhampton
Wolverhampton, United Kingdom

Researcher
National Institute of Dance Medicine and Science
Birmingham, United Kingdom

**Amy X. Yin, MD**
Sports Medicine
Department of Orthopedics, Podiatry,
     and Sports Medicine
Kaiser Permanente San Leandro Medical Center
San Leandro, CA, United States

**Kate LaRiviere Homer, MM**
University of Michigan Medical Center
Ann Arbor, MI, United States

**Meghan L. Keating, MPAS, PA-C**
Physician Assistant
Boston Children's Hospital
Boston, MA, United States

**Allyson L. Parziale, BS**
Clinical Research Assistant
Boston Children's Hospital
Boston, MA, United States

# Preface

Although performing artists spend hours of time fine tuning their body to achieve a high level of physical function, they often do not see themselves as athletes because their end goal is the production of art. As a result, many of the concepts of performance enhancement including cross-training, periodization, specificity, and overload may not be applied to their training, predisposing them to injury. Competition and culture interfere with the artists' utilization of the medical field when they do have symptoms; they believe that physicians do not understand the challenges and the consequences of disclosing an injury. The successful treatment of the performing artist requires the understanding of the emotional vulnerability of the patient as well as the utilization of a team to comprehensively address the psychosocial aspects of rehabilitation as they apply to the individual.

Treating the performing artist can be extremely rewarding. They are extremely motivated to not only attain their previous level of function, but to strive for improvement. This book provides treatment approaches for physicians that encounter this special population.

I am honored to bring together experts from the Performing Arts Medicine Community to share principles on optimizing management of the performing artist. Randy Dick, champion of the Athletes in the Arts movement, introduces us to the cross-pollination of the sports and performing arts fields. The reciprocal sharing of knowledge is leading to advances in the prevention, diagnosis, treatment, and rehabilitation of performing arts injuries and to the improvement of kinesthetic awareness and training strategies for athletes. Chapters 2 and 3 provide context and examples of strategies to ensure that the needs of the artists are met. Musculoskeletal and neurological syndromes seen in musicians are presented in Chapter 4 with attention to specific considerations for treatment and rehabilitation for this population. Chapter 5 demonstrates the importance of the biopsychosocial model in treating and rehabilitating musicians. A common, but not often discussed, occupational risk for musicians is hearing loss. Information and education regarding prevention and treatment

of auditory symptoms can be found in Chapter 6. Chapter 7 addresses the unique injuries that arise in the marching musician. Region specific pathologies seen in dancers, including their predisposing risks, diagnosis, and management are described in Chapters 8–10. Dance injuries are extremely prevalent in the adolescent dancer due to biomechanical changes and social pressures. These are addressed in depth in Chapter 11. Screening is a hot topic in the sports medicine world—if risks that predispose an individual to injury can be eliminated, valuable time and money can be saved. Chapter 12 discusses the current thoughts surrounding the utility of screening professional dancers and gives an up-to-date account of the literature and practice recommendations from Dance USA, the governing body of professional dance companies in North America.

Due to the aesthetic demand for lean dancers, bone health is often compromised in professional ballet dancers. The risks for injury and implications in treatment are reviewed in Chapter 13. Dr. Matthew Wyon, one of the eminent researchers on dance and physiology addresses the importance of and strategies for cross-training in dancers. Perhaps one of the most important concepts in working with dancers is the "can-do" approach for rehabilitation. Dancers always need to be given proactive activities that can keep them engaged throughout the rehabilitation process. Chapter 15 is a guide for dance rehabilitation. In Chapter 16, psychiatric diagnoses common in performing artists and initial treatment steps and recommendations are reviewed. Lastly, in Chapter 17, common symptoms affecting the vocal artist are discussed along with management strategies.

I want to thank the authors for sharing their expertise and passion for the care of the performing artist.

**Lauren E. Elson, MD**
*Director of Dance Medicine*
*Physical Medicine and Rehabilitation, Sports Medicine*
*Harvard Medical School*
*Boston, MA, United States*
*Spaulding Rehabilitation*
*Charlestown, MA, United States*

# Contents

## CHAPTER 1

# Sport or Art? The Intersection of Sports and Performing Arts Medicine

RANDALL W. DICK, MS, FACSM

Performing artists are athletes (see https://vimeo.com/67806662 for visual confirmation).

Just like sport athletes, they:
- practice or perform almost every day,
- face extreme competition,
- play through pain,
- compete in challenging environments,
- experience little "off-season,"
- face the risk of mental burnout, physical overuse, and other career-threatening injury.

Consider the work schedules of a professional performing artist and a baseball player. Both perform/play in the evening (8–11 p.m. or later) with a schedule that may repeat over 150 games/performances a season. Their routine becomes habitual with disturbed eating and sleeping habits such as sleeping late into the morning/early afternoon, skipping breakfast or not eating at all. A "Day in the Life" of either profession might include:
- Sleep late (arise at 10 a.m.)
- Breakfast (possibly)
- Free time until midafternoon if not taking extra batting practice or training an understudy
- Arrive at venue midafternoon for sound check/batting practice
- Pre-event meal
- Further warm-up/video review
- Start at 7 p.m.
- End at 11 p.m.
- Postevent meal
- Recovery/unwind
- Travel to new city

In this scenario, the professional baseball player has access to nutrition information to help him understand what and when to eat, medical support for injury prevention and rehab, film review to modify posture and mechanics, pitch counts to reduce the risk of overuse injuries, and a sport psychologist to help with mental fatigue or a batting slump. The performing artist has few if any of these resources, yet many of the same needs to optimize performance.[1]

Performing artists are an underserved population related to medical coverage, care, injury prevention, performance enhancement, and wellness. This book provides an outstanding opportunity to learn how medical professionals can fill this gap by both applying existing knowledge of treating sport athletes (e.g., nutrition, injury prevention, rehabilitation) and gaining a better understanding of performers' unique issues (hearing loss, focal dystonia, biomechanical compensations). By better understanding the needs of a very diverse performing arts population (professional to street performers, youth to elderly, dynamic drum corps to stationary orchestra), and various instruments/activities (strings, horns, guitars, percussion, or keyboards to vocals, dance, or acting) and applying existing concepts and knowledge, sports medicine professionals can expand their impact to a new patient base that desperately needs their support.

*You play in a bar room, people are smoking, there are long hours, practicing, you carry equipment to your gig. The idea of all of this (health needs) is foreign to the music community, from the conservatory level to the level of street performers and everything in between.*

**JONATHON BATISTE, PROFESSIONAL MUSICIAN.**

## WHAT IS THE ISSUE?

While there is significant published research on sport athlete injury type, mechanism, and prevalence, only small pockets of such information exist in the performing arts world.[2-4]

- Orchestra—Up to 88.6% of orchestral musicians reported pain during the previous year, and an average of 84.2% of orchestral musicians indicated pain interfering with playing during their lifetime[5]
- Orchestra—75% of orchestra instrumentalists will develop at least one musculoskeletal disorder from playing during their lifetimes[6]
- Marching band—Over 60% of a sample of world-class drum corps reported at least one stress fracture during their 2013 season (unpublished survey—Drum Corp Medical Project). Such performances typically require performers to play music while executing intricate marching maneuvers and choreography at speeds that can exceed 200 beats/min.
- Instrumental, voice—67% of school-aged musicians,[7] 70.6% of undergraduate students, 64.4% of graduate students, and 54.9% of professors[8] reported playing or singing-related pain.
- Dance—67% to 95% of pro ballet and modern dancers suffer injuries annually (2-7 injuries per dancer)[9,10]
- Music—50% of undergraduate music majors reporting pain while playing sought out their music teacher for assistance, 30% report going to nobody, and only 11% report going to a medical professional[8]
- All—45% of student musicians have noise-induced hearing loss compared with 11.5% in the general population[11]

These limited data highlight a real concern about the health and safety risks of these populations and underscore the opportunity for medical personnel to make a real difference in the lives of performing artists. The following chapters will expand on that opportunity. However, a foundation of basic health education is an important component to emphasize when dealing with performing artists:

*At the root of the problem is that our performers have poor health seeking patterns. Approximately 67% of New Orleans Musician's Clinic (NOMC) patients do not have a regular health provider. What brings them to the NOMC is generally an occupationally complaint—however what the NOMC medical team battles every day is death by lifestyle as the majority of our patients suffer from one or more chronic conditions which demand prevention strategies and on-going care. Depression, Hypertension, Diabetes, Obesity, Asthma being most prevalent. And when you look at the high suicide rate amongst the creative community—it is clear that mental illness goes hand and hand with many of the medical problems—but treatment resources are few*

**BETHANY BULTMAN, COFOUNDING DIRECTOR AND CHAIR, NEW ORLEANS MUSICIANS ASSISTANCE FOUNDATION.**

Specific topics that should be considered when dealing with performing artists include:

- *"Common" Sports Medicine Issues*: Nutrition, overuse, injury prevention, cross-training, mental health, substance abuse, and acclimatization strategies.
- *"Unique" Issues*: The 6-8 h of daily practice many music and dance students believe is the path to success expose them to hearing issues and overuse/repetitive trauma.
  - *Hearing Loss*: Noise-induced hearing loss is a flagship issue that affects up to 50% of musicians and may be the "concussion" of the performing arts world. Many musicians practice 6-8 h/day. Dynamic range of music, live or recorded, can peak at or above 95 dB. Hearing damage can occur when exposed to these volumes daily for 60 min or less, and many performing artists have some form of hearing loss as a result. Music itself is not the issue; loudness and its duration are the concern. Permanent noise-induced hearing loss is irreversible.
  - *Repetitive Motion/Overuse*: Established research tells us how many pitches are thrown in a baseball game, how many steps one would take in a marathon or the number of miles a soccer player might run in a match. Such information can help medical professionals understand the loads, energy, and strain involved in these sport activities and help in developing diets, recovery, or prevention prescriptions. However, there is very little information available to help the medical professional assess overuse in the performing arts. For example, how many dance steps are in a Broadway show, violin bow strokes in a movement, or notes sung in an opera?
- *Injury Prevention and Recovery*: While most health professionals know how to strengthen or rehab a quadriceps muscle, many may not know (for example) about training and recovery for the small muscles around the mouth (the embouchure) which are so critical to a wind or reed player.
- *Practice and Performance*: What is the volume and type of practice needed to optimize health and performance? When do additional practice hours hurt rather than help?

- *Preparticipation Exam*—A sports preparticipation exam or screening is a foundation of sport participation at any level. Such a document or mindset does not exist in most of the performing arts community.

## PRACTICE AND PERFORMANCE IN PERSPECTIVE

In most sports, there are objective measures that can be used to show individual improvement. These include variables measured by time (speed, agility, pitch velocity) or distance (jump height or length, throw length). Pre- and posttraining measures of these variables can indicate improvement. Even team sports have a metric—the final score.

Defining improvement in performing arts is more subjective (similar to sports such as gymnastics and diving). The audience or critics become the judges. The element of creativity is even more pronounced in the arts and even harder to define. Yet performing artists spend countless hours practicing to get better; a "better" that may not be able to be objectively measured. The medical professional must understand the challenging of "measuring" optimal performance in a performing artist population.

In addition, the work of Ericsson and colleagues[12] on training patterns of elite musicians has set the standard for many young aspiring performers in musical, athletic, and academic arenas. These researchers report that 10,000 h of "deliberate practice," training focused on improvement as opposed to enjoyment, is the threshold that distinguishes good from expert-level performers.

So what is the optimal number of hours to practice? At what point do additional hours of practice hurt rather than help performance? There is much to learn in this area; however, the sport athlete world provides some guidance:

- At the college level, NCAA sport athletes may participate in no more than 20 h of practice a week, with 1 day per week completely off. These rules are in place to allow student-athletes time to be students, but also for health and safety reasons. Ironically, at many of these same institutions with performing arts programs, many music and dance students are practicing 6—8 h a day.
- Baseball pitchers of all ages are monitored for pitch counts.[13] As pitchers rise in level of competitiveness, the pitch counts increase gradually as their physical development and training increases. Individuals at risk or returning from an injury may be monitored closely as well.
- Many sport athletes cross-train to maintain aerobic fitness while minimizing the mental and physical stress associated with their principal activity. Soccer players play basketball, swimmers do running workouts, and vice versa.
- Young athletes often are ill-equipped physically, socially, and psychologically to handle the rigors of intense training and make informed decisions about their training path. Daily training demands in addition to academic and other social activities can exhaust children. Youth in today's culture are driven to train early and extensively. Early specialization and extensive training creates well-documented risks of overuse injury, burnout, stress, and less enjoyment in youth sports.[14—17]
- Organizational policy and guidelines have the potential to enhance education, and when needed, behavior modification. Sports medicine guidelines from the NCAA (e.g., preparticipation physical exams[18]), position stands from the American College of Sports Medicine (e.g., participation in extreme environments[19]), and recommendations from the American Academy of Pediatric[14] have been successful in enhancing health and safety in sport.

These findings from the world of sports intuitively have application to performing artists and should provide a framework around which to consider the information in the subsequent chapters. For example:

- Encourage performing artists to establish a relationship with a medical professional before the need for acute care. This involves medical staff supplementing traditional health screening by adding performance-specific screenings (such as hearing) and pre-participation exams and wellness counseling.
- Understand the performing artist's ultimate goal and how long and how intense (per week) they are working to achieve it. Discuss a typical week and length, start-end times and intensity of all activities as well as external factors such as travel, teaching, and existing health issues.
- Observe their performance in your office (or via video). Understand specifics of the activity and evaluate posture, ergonomics, and repetitive motion.
- Discuss what metrics are used to measure performance. The ability to identify and objectively measure improvement in each aspect of the performing arts is essential to better understand the type and volume of practice necessary to optimize performance and minimize injury risk.
- Discuss *focused* practice segments with different goals in each session. Rote repetition for extended periods of time has not proven successful in the sport athletic world.

- Create a plan to gradually increase practice volume and intensity. Large *acute* increases in the time spent physically practicing/performing have been shown to increase risk of injury.
- Employ a mental or physical activity that allows the person to occasionally focus on something different than their primary activity (cross-train).
- Define and emphasize rest and recovery when possible.
- Introduce the concept of "Exercise is Medicine." Help them understand how much their instrument weighs and the strength needed to hold it during long stretches of practice, how many repetitive strokes they take a day, and how much their posture is dependent on core strength. Encourage them to invest in themselves, in order to enhance their ability and longevity to play or perform.
- The National Association of Schools of Music (NASM), representing over 600 schools of music, has an existing health and safety standard that reads, in part:

*It is the obligation of the institution that all students in music programs be fully apprised of health and safety issues …inherent in practice, performance, teaching and listening… Students enrolled in music unit programs and faculty and staff with employment status in the music unit must be provided basic information about the maintenance of health and safety within the contexts of practice, performance, teaching, and listening.[20]*

In addition, Texas recently adopted the Texas Essential Knowledge and Skills in Fine Arts standards for the 2.7 million middle and high school students requiring education in "health and wellness concepts related to music practice such as body mechanics, repetitive motion injury prevention, first-aid training, hearing protection, vocal health, hydration, and appropriate hygienic practices."[21]

While these standards apply to every NASM and Texas middle and high school, most institutions do not have the knowledge or resources to address these issues. There is a great opportunity (and need) for medical personnel to collaborate with their local schools (some of which may exist on the same high school or college campus you currently support) through these standards. Collectively, this effort can enhance the knowledge and wellness of millions of music students annually and the future generations they touch, through both performing and teaching.

*The conservatory environment is very different. I went six years and never in any of my lessons was there any instruction about nutrition or any sort of quantifiable method to determine the pros and cons of playing long hours. If I missed a note, I was just told to do it again, to practice more.*
**JONATHON BATISTE, PROFESSIONAL MUSICIAN.**

## ATHLETES AND THE ARTS—A NATIONAL COLLABORATIVE AND CHANGE AGENT

Launched at the May 2013 ACSM meeting, Athletes and the Arts (AATA) is a multiorganizational collaboration focused on linking the sport athlete and musician/performing artist communities through collaborative exchange and application of wellness, training, and performance research and initiatives.[22] This program is committed to the belief that athletes exist throughout the performing arts community and that established practice, wellness, and injury prevention research for sport athletes also is applicable to performing artists (see Table 1.1 for collaborating organizations and www. athletesandthearts.com for educational resources).

| TABLE 1.1 Athletes and the Arts (AATA) Collaborating Organizations as of August 1, 2018 |
|---|
| ***American College of Sports Medicine (ACSM)*** |
| ***Center for Music Arts Entrepreneurship, Loyola University (New Orleans)*** |
| ***Performing Arts Medical Association (PAMA)*** |
| *American Academy of Podiatric Sports Medicine* |
| *American Medical Society for Sports Medicine (AMSSM)* |
| *American Osteopathic Academy of Sports Medicine (AOASM)* |
| *Association for Applied Sport Psychology (AASP)* |
| *Drum Corp International (DCI)* |
| *Healthcare for Artists* |
| *International Association for Dance Medicine and Science (IADMS)* |
| *MusiCares* |
| *Music Teachers National Association (MTNA)* |
| *National Association for Music Education (NAfME)* |
| *National Association of Teachers of Singing (NATS)* |
| *National Athletic Trainers' Association (NATA)* |
| *National Hearing Conservation Association* |
| *New Orleans Musician's Clinic* |
| *The Voice Foundation* |

Founding Organizations in Bold

AATA Mission—Integrating the science of sports and the performing arts for mutual benefit by:

- creating opportunities for performing artists and sport athletes to access and benefit from the established research, training, and education of the other discipline,
- providing medical personnel, music and dance educators, and performing artists access to resources that meet the unique wellness, healthcare, and performance needs of performing artists,
- uniting organizational efforts to create a sustainable national initiative that addresses the needs of performing artists through multiple channels.

Through the efforts of AATA partners, many initiatives have been or are in the process of being developed to enhance support of performing artists. Three examples are presented to raise awareness of opportunities for medical personnel to get involved:

- **Dancer, instrumentalist, vocalist, and actor (DIVA) Preparticipation screening for performing artists tool**

  Preparticipation medical screening of sport athletes has become mandatory at many levels with a standard preparticipation physical exam having been developed by various medical organizations. More recently concussion baseline testing has been added to this package. However, as noted above and in the subsequent chapters, performing artists often have active and long annual schedules and injury risks at least comparable with sports athletes. Unlike sport athletes, performing artists are not usually screened annually before active participation, and accepted evaluation tools for this population do not exist.

  The dancer, instrumentalist, vocalist, and actor (DIVA) preparticipation screening tool has been in development since the summer of 2015 under the guidance of Bronwen Ackermann and the Performing Arts Medicine Association and represents a current best-practice approach. It includes a selection of the most reliable and clinically relevant tools that fit with the pragmatic goal of the test being administered in one sitting. The tool is designed for all performing artists (dancers, instrumentalists, vocalists, and actors) and is divided so that relevant sections can be used at the discretion of the health professional. Publication is planned for 2018 in the *Medical Problems of Performing Artists*. For more information, contact Bronwen Ackermann at bronwen.ackermann@sydney.edu.au or Julie Massaro at executive@artsmed.org.

- **Performing Arts Medicine certification**

  The Essentials of Performing Arts Medicine is a multidisciplinary continuing professional development course designed to meet the professional interests and career goals of clinicians as well as developing components targeting performing arts educators and performing artists. Created by the Performing Arts Medicine Association (PAMA) Education Committee in 2016, this course addresses specific opportunities and techniques for education, assessment, prevention, and treatment in response to various arts-specific health concerns. Collectively, research-informed lectures engage participants on specific health concerns relating to problems that are unique to performing artists.[23] For more information, contact Julie Massaro at executive@artsmed.org.

- **Grammy MusiCares**

  The Recording Academy's charity MusiCares provides a safety net of critical assistance for music people in times of need. MusiCares also focuses the resources and attention of the music industry on human service issues that directly impact the health and welfare of the professional music community.

  To better address the ever-growing number of music professionals without basic medical coverage, high deductibles, or limited catastrophic coverage, MusiCares works closely with a dedicated group of volunteer healthcare professionals through the MusiCares Medical Network to provide the valuable and often life-changing services that some clients require but simply cannot afford. The network is comprised of providers who recognize this reality and generously donate their time and expertise to treat MusiCares' referrals that are uninsured and lack the means to pay for services. Through the efforts of these professionals, clients are able to access specialty care that may not otherwise be available to them. MusiCares vets the client's eligibility and refers to the providers in the network when appropriate; providers are not contacted directly.[24]

  Medical Network providers are needed in a variety of specialty areas nationwide, including internal medicine, anesthesia, orthopedic surgery, general surgery, physical therapy, ophthalmology, dentistry, occupational therapy, podiatry, urology, otolaryngology, dermatology, addiction medicine, and family medicine.

MusiCares also has developed a range of nationwide clinics, workshops, and programs to address the health and wellness needs of music professionals. For more information, see https://www.grammy.com/musicares

## CONCLUSION

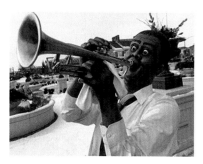

Imagine the following scenario for a trumpet player:

- Regular morning exercise program for wellness and to increase aerobic capacity
- Annual hearing tests
- Modify practice time and substitute with other cross-training activities
- Swim to strengthen arms and shoulders to account for the extending support of a 4-pound instrument
- Core strengthening to enhance posture, diaphragm, and breath control
- Modify nutrition (less fried foods)
- Modify hydration (volume and type)

While this book focuses on the health care professional, it is important to understand that this information is also very relevant to both the performing artist and the music/dance teacher/choreographer (the coach in the sport scenario). Just as in the sports world, these groups must work in conjunction with the medical team to understand and effectively enact any recommendations.

Some key messages to remember:

- Know if you are seeing a performing artist and encourage them to include you on their "team" before they have an issue.
- Ask them to play/dance for you and to document a week's worth of activity so you can understand the ergonomics and volume of the activity.
- Understand that the volume of practice/performance hours and number of repetitive motions may far exceed anything experienced in a comparable skilled sport athlete.

- Understand what optimal performance means and how it is measured in their world.
- Educate about and test for noise-induced hearing loss.
- Discuss rest and recovery, foreign subjects to most performing artists.
- Consider a preparticipation physical exam for performing artists (see DIVA).
- Discuss possible benefits of aerobic, core, or targeted area strength conditioning.

Performing artists are an underserved population. Sports medicine health professionals can be a valuable resource for filling this gap by applying their existing knowledge of treating sport athletes while gaining a better understanding of the performer's unique needs and environment.

This book, AATA and its collaborative organizations are positioned to assist medical personnel, performance arts educators, and the performers themselves in optimizing health and performance. By integrating the science of sport concepts into the performing arts population, sports medicine professionals can expand their impact to an entirely new patient base that desperately needs their help. Take advantage of this opportunity.

*Music is healing and if you want to heal other people, you've got to heal yourself first. The healthier we are as musicians and the arts community in general, the better the world will be.*

**JONATHON BATISTE—AMBASSADOR, ATHLETES AND THE ARTS.**

## REFERENCES

1. Dick RW, Berning JR, Dawson W, Ginsburg RD, Miller C, Shybut GT. Athletes and the arts—the role of sports medicine in the performing arts. *Curr Sports Med Rep.* 2013; 12(6):397−403.
2. Schaefer PT, Speier J. Common medical problems of instrumental athletes. *Curr Sports Med Rep.* 2012;11(6):316−322.
3. Kenny D, Driscoll T, Ackermann B. Is playing in the pit really the pits?: Pain, strength, music performance anxiety, and workplace satisfaction in professional musicians in stage, pit, and combined stage/pit orchestras. *Med Probl Perform Art.* 2016;31(1):1−7.
4. Ackermann B, Driscoll T, Kenny D. Musculoskeletal pain and injury in professional orchestral musicians in Australia. *Med Probl Perform Art.* 2012;27(4):181−187.
5. Silva AG, Lã FM, Afreixo V. Pain prevalence in instrumental musicians: a systematic review. *Med Probl Perform Art.* 2015;30(1):8−19.
6. Leaver R, Harris EC, Palmer KT. Musculoskeletal pain in elite professional musicians from British symphony orchestras. *Occup Med.* 2011;61(8):549−555.

7. Ranelli S, Smith A, Straker L. Playing-related musculoskeletal problems in child instrumentalists: the influence of gender, age and instrument exposure. *Int J Music Educ.* 2011;29(1):28−44.

8. Stanek JL, Komes KD, Murdock Jr FA. A cross-sectional study of pain among us college music students and faculty. *Med Probl Perform Art.* 2017;32(1):20.

9. Garrick JG, Requa RK. Ballet injuries. An analysis of epidemiology and financial outcome. *Am J Sports Med.* 1993; 21(4):586−590.

10. Allen N, Nevill A, Brooks J, Koutedakis Y, Wyon M. Ballet injuries: injury incidence and severity over 1 year. *J Orthop Sports Phys Ther.* 2012;42(9):781−790.

11. Phillips SL, Henrich VC, Mace ST. Prevalence of noise-induced hearing loss in student musicians. *Int J Audiol.* 2010;49(4):309−316.

12. Ericsson KA, Krampe RT, Tesch-Romer C. The role of deliberate practice in the acquisition of expert performance. *Psychol Rev.* 1993;100:363−406.

13. Little League International Baseball. Softball Web site; 2018 [Internet]. https://www.littleleague.org/partnerships/pitch-smart/

14. American Academy of Pediatrics Committee on Sports Medicine and Fitness. Intensive training and sports specialization in young athletes. *Pediatrics.* 2000;106:154−157.

15. Butcher J, Lindner KJ, Johns DP. Withdrawal from competitive youth sport: a retrospective ten-year study. *J Sport Behav.* 2002;25:145−163.

16. Côté J, Baker J, Abernethy B. Practice and play in the development of sport expertise. In: Tenenbaum REG, ed. *Handbook of Sport Psychology.* Hoboken, NJ: Wiley; 2007:184−202.

17. Côté J, Lidor R, Hackfort D. ISSP position stand: to sample or to specialize? Seven postulates about youth sport activities that lead to continued participation and elite performance. *Int J Sport Exerc Psychol.* 2009;9: 7−17.

18. National Collegiate Athletic Association (NCAA). *Sports Medicine Handbook.* Indianapolis, Indiana: The National Collegiate Athletic Association; July 2016:46206−46222. Twenty-seventh edition www.NCAA.org.

19. American College of Sports Medicine Position Stand. Exertional heat illness during training and competition. *Med Sci Sports Exerc.* 2007;39:556−572.

20. National Association of Schools of Music (NASM). *Handbook: Health and Safety Standard.* 11250 Roger Bacon Drive, Suite 21, Reston, Virginia: National Association of Schools of Music; 2012−13:20190−25248. Pub Jan 24, 2013 http://nasm.arts-accredit.org. p. 67.

21. Texas Essential Knowledge and Skills in Fine Arts Web site [Internet]. Dallas, TX: Texas Education Association. Available from: http://ritter.tea.state.tx.us/rules/tac/chapter117/ch117b.html, http://ritter.tea.state.tx.us/rules/tac/chapter117/ch117c.html.

22. Athletes and the Arts Web site [Internet]. Denver, CO: Athletes and the Arts. Available from: http://www.athletesandthearts.com.

23. Performing Arts Medicine Association Web site [Internet]. Denver, CO: Performing Arts Medicine Association. Available from: http://www.artsmed.org/.

24. Grammy MusiCares Web site [Internet]. Los Angeles, CA. Available from: https://www.grammy.com/musicares/programs.

## CHAPTER 2

# Treating the Performing Artist: Special Considerations

SELINA SHAH, MD, FACP

## INTRODUCTION

The performing arts is a broad term that encompasses dance, music, theater, and circus arts. All share a common ground of combining aesthetics, whether visual or auditory, and repetitive stress of muscle groups that are utilized in their respective genres. As both an artist and athlete, performing artists experience physical and psychological stressors of both realms.

At the professional level, performances can last a few hours, similar to a sports game such as American football or a tennis match. Although performing artists are athletes, they are different in that there is an emphasis of artistry with the goal of presenting a pleasing performance for the audience. As an audience member of a sports competition, one can often see the work and fatigue of the athlete demonstrated by gesturing or grunting. Although similar fatigue can occur in artists, it is rarely demonstrated in performance. Imagine sitting in the audience of the Swan Lake Ballet and seeing the principal dancer performing the Swan solo grunt on stage. Not many would likely attend another performance!

To understand how to care for a performing artist, it is important to understand what they do.

## BACKGROUND ON DANCE

The common dance studio styles include ballet, jazz, modern (lyrical and contemporary), hip hop, and tap. Other styles, found less frequently, include Irish, African, Bollywood, Flamenco, Belly Dancing, ballroom dance, and more.

Ballet is the basis for much of the dance studio styles. It originated in aristocratic Italy in the 14th century where the nobles were the performers and was popularized by Louis the IVX in France when he started the first ballet school called the Royal Academy of Dance in 1661.[1] Pierre Bauchamps defined the five basic positions of dance as we know it today.[2] Ballet is a rigid style requiring mastery of specific positioning and placement. Ballet "defies" gravity.

Ballet is danced in two different types of shoes: flat flexible ballet slippers or pointe shoes. Pointe shoes allow dancers to relevé, dance on the tips of their toes, and balance mostly on the great toe (Fig. 2.1). Ballet Slippers, on the other hand, allow dancers to relevé by weight-bearing on the metatarsal heads. Ballet slippers are usually made of canvas or leather (Fig. 2.2). Pointe shoes are made with a satin fabric that encloses the toe box that is made of layers of fabric and glue. Pointe shoe soles are made of a shank that usually comprises shoulder leather.[3] To this day, pointe shoes are primarily handmade. Professional dancers often have custom-made pointe shoes and will use multiple pairs in one performance. Preprofessional and professional dancers usually have multiple pairs of shoes that they use in class. Dancing on pointe requires

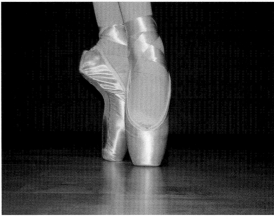

FIG. 2.1 Relevé in pointe shoes. (Courtesy of Selina Shah, MD.)

Performing Arts Medicine. https://doi.org/10.1016/B978-0-323-58182-0.00002-X

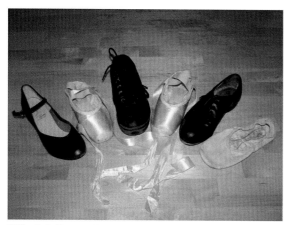

FIG. 2.2 Dance shoes from left to right: tap shoe, pointe shoe, jazz sneaker, pointe shoe, jazz shoe, ballet slipper. (Courtesy of Selina Shah, MD.)

adequate technique, strength, flexibility in the foot and ankle complex, core strength, maturity, balance, proprioception, and skill.[4]

Modern Dance originated at the turn of the 20th century in defiance of the rigidity of ballet.[1] The new genre almost parallels the transition to modernism in fine arts. Different from ballet, Modern dance utilizes gravity in movement. There are now several modern dance styles. Modern is usually danced barefoot but some dancers wear a small sole to cover the metatarsal head region to help ease turns.

Jazz is more structured than modern but less rigid than ballet. Jazz shoes consist of two types: a flat shoe made of leather similar to ballet slippers or a jazz sneaker that has some cushioning for shock absorption for jumps (Fig. 2.2).

Tap is a dance form that uses the feet as percussion instruments to create rhythms that may complement or replicate the beat of the music. It is usually danced in an oxford style shoe to which metal plates are attached to the toe and heel (Fig. 2.2).

Hip Hop encompasses a vast variety of subcategories that has its origins on the streets of New York City in the late 1960s. It is often performed in street shoes. Some styles emphasize quick, pulsating movements made of muscle group isolation.

Irish combines the rhythmic qualities of tap with the expressiveness of jazz and artistry of ballet. Its origins trace back to 1300 and became popularized in 1994 with the *Riverdance* production. Shoes are soft leather lace up slipper with fiberglass tips and heels.[5]

Bollywood dancing originated with the film industry in India. Traditionally, Indian movies from "Bollywood" are musicals with an emphasis on elaborate music videos that usually involve Bollywood dancing. Bollywood is danced barefoot and combines rhythmic movements using the arms and legs with an emphasis on jumping. Its roots are based on classical Indian dance forms.

## DANCE CLASS STRUCTURE

Often, dancers with injuries can participate in portions of class depending on the injury so it is important to have a basic understanding of dance class progression. Ballet class is structured so that the first part of class starts with the dancers using a barre that is held for support to work on basic technique, fine motor coordination, strength, balance, and stretching, followed by technique work in the center and ending with jumps.[3] The majority of other dance classes perform a warm-up in the center, followed by technique work doing repetitive movements across the floor, followed by a short choreographed routine. Styles that require relevé such as ballet, modern, and jazz will ease into single-leg relevé balances during warm up.

## BACKGROUND ON THEATER

Every society has had some type of theatrical form of entertainment with most sources dating the origin to several thousand years ago. Theatrical performances range from plays, to operas, to Broadway in New York City and West End in London, Circus Arts, and more. Actors, singers, acrobats, and dancers all can share a stage often with elaborate costumes, sets, and lighting.

## BACKGROUND ON MUSIC

Similar to theater, music has been a part of every society each with its own unique set of instruments. During the Middle Ages (AD 450–1450), in Europe, the cathedral was a central focus of life. Music was primarily associated with the church and, during the first part of the Middle Ages, was mostly vocal. After 1100, instruments were used increasingly in the church. During the Renaissance (1450–1600), the invention of printing widened the circulation of music.[6] Every instrument has its unique technical aspects requiring repetition of motion, often in unnatural positions.

### Epidemiology

As artists, professionals in the performing arts specialize in their genre in their youth. Female dancers begin classes between ages 4 and 9 while male dancers start dancing between ages 12 and 16.[4] Professional orchestra musicians start playing their respected instruments between ages 7 and 9.[7] Broadway actors begin training at an average age of 14−16.[8]

When treating performing artists, it is important to consider the instrument used as a contributing factor to injury and career longevity. A musician's instrument is obvious, while a singer or actor's instrument is the voice and a dancer's instrument is the body. The hours of training and performing take a toll as performers age so those that utilize extreme range of motion or power within the body as an instrument have shorter duration careers. The average age of professional dancers is 26−27 years[9] and most complete their careers by late thirties. Musicians and actors can continue performing professionally well into the late decades of life.

Most injuries in performing artists are related to overuse. Injury definitions vary between studies with some reporting any musculoskeletal complaint and some focusing only on time loss injuries. Studies that include musculoskeletal complaints more accurately reflect the overall burden of disease, while time loss studies emphasize more serious injuries.

In dance, ballet has been studied the most with initial studies primarily based on retrospective data and few based on prospective data. Between 75% and 95% of ballet dancers suffer at least one injury per year with a prevalence of 2.7−3.2 injuries per dancer per year.[5,9] Among ballet and modern dance professionals, 57% of injuries are due to overuse.[9,10] In ballet, females suffer a greater percentage (64.4%) of overuse injuries compared to males (50.1%).[9] Up to 82% of modern dancers suffer at least one injury per year with an annual incidence of 1.7 injuries per female and 1.2 per male modern dancer.[10] About Up to 60% of professional Irish dancers have suffered injuries with 79.6% categorized as overuse.[5]

Injury rates per 1000 h of dancing have been calculated in more recent studies (Table 2.1). Professional female ballet dancers suffer 1.06 injuries per 1000 dance hours while males suffer 1.46 injuries per 1000 dance

hours with an average of 1.24 injuries per 1000 h overall.[9] Professional female modern dancers suffer up to 0.67 injuries per 1000 h while professional male modern dancers suffer 0.46 injuries per 1000 h averaging 0.59 injuries per 1000 h.[10] One company was able to improve their injury per 1000 h of dance exposure from 0.41 to 0.25 with a robust medical intervention program.[11]

As expected, the most common location of injuries in dancers is the lower extremity. In professional dancers, the foot and ankle complex comprise the majority of injuries (14%−57%). The knee accounts for anywhere from 14% to 24% of injuries, the spine 10%−20.5% of injuries, and the hip 7%−14.5% of injuries.[5,9−12]

One recent study on ballet evaluated injuries based on age and professional level. The younger professional dancers suffered a higher prevalence of injuries compared to more experienced professionals. Patellofemoral syndrome, os trigonum syndrome, second metatarsal stress fracture, and snapping hip syndrome were more common in younger professionals while Achilles tendinopathy was equally distributed among all professional level groups. Chondral injuries of the knee and lumbar disc disease prevalence increased with increasing age.[13]

Although most injuries are related to overuse, a recent study showed an estimated 240,037 dancers over the age of 10 presented to emergency departments between the years 2000 and 2013 in the United States with dance injuries. This accounts for an annual incidence of 17,145 injuries or 6.6 injuries per 100,000 population. Females accounted for 80.8% of the injuries and those aged 10−18 for 65.4% of the injuries. Ankle sprains were the most common injury as is typical of most sports. Knee sprains were second followed by foot sprains. Interestingly, about 464 dancers suffered concussions each year. Males suffered a greater proportion of shoulder sprains and facial lacerations compared to females who suffered a greater proportion of ankle sprains and foot injuries.[14]

| TABLE 2.1 Injury Rate per 1000 | | | | | |
|---|---|---|---|---|---|
| Performance Category | Ballet | Modern | Broadway Actors | Broadway Dancers | Circus Musculoskeletal Complaints |
| Injury rate/1000 h | 1.24 | 0.67 | | | |
| Injury rate/1000 artist exposures or performances | | | 3 | 8.4 | 7.37−9.7 |

Please note it is difficult to compare these given the differences in injury definitions (complaints vs. time loss) and artist exposure definitions.

Although the prevalence of injuries is high, most dancers likely dance through the pain and will avoid missing performances whenever possible. Unfortunately, ignoring the pain may put dancers at risk for worsening or additional injury. For example, one study found that although 91% of dancers had symptoms for >1 week, yet 84% of the dancers reported missing no performances. Additionally, 81% of dancers have reported that pain did affect their dancing yet the majority did not limit their dancing.[10]

Most professional dance companies do not have the same level of care as professional athletes in the United States. Teams such as American football and basketball usually have access to a dedicated training room and a robust team of athletic trainers, physical therapists, physicians of various specialties, and more. Generally, dance companies with the largest operating budgets may have a healthcare provider, usually a physical therapist, on staff that dancers have regular access to. Some companies may have a physical therapist, a physician, or other healthcare provider who provide voluntary support. One modern dance company followed their injury trends before and after instituting a robust medical and physical therapy program that resulted in 34% decline in total injury incidence, 66% decrease in worker's compensation claims, and 56% decrease in days lost from work.[11]

Work-related musculoskeletal disorders among musicians range from 73% to 88%. Lifetime musculoskeletal symptom prevalence among professional musicians has been reported to be as high as 62%–93%. Similar to dancers, females have a higher number of musculoskeletal problems compared to males. Different from dancers, the majority of injuries are upper extremity with at least 75% of musicians experiencing some type of upper extremity symptom at some point in their careers. In musicians, overuse syndrome is a major cause of playing-related musculoskeletal disorder (PRMD). The syndrome is a result of fatigue from cumulative physical stress by the overuse of particular parts of the body required to play the instrument.[7]

Broadway performers include dancers, actors, and singers many of whom are required to perform all three. Dancers sustained 5.1 injuries/1000h of performances and 8.4 injuries/1000h of performing on stage. Actors sustained 3 injuires/1000h of performances and 2.8 injuries/1000h of performing on stage, respectively (Table 2.1). For dancers and actors, 37% and 28.8% of injuries resulted in at least one missed performance, respectively. Both dancers and actors location of injury primarily involved the lower extremity with most suffering sprains/strains.[8] Broadway shows usually have a physical therapist on staff.

Circus artists encompass a wide range of disciplines and can generally be divided into three groups: acrobats, nonacrobats and musicians. Based on the differing technical demands of each discipline, injury patterns will vary. Similar to dance, studies on injuries have been based on either musculoskeletal complaints or time-loss injuries. Rates of injury are difficult to compare given the variety of methods used to calculate them among the various studies but range from 0.13 to 0.62/1000 artist exposures or performances when using time loss as a definition or 7.37–9.7/1000 artist exposures when using musculoskeletal complaint as the definition of injury (Table 2.1). Risk of injury is highest for acrobats followed by nonacrobats, followed by musicians. The spine and ankle are the most common regions affected. Muscle strains were the most common type of injury followed by ligamentous injuries. Similar to dance, most circus artists with injuries report missing no performances with one study reporting that 70% missed no performances. One study found that more than 80% of injuries were considered minor.[15] *Cirque du Soleil* has a robust medical program including physical therapists that are on site and routinely review emergency procedures.

Performing artists primarily suffer from overuse injuries related to overuse of the muscles and joints involved in their respected categories of performance. The majority of injuries involve the lower extremity in dancers, actors, and circus artists while musicians primarily suffer from upper extremity complaints. The majority of injuries involve muscles, tendons, or ligaments and result in few missed performances either because the injuries are minor or because the performers simply ignore the pain.

## RISK FACTORS FOR INJURY

As both an artist and athlete, performing artists experience physical and psychological stressors of both realms that contribute to injuries. These risk factors can be divided into two main categories: extrinsic and intrinsic.

Several studies in dance have looked at risk factors for injury. Much of the research is based on self-report of what the dancers perceive as the cause for injury.

Extrinsic risk factors for injury reported by dancers include demands of the role, demands of the choreographer, choreography, flooring, unsuitable stages, cold conditions, and footwear.[5,10,16] Dance floors usually consist of wood planks or rubber flooring on top of springs to allow for resilience and shock absorption. However, some rehearsal spaces and studios have wood floors on top of concrete that can lead to increased ground reaction forces that may increase the risk for injuries such as stress fractures. Some stages are raked (angled toward the audience) creating a dangerous environment for dancers, especially those on pointe (dancing on the tips of the toes). The slope makes maintaining balance, especially when performing multiple turns, difficult.

Intrinsic risk factors for injury perceived by dancers include self-pressure, anatomic structure, inadequate strength, inadequate flexibility, inadequate turn-out (external rotation of the feet), inadequate warm-up, inadequate sleep, inadequate nutrition, ignoring pain, weakness, fatigue, and poor physical condition.[5,10,16]

Turnout is one of the major components of ballet and also important for jazz and modern. The visual aesthetic goal is 180° of external rotation of the feet. Turnout primarily comes from hip external rotation but also requires contribution from tibio-femoral (knee joint) rotation, tibial torsion (twisting of tibial shaft along its long axis), and external rotation of the feet.[17] Until recently, many dancers had a difficult time obtaining a role in a professional ballet company without the 180° of turnout. This trend may be changing.

Many dancers use incorrect technique to try to obtain the 180° of turnout, which has long been an emphasis in ballet. Unfortunately, cheating turnout is a major contributor to injuries. Dancers may pronate excessively that can lead to problems such as posterior tibialis tendinopathy, flexor halluces longus tendinopathy, and iliopsoas tendonitis that can result in painful or nonpainful snapping hip syndrome. Excessive tibial torsion and tibio-femoral rotation can lead to stress on the anterior hip and medial knee structures and make a dancer less stable on relevé (dancing on the metatarsal heads or on the tips of the toes in full pointe). Excessive lumbar lordosis and pelvic tilt can lead to excessive stress on the anterior hip and low back resulting in injury.

Musicians, similar to dancers, perform repetitive motions in often unnatural positions that can lead to overuse injuries. Musicians' intrinsic risk factors for injury are related to the position of playing the instrument as well as psychological demands. Neck and shoulder symptoms, including cervical dystonia, are more common in instruments that require an elevated arm position such as violin, viola, flute, and trumpet. Elbow pain is more common with the oboe, bassoon, and trombone.[7] Wind instrumentalists may have problems of pain, fatigue, and loss of control or power over the lips and facial muscles. Ideally, wind instrumentalists have functional embouchure: efficient playing to create the intended tone without causing physical discomfort.[18] Psychological demands such as performance anxiety and stage fright can produce psychosomatic symptoms including dry mouth, elevated heart rate, hand tremor, and irritable bowel symptoms to name a few that can negatively impact performance.[7] Extrinsic risk factors include noise levels of the music, performance venues, performance schedules, and complexity and repertoire of the music. One study of orchestra musicians found that percussionists are at the most risk of excessive noise exposure with a decibel level that can reach as high as 135 dB. String instrumentalists experienced up to 89 dB, woodwinds up to 97 dB, and brass up to 95 dB[19] Musicians often play in crowded environments such as small stages or orchestra pits that can compromise positioning of playing. Musicians may have erratic, unpredictable schedules that can make maintaining good health habits such as eating properly and sleeping adequately difficult putting them at risk for injury. Late night performances and early rehearsals can be difficult to manage.

Theatrical performers' extrinsic risk factors include costumes, lighting, sets, demands of the role, tour schedule, and demands of the director. Costumes can be quite elaborate with heavy head pieces that can cause neck and upper body problems. Illnesses such as upper respiratory tract infections can interfere greatly with an actor and especially a singer's ability to perform. Increased BMI and lack of exercise have been shown to contribute to increased incidence of injuries in Broadway actors.[8] Intrinsic risk factors for theatrical performers include health habits, fatigue, inadequate sleep, inadequate nutrition, and vocal cord difficulties.

Risk factors for injury in circus artists vary depending on the roll. Falling was the most common mechanism of injury in one study.

## CONCLUSION

Performing artists are a unique population to care for because they are both athletes and artists with risk factors for injury based on their specific genre. They specialize in their respected category of performance early. There is a high prevalence of injury, mostly overuse. However, most do not miss performances either because injuries tend to be minor or because they ignore pain, or a combination of the two. They tend to seek care when their ability to practice or perform is inhibited. Because they delay care rather than seeking care at symptom onset, performers often have multiple musculoskeletal problems along the kinetic chain that have resulted from compensation for the original problem making diagnosis of the original problem difficult. The key to delineating the original injury is obtaining a thorough history and exam and understanding the artists' activity and what movement causes pain.

The key to understanding how to care for a performing artist is to understand what muscle groups are used and what the repetitive movements are for their specific genres. Knowing terminology helps build trust. Allowing the artists to keep practicing or performing even in a limited capacity, whenever safely possible is best. To be able to provide this guidance on limitation, the healthcare provider must understand the elements of practice, rehearsal, and performance for the performance genre.

## REFERENCES

1. Quirk R. Injuries in classical ballet. *Aust Fam Physician.* 1984;13(11):802–804.
2. Hardaker WT, et al. Dance medicine: an orthopaedist's view. *NC Med J.* 1993;43(2):67–71.
3. Shah S. Caring for the dancer: special considerations for the performer and troupe. *Curr Sports Med Rep.* 2008; 7(3):128–132.
4. Shah S. Determining a young dancer's readiness for dancing on pointe. *Curr Sports Med Rep.* 2009;8(6): 295–299.
5. Young C, Shah S, Gottschlich L. Dance. In: Madden C, Putukian M, McCarty E, Young C, eds. *Netter's Sports Medicine.* Philadelphia, PA: Elsevier, Inc; 2018:693–699.
6. Kamien R. *Music an Appreciation.* 5th ed. New York: McGraw-Hill, Inc; 1992.
7. Viljamaa K, Lira J, Kaakkola S, Savolainen A. Musculoskeletal symptoms among Finnish professional orchestra musicians. *Med Probl Perform Art.* 2017;32(4):195–200.
8. Evans R, Evans R, Carvajal S, Perry S. A Survey of injuries among Broadway performers. *Am J Pub Health.* 1996; 86(1):77–80.
9. Smith P, Gerrie B, Varner K, et al. Incidence and prevalence of musculoskeletal injury in ballet: a systemic review. *Orthop J Sports Med.* 2015;3(7):1–9.
10. Shah S, Weiss D, Bourchette R. Injuries in professional modern dancers: incidence, risk factors, and management. *J Dance Med Sci.* 2012;16(1):17–25.
11. Ojofeitimi S, Bronner S. Injuries in a modern dance company: effect of comprehensive management on injury incidence and cost. *J Dance Med Sci.* 2011;15(3):116–122.
12. Cahalan R, Purtill H, O'Sullivan K. Biopsychosocial factors associated with foot and ankle pain and injury in Irish dance. *Med Probl Perform Art.* 2017;32(2):111–117.
13. Sobrino F, Guillen P. Overuse injuries in professional ballet: influence of age and years of professional practice. *Orthop J Sports Med.* 2017;5(6):1–11.
14. Vasallo A, Hiller C, Stamatakis E, Pappas P. Epidemiology of dance-related injuries presenting to emergency departments in the United States, 2000–2013. *Med Probl Perform Art.* 2017;32(3):170–175.
15. Wolfenden H, Angioi M. Musculoskeletal injury profile of circus artists: a systemic review of the literature. *Med Probl Perform Art.* 2017;32(1):51–59.
16. Bowling A. Injuries to dancers: prevalence, treatment, and perceptions of causes. *BMJ.* 1989;298:731–734.
17. Grossman G, Waninger K, Voloshin A, et al. Reliability and validity of goniometric turnout measurements compared with MRI and Retro 0 reflective markers. *J Dance Med Sci.* 2008;12(4):142–152.
18. Rodrigues M, Freitas M, Neves M, Silva M. Evaluation of the noise exposure of symphonic orchestra musicians. *Noise Health.* 2014;16(68):40–46.
19. Woldendorp K, Boschma H, Boonstra A, et al. Fundamentals of embouchure in brass players: towards a definition and clinical assessment. *Med Probl Perform Art.* 2016; 31(4):232–243.

## CHAPTER 3

# Coordinating the Care Team for the Artist

JOANA L. FRASER, MD, RYT

## INTRODUCTION

The comprehensive care of the performing artist often requires coordination and communication between multiple different providers, all of who must have a deep understanding of the needs and demands of the artist's discipline. Performing artists, who may also be considered as artistic athletes, are similar to traditional sports athletes in the intensity of their practice, their willingness/ability to push through pain, the intensely competitive environment they face, minimal "off time," risk of mental health disorders and substance abuse, and the real and constant threat of a career limiting or ending injury. The demands of their discipline can also impact sleeping and eating habits, social interaction, and academics.

Each type of performing artist will exhibit different injury patterns depending on the system most taxed—hips, knees, and ankles in the dancer, vocal cords in the singer, and hand and wrist in the instrumentalist. In addition, both medical and nonmedical providers may be involved in the rehabilitation and care of the artistic athlete, and close coordination and communication between providers are beneficial.

This chapter will outline the different medical and complementary providers, who may play a role in the care of the performing artist, and how these teams can work together to ensure complete and holistic care is provided for all of their specialty needs.

## PROVIDERS AND THEIR ROLES

### Physician

Medical providers that may have a role in caring for the performing artist may span across multiple specialties (Table 3.1). Primary care physicians are often the first port of call for many issues. Injuries—whether acute or chronic—often require the additional care of an Orthopedist, Rehabilitation Medicine specialist, or Sports Medicine physician, and seeking a provider with prior knowledge of the demands of the artist and specific injuries that can be seen is highly beneficial. For example, instrumentalists may suffer from skin disorders including abrasions, ulcers, or eczema (allergy to bow resin), and these complaints have been found in up to 1/3 of string players.[1] Concern for nerve entrapments syndromes may require EMG for diagnosis, often done by a Neurologist or Rehabilitation Medicine specialist. Dancers suffer from very specific conditions of the foot and ankle, such as an os trigonum or flexor hallucis longus (FHL) tendinitis. In addition to having the knowledge to be able to recognize and treat these conditions, providers who are familiar with the demands and training regimes of the performing artist are able to give recommendations regarding what level of participation is safe and guide their full return, to avoid the artist being removed from their discipline completely. The vast majority of the time, complete rest is not necessary to heal an injury, but it requires the skill and experience of a specialized provider to know how to strike a balance between participation and recovery.

Given the demands placed on the performing athlete, mental health issues are not uncommon. These can include performance anxiety, generalized anxiety disorder, adjustment disorder, and major depression. Input from counselors, sports psychologists, or, if severe, intervention from a psychiatrist, can be helpful. A heightened awareness for these conditions should be present especially if an artist is dealing with a prolonged recovery or chronic injury, which can put increased stress on their coping skills.

Medical providers must also be aware that performing artists may develop disordered eating and abnormal body image perception. This is especially true in dancers, whose physique is constantly on display and who may face outside pressure to maintain a certain

Performing Arts Medicine. https://doi.org/10.1016/B978-0-323-58182-0.00003-1

**TABLE 3.1**
**Examples of Specialized Issues in Performing Artist and Suggestions for Medical Intervention**

| Discipline | Injury(ies) | Medical Intervention(s) |
|---|---|---|
| Dance | **Musculoskeletal injury**<br>• Hallux valgus, bunions, hammer toe(s)<br>• Stress fractures, acute trauma<br>• Ligament strain, tendinitis<br>**Endocrine disorders**<br>• Delayed menarche, low bone density<br>**Mental health issues**<br>• Performance anxiety, depression<br>• Disordered body image/eating disorders | Podiatry evaluation<br>Sports Medicine referral<br>Imaging with X-ray and/or MRI/CT<br>Referral to PT, antiinflammatories<br>Referral to Endocrinologist<br>Referral to sports psychologist and/or psychiatrist<br>Evaluation by RD for dietary counseling and weight maintenance |
| Vocal Artist | **Upper airway ENT issues**<br>• Eustachian tube dysfunction, otitis media, sinusitis, allergic rhinitis<br>**Lower airway ENT issues**<br>• Vocal nodules<br>• Reflux laryngitis | Prescription of antibiotics when indicated; advice on symptom management<br>Referral to ENT specialist if chronic or severe<br>Referral to ENT specialist if chronic or severe<br>Speech therapist evaluation<br>Counseling on symptom management, prescription of antacids if indicated |
| Instrumental Musicians | **Skin disorders**<br>• Bruises, calluses, ulcers, eczema, hyperhidrosis<br>**Musculoskeletal injury**<br>• Overuse disorder(s)<br>• Nerve entrapment disorders<br>• Focal dystonia ("Cramp")<br>• Early arthritis | Skin hygiene counseling<br>Dermatology consultation if severe<br>Sports Medicine referral<br>Neurology/Physiatrist referral for EMG testing<br>Occupational therapy |

weight. If there is concern for disordered eating, sudden changes in weight, or unhealthy body image, this should be addressed quickly and the emphasis placed on healthy fueling of the body. Stressing that this is beneficial for performance can be helpful in encouraging the artist to maintain a healthy weight. In addition to enlisting the help of a registered dietician (RD), more severe cases (reduced or stopped menstrual cycles, concern for bone health, low heart rate, and/or blood pressure) should also be seen by an Endocrinologist who can help guide laboratory studies, bone health evaluation, and counsel regarding healthy weight gain.

Artists who are living away from home present a particular challenge. Barriers may exist in terms of access to care and/or insurance coverage. Depending on the situation, it may be in the artist's best interest to return home for a period to obtain the appropriate care and provide a more supportive environment for healing, away from the stresses of school and seeing their fellow students continue to progress and practice

while they cannot. These discussions should involve the athlete and their parents. Although there is usually a concern that missing part of a season may have potential negative implications for the athlete's career, the successful rehabilitation of an injury is the top priority, as career progression can also be significantly altered—at times more so—by a chronic injury. The physician can often serve as the "gatekeeper" for the artist, especially in situations where they may feel guilty about taking time off. When this is medically directed, the stress of making this decision is taken away and the artist can fully focus on healing from their injury.

### Physical Therapist

Although some dance and performing arts schools are sufficiently fortunate to have an on-site physical therapist, this is by no means the norm. However, a physical therapist (PT) with in-depth knowledge regarding the discipline of the athlete they are caring for is invaluable. Often they are seeing the athlete more frequently than any other provider, and the athlete may develop a close relationship with their PT. An experienced and supportive PT can also function as an impartial support system that the athlete can confide in, as opposed to their fellow athletes or coach/artistic director who may impart—intentionally or not—stresses to perform or recover from injury too quickly.

Therapists who are in-house or closely affiliated with a dance company may also implement a dance-screening program such as that outlined by the International Association for Dance Medicine and Science (IADMS).[2] The screening incorporates a physical assessment, as well as collecting information regarding the dancer's health history, nutritional well-being, and psychological well-being. This information can then be used to ensure the most appropriate care is being provided and to identify risk factors for injury, mental health conditions, or eating disorders. A specialized PT is key in helping the athlete progress safely back to full participation after an injury. In coordination with the treating physician, the specific limitations required at each stage of recovery can be maintained while still allowing the highest level of participation possible without unduly increasing the risk of worsening and/or repeat injury. The importance of allowing the athlete to continue at some capacity, even if limited, cannot be stressed enough leads to increased compliance with decreased risk of reinjury.

### Registered Dietician

Adequate and appropriate nutrition is vital to maintaining the stamina and strength for the intense training and performance schedule of the performance athlete. In dance athletes, in particular, disordered eating and eating disorders are common, and can increase their risk of injury.[3] A high index of suspicion may be required to identify these disorders but certainly signs such as weight loss, easy fatigability, recurrent injuries, abnormal fixation on body shape/appearance, and restrictive eating behaviors should alert the healthcare provider or teacher to the possibility of an eating disorder. Often the athlete simply underestimates the caloric needs required for their training schedule, a condition known as "Relative Energy Deficiency in Sport" or RED-S. A dietician can help identify this condition and prescribe an eating plan to meet the athlete's requirements while still providing well-balanced and complete nutrition.

When an eating disorder is present, it is very helpful for multiple different providers to be checking in and monitoring the athlete. Not only can support be provided from various individuals, but also any lapses or complications in the treatment plan can be identified and addressed quickly. If activity levels are being restricted to reduce calorie expenditure, several different individuals can also monitor this more effectively.

### Psychological Support

The internal and external stressors that performing artists face place them at high risk of psychological disorders including depression, anxiety, compulsive behaviors, and eating disorders. Early recognition and treatment of these is paramount to maintaining the overall health of the artist and ensuring their successful career. In one study, >50% of injured dancers screened using the brief symptom inventory (BSI), a screening tool for psychological distress, met criteria for a referral to a psychologist or psychiatrist.[4]

When such a disorder is suspected, the artist should be encouraged to seek intervention. Depending on their age and level (amateur, preprofessional, professional, etc.), this can be coordinated through the primary care physician or sought out directly by the artist. Although minors should be encouraged to disclose their feelings to parents/guardians (and often this is necessary for accessing care), confidentiality is key, unless the artist poses a significant risk to themselves or others, in which case referral to emergency psychiatric services is warranted.

### Alternative Therapies

The role of alternative therapies should not be overlooked. Unfortunately, little research has been conducted in this area but there is anecdotal evidence for its benefits. Specifically, acupuncture can be used to target areas of muscle strain/tension, musician's dystonia, and for stress reduction and relaxation. Somatic therapy is a form of mind—body therapy that aims to increase self-awareness, and self-control and how to use these tools and apply them to the artist's personal growth.[5] Sessions take place away from the studio and have a meditative feel, and the importance of rest between intervals of physical activity is emphasized.

## COMMUNICATION BETWEEN PROVIDERS AND CARE GIVERS/PARENTS
### Consent

Traditionally, the law considers minors to be incompetent to give consent to medical treatment, with the exception of emergencies where treatment can be given without consent of a parent or guardian. In some cases, minors of a certain age may give consent for specific types of treatment in some states. Examples of this include obtaining birth control or treatment for a sexually transmitted disease. With the exception of these confidential situations, a parent does still have access to their child's medical records with a few exceptions[6]:

1. When the minor consents to care and the consent of the parent is not required under State or other applicable law
2. When the minor obtains care at the direction of a court or a person appointed by the court; and
3. When, and to the extent that, the parent agrees that the minor and health care provider may have a confidential relationship.

An emancipated minor is one who has gained the legal authority to consent for or refuse their own treatment, and laws governing this status also vary by state to state. However, most states consider a minor to be emancipated if married, economically self-supporting and not living at home, or on active-duty status in the military.[7] In some cases a minor who is pregnant may also be considered emancipated.

For adolescent artistic athletes living away from home, it is recommended that the parent/guardian complete a consent form that allows them to be seen on their own if injured or ill. When medical intervention is needed and this does not fall under one of the confidential criteria above, the parent/guardian of the child must be informed. However, some or all of the medical information may be withheld from teachers, instructors, or other individuals at the artist's request. This may be preferred to minimize the stress and pressure on the artist when recovering from an injury or illness.

## CONCLUSION

Comprehensive care of the performing artist requires a complex skill set and often a team of multiple providers. Open communication between the providers can help to facilitate their recovery, with sensitivity to the fact that an injury or illness in this population can have dramatic and often career-altering effects. Building a strong relationship with the artist and a sense of trust is important to ensure that injuries are disclosed in a timely manner, rather than ignored, which could result in worsening or chronic issues. The performing artist is unique and so should the team be that cares for them.

## REFERENCES

1. Ostwald PF, Baron BC, Byl NM, Wilson FR. Performing arts medicine. *West J Med.* 1994;160:48−52.
2. Potter K, Kimmerle M, Grossman G, Rijven M, Liederbach M, Wilmerding V. *Screening in a Dance Wellness Program.* International Association of Dance Medicine & Science; 2008. https://www.iadms.org/page/174.
3. Russell JA. Preventing dance injuries: current perspectives. *Open Access J Sports Med.* 2013;4:199−210.
4. Air M. Psychological distress among dancers seeking outpatient treatment for musculoskeletal injury. *J Dance Med Sci.* 2003;17(3):115−125.
5. Batson G. *Somatic Studies and Dance.* International Association for Dance Medicine and Science; 2002. https://c.ymcdn.com/sites/www.iadms.org/resource/resmgr/imported/info/somatic_studies.pdf.
6. Does the HIPAA Privacy Rule Allow Parents the Right to See Their Child's Medical Records? Department of Health and Human Services; 2002.
7. Sirbaugh P, DS D. AAP Policy Statement: consent for emergency medical services for children and adolescents. *Pediatrics.* 2011;128(2).

CHAPTER 4

# Musculoskeletal Pathologies and Their Treatment in Instrumental Musicians

SCOTT HOMER, MD, BM JAZZ STUDIES • KATE LARIVIERE HOMER, MM

## INTRODUCTION

Due to the high-level demands on instrumental musicians, they often face unique challenges when dealing with common musculoskeletal disorders and peripheral nerve entrapments. Familiarity with these demands and challenges is essential for optimal care. Patient buy-in is facilitated when patients sense that the provider empathizes with their goals and has some understanding of the emotional and financial implications of injury.

Given the extraordinary physical and psychological demands placed on an instrumentalist musician to perform at an elite level, it is not surprising that in some cases the musculoskeletal system can be stressed beyond its physiologic limits, resulting in pain and dysfunction. It has been estimated that instrumental musicians spend at least 16 years and 10,000 hours to reach their performance peak.[1]

According to studies of pianists, many musicians believe that pain is a normal part of playing a musical instrument and a culture of playing through pain exists.[2,3] This perception may lead to worsening of symptoms before the musician seeks medical attention.

## PREVALENCE AND RISK FACTORS

Studies have repeatedly shown a high prevalence of playing-related musculoskeletal disorders (PRMDs) among instrumental musicians.[4-7] In fact, it appears that a large majority (up to 87%) of university musicians have or will experience playing-related injuries at some point during their careers.[8] PRMDs are also common in professionals, amateurs, and younger students. A systematic review of adult musicians found a prevalence of 39%–87%.[8] Performance-related injuries are seen with essentially all instrument categories,[9] with some proclivities for specific instruments.

Efforts have been made over the years to determine the predisposing factors for injury. One of the most salient findings is the combination of long hours of practice and a sudden increase in playing time.[1,10] One study found an increased prevalence of injuries in pianists who practiced greater than 4 hours per day,[4] although many professional musicians practice or play up to 8 hours per day on an ongoing basis.[11] **Sudden increases in playing time** often occur in the setting of preparation for performances and auditions, summer camp, or returning to school or rehearsal after an extended break. In one study, 81% of those who significantly increased practice times developed new playing-related complaints, and all of the musicians who at least tripled their practice time developed new problems.[12] This phenomenon has also been observed in athletes, where the measure of acute-to-chronic workload ratio was found to be a significant risk factor for injury.[13]

Poor practice habits such as insufficient breaks, excessive tension, and postural problems can increase the risk of injury. Other risk factors identified in some studies include age, gender,[14-16] and joint hypermobility,[17,18] which was further defined by Brandfonbrener to reflect the peculiar demands of instrumentalists at the metacarpophalangeal and proximal interphalangeal joints.[19]

## MUSCULOSKELETAL EVALUATION

In evaluating the musician patient, to have an effective therapeutic relationship, it is important to communicate (1) a genuine interest in understanding the significance of the situation for the patient, and in less straightforward cases (2) a deliberate and detailed explanation of the potential complexities of the diagnosis rather than rushing to the closest traditional diagnostic

Performing Arts Medicine. https://doi.org/10.1016/B978-0-323-58182-0.00004-3

category. This is especially true if the patient has been seen by multiple providers with conflicting diagnoses or failed treatment strategies.[20,21] Symptoms that might be easier for a nonmusician to accommodate may present recalcitrant functional impairment in the life of a musician. Musicians failing to improve may repeatedly reconsider the diagnosis or treatment plan. In these situations, additional explanation and assurance may be required to avoid an unsettled journey through numerous providers in search of a "better" diagnosis.[20,21]

In addition to the usual history, it is helpful to gather specific information related to **playing habits** within the larger context. This includes recent changes in playing time and intensity, new instruments, change in technique, new repertoire, highly repetitive practice, upcoming performances, total daily and weekly playing hours, frequency of breaks, performance settings, financial dependence on music, and ability to take time off. It is also helpful to get a sense as to whether technique has been adequately assessed and optimized with a teacher, and whether the patient is aware of any suboptimal posture or excessive tension. Many musicians are already aware of aspects of their techniques that need improvement. In addition, it may shed some light to inquire about recent psychological stressors[22] (including the injury itself) as well as general health, fitness, diet, sleep, and use of recreational drugs.[23]

Examination is tailored to the specific symptoms, but may benefit from routine assessment of spine and shoulder girdle **posture** and range of motion, because these serve as a foundation for the upper extremity. Neck- or shoulder-forward posture may need to be addressed in the treatment plan. Joint hypermobility can be assessed, in particular looking for a 10-degree excess beyond 0 degrees extension at the proximal interphalangeal joint or 90 degrees extension at the metacarpophalangeal joint.[19] Assessment should include **observation of the patient playing** his or her instrument. Poor technique may be difficult for the physician to identify and may require collaboration with a music teacher or knowledgeable physical or occupational therapist, because the technical nuances involved in performing music at a high level vary greatly by instrument and, for the same instrument, more subtly by school or teacher. However, idiosyncrasies of positioning (including excessive tension or unnatural ergonomic positions) that have become commonplace to the musician may at times be easily detectable by the provider.[24] Biofeedback can visually and audibly amplify perception of tension and the effects of ergonomic adjustments, and is addressed in detail in the next chapter.

Pain, fatigue, stiffness, numbness, weakness, or subtle decreases in coordination should be investigated via observation, palpation, range of motion, resisted activation, strength and sensation testing, and/or focal maneuvers as appropriate. Asymmetries merit closer examination, although a degree of shoulder asymmetry can be normal in some instrumentalists, such as violinists. Palpation should attempt to define consistent areas of maximal tenderness, focal swelling, muscle atrophy, or cysts/masses, as appropriate. Keeping in mind potential predisposing biomechanical factors, a reasonable attempt should be made to find a **focal anatomical diagnosis** where possible. However, a diagnosis should not be forced when not forthcoming. Passive range of motion can reveal pain, instability, laxity, stiffness, spasticity, subluxation, or neurovascular compression, and active range of motion can reveal pain, weakness, mechanical disruption, or subluxation. Resisted activation can help identify or confirm pain sources. Strength testing can help identify moderate-to-severe motor nerve compression, but weakness can also reflect pain inhibition or incomplete effort. One performing arts clinic routinely performs repeat strength testing after the instrument is played for 5 min, to assess for the development of weakness associated with dynamic nerve entrapment. **Sensory testing** can help identify moderate-to-severe sensory nerve compression and is most useful when direct comparisons are made between adjacent dermatomes and peripheral nerve distributions. Sensory testing relies on what can often be a difficult subjective distinction and may not always be reliable. In some cases, two-point discrimination and Semmes-Weinstein monofilament testing can be used to increase objectivity. Distinct sensory impairment often reflects more advanced nerve injury in the case of nerve compression and may inform the decision of when to proceed with surgical decompression to reduce the risk of permanent deficit.[25] Focal maneuvers or "special tests" are often taught as a focused evaluation of specific tissue structures but are usually limited in sensitivity and specificity and should be evaluated in context. For instance, a negative Tinel sign or Phalen test does not rule out the possibility of carpal tunnel syndrome, particularly if the history is appropriately suggestive. Conversely, its presence alone is insufficient to establish the diagnosis.

## ANATOMIC INJURIES BY JOINT LEVEL

Musicians are subject to the same upper extremity disorders as the general population, and thus it is beneficial for the provider to be aware of pertinent common conditions. In addition, a thorough working knowledge of upper extremity musculoskeletal and peripheral neurologic anatomy is essential to the formulation of a focused anatomical diagnosis.

## Hand/Wrist Pathology

### Thumb

A common area of tendon stress occurs at the first dorsal compartment, a condition known as **de Quervain tenosynovitis**. It presents as radiating pain along the radial styloid toward the base of the thumb, with local tenderness of the tendons at the radial styloid and sometimes visible swelling. If Finkelstein maneuver does not reproduce pain at the radial styloid, the diagnosis should be questioned. If severe or not resolving with rest, activity modification, and splinting, steroid injections can be particularly effective and sometimes curative. **Ultrasound** can be useful to identify fluid in the compartment as well as a separate EPB subsheath, which may lead to an increase in the efficacy of injection.[26,27]

Pain in a middle-aged or older patient just distal to the radial styloid, usually wrapping around the base of the thumb, often represents **first CMC osteoarthritis**. This almost never radiates proximally in the region of the first dorsal compartment. There is usually tenderness to palpation at the dorsal and volar aspect of the joint, which can be reliably located by palpating proximally along the thumb metacarpal to its base. Tenderness over the radial aspect of the joint can be nonspecific because the first dorsal compartment tendons pass through this area. Conservative measures can be helpful, and steroid injections can provide effective, but of limited duration, pain relief. **Ultrasound guidance** may assist in confirming accurate placement, particularly in narrow joints, and may help to avoid unnecessary needle-to-bone contact. Many surgeons delay surgery until severe pain has developed, because trapeziectomy can be painful with an extended time course for recovery. Musicians considering trapeziectomy or fusion will need to consider the mechanical implications for future playing needs.

**Trigger thumb** can present as obvious painful mechanical locking of the IP joint, or more subtly as pain and tenderness at the volar MCP joint radiating into the IP joint. Less commonly, the only symptom will be pain or even stiffness at the IP joint, which can be diagnostically confusing. Tenderness to palpation at the volar MCP joint (where the A1 pulley lies over the FPL tendon) is a reliable examination finding essential to the diagnosis. Splinting can be helpful in mild cases, although it can be functionally limiting. Steroid injection is typically rapidly effective and can sometimes be curative.

Less well defined is **pain in the thenar eminence** in the region of the thenar musculature and FPL tendon, proximal to the site of tenderness seen in trigger thumb. This may be myofascial in nature or a form of overuse tendonitis. **FCR tendonitis** is also known to radiate into the thenar eminence in some cases.

### Hand/Fingers

The most common digit affected by **triggering** is the ring finger, but triggering can be present in any digit.[28,29] Triggering (minus the pain) can be mimicked by **extensor subluxation/dislocation**, which is the result of **sagittal band insufficiency**, allowing the tendon to slide into the notch between adjacent knuckles. In such cases, MCP extension is difficult to initiate from a flexed position because the extensor tendon is displaced to a mechanically disadvantageous position, but the tendon can easily maintain extension once passively extended. Thus, an as-needed splint, if tolerated, can functionally minimize its effects. Curative treatment can be attempted with 4–6 weeks of MCP extension splinting, which is most successful if started early after injury.[30] Sometimes surgical repair is required. Any digit can be affected by **interphalangeal joint osteoarthritis**, which is often diffuse but not always painful. Less commonly, MCP joints can also be affected, but **MCP arthritis** in the absence of DIP involvement should prompt consideration of inflammatory conditions such as **rheumatoid arthritis**. Given its diffuse nature, IP osteoarthritis is difficult to treat other than with symptomatic management, such as modalities. If a particular joint is causing difficulty with instrument performance, consideration could be given to splinting, steroid injection (which usually has a limited duration of effect), or surgical intervention. DIP involvement can sometimes be associated with **mucous cysts**, which are small dorsal digital ganglion cysts. Tiny **flexor tendon sheath ganglion cysts** can also occur on the volar aspect of the finger or distal palm, which feel like little BBs and can be tender during gripping activities. Aspiration or puncture can be attempted but the cyst can recur. Painless wrinkling skin nodules or cords in the palm, with or without extension across the MCP and PIP joints, represent **Dupuytren disease**, which is a contracture of the palmar fascia.[31] As the condition progresses, MCP or PIP joint contracture can develop, which should only be treated when it begins to limit function (usually around 30 degrees for nonmusicians). Traditional open surgical or minimally invasive surgical treatments are available, and, more recently, injectable collagenase enzymatic treatments with subsequent manual manipulation have become more widespread. Injection treatment offers convenience, with the most notable but rare risk being flexor tendon rupture, particularly if misdirected. Nothing has been shown to prevent recurrence of contracture in prone individuals, and multiple treatments may be required over the years. **Boutonniere deformity** manifests as a flexion posture of the PIP joint with hyperextension of the DIP joint and is typically caused by a loss of integrity of the extensor tendon apparatus central slip.[32] Thus, extension of the middle phalanx is compromised and the lateral bands migrate volarly, contributing to PIP flexion instead of extension and exerting an increased extension force on the distal phalanx. If a central slip injury occurs acutely, it may be possible to manage nonsurgically. A passively correctable boutonniere can also be managed with a ring splint while playing if this adequately restores function; otherwise, surgical corrections are available. **Swan neck** deformity is characterized by hyperextension at the PIP and loss of full extension at the DIP and primarily occurs due to loss of PIP volar plate integrity or as a sequela of chronic untreated mallet finger. If the joints are passively correctable, a ring splint can be used while playing; surgical corrections are also available.[33,34]

### Wrist

Synergistic contraction of wrist flexors and extensors occurs when the wrist extends to bring the finger flexors into a position of mechanical advantage for grip; thus, a high **radial nerve injury** can indirectly cause severe grip weakness. In radial and ulnar deviation (a common motion in drumming, strumming, and bowing), the radial wrist flexor and extensor fire together, and the ulnar wrist flexor and extensor fire together.

Wrist disorders can be loosely divided into volar, dorsal, radial (lateral), and ulnar (medial) regions, which can be a useful distinction to organize and narrow the differential diagnosis.

*Volar:* The flexor carpi radialis tendon occupies a small sheath extending over part of the scaphoid and trapezium bones, where it is subject to tendonitis or even attritional **rupture due to severe STT arthritis**. **FCR tendonitis** manifests as pain at the radial side of the volar wrist, often radiating into the thenar region. Just radial to this is a common site of **ganglion cyst** formation,[35] often directly adjacent to the radial artery, causing some providers to be reluctant to aspirate without ultrasound guidance. Sometimes pain occurs more broadly at the volar wrist and is attributed to diffuse **flexor tendonitis/tenosynovitis**.

*Dorsal:* Diffuse dorsal wrist pain with activity is often attributed to **extensor tenosynovitis**, which, in a minority of cases, can be associated with increased peritendinous fluid and visible swelling. **Dorsal ganglion cysts** can be associated with the radiocarpal joint, scapholunate ligament, or midcarpal joint, and while they can cause pain, they can also be incidental findings. The presence of a cyst does not necessarily imply clinically significant joint pathology. **Radiocarpal** or other **wrist arthritis** typically occurs in the setting of prior trauma or inflammatory arthritis, and is relatively rare in the general population. It is treated symptomatically with activity modification, over-the-counter pain medication, splints, steroid injections, and, in severe recalcitrant cases, salvage operations that trade pain relief for limited motion.

*Radial:* The main use-related causes of radial-sided wrist pain are mentioned above in the thumb section. In addition, slightly more proximally and dorsally, a relatively rare condition occurs at the crossing of the APL and EPB musculotendinous junctions over the ECRL and ECRB tendons, called **intersection syndrome**. This location is easy to pinpoint with ultrasound evaluation.

*Ulnar:* Ulnar-sided wrist pain is commonly caused by **ECU tendonitis** with or without painful tendon **subluxation or dislocation** during wrist supination. Ultrasound can be of assistance in assessing the dynamic location of the tendon, especially if there is swelling or thick subcutaneous tissue obscuring the physical exam. A dislocating tendon can be treated with surgery or at times with prolonged casting in pronation (point of care ultrasound can verify that the tendon is fully reduced before application). **TFCC sprain** or tear can be acute or chronic. In some cases, it can be associated with positive ulnar variance causing increased loading forces to the lunate (**ulnar impaction syndrome**). The flexor carpi ulnaris tendon, subject to **FCU tendonitis**, travels with the ulnar nerve until it attaches to and passes over the pisiform bone, which develops as a sesamoid within the tendon. **Pisotriquetral arthritis** can be tested by pressing on and displacing the pisiform from ulnar to radial.[36]

### Elbow Pathology

Elbow pathology can also be divided into lateral, medial, posterior, and anterior.

*Lateral:* **Lateral epicondylitis**, commonly known as tennis elbow, has acquired various names in recent years in an attempt to more accurately describe its pathophysiology, including common extensor tendinopathy, lateral epicondylosis, and lateral epicondylalgia.[37] Given its ubiquitous nature, much has been written on the variable efficacy and incomplete evidence base for current treatment options,[38] and some advocate a hands-off approach in the hopes that the natural history will lead to resolution of pain for most patients within about a year.[39] Certainly, even the most conservative approach needs to take into account the patient's need to continue living life in the meantime, and for musicians, this includes counsel regarding activity modification, relative rest, and prognostic expectations. Sometimes pain extends into or occurs exclusively in the proximal dorsal forearm, raising the possibility of an alternate anatomic site of pathology, such as the controversial **radial tunnel syndrome** hypothesis or concomitant **extensor myofascial trigger points**.[40,41] In cases when the diagnosis of lateral epicondylitis is in question, important examination findings include focal tenderness at the distal aspect of the lateral epicondyle as well as pain in this area with resisted supination, resisted middle finger extension, and/or resisted wrist extension, all with the elbow extended. For difficult-to-evoke symptoms, even more stress can be applied with the chair test, in which a patient attempts to lift a chair back with an outstretched pronated forearm. Imaging rarely impacts management to a large degree, as a range of findings from enthesopathic calcification to normal tendon to tendinosis and even tears, as well as associated mild radial collateral ligament abnormalities, all fall within the range of nonoperative management. However, imaging can assess for underlying elbow **osteoarthritis**, **osteochondral lesions**, or, in the case of elbow instability, complete **tears of the lateral collateral ligament complex**.

*Medial*: **Medial epicondylitis**, known as golfer's elbow, mirrors lateral epicondylitis and is treated similarly, with the additional factor that in a subset of cases it can be associated with ulnar neuritis, resulting in both medial elbow pain and small/ring finger paresthesias. Caution should be employed when injecting near the medial epicondyle due to the proximity of this nerve. In cases of elbow instability, imaging can be useful to identify complete **tears of the anterior band of the ulnar collateral ligament**.

*Posterior*: **Triceps tendonitis** can be less straightforward to diagnose than epicondylitis, as the tendon is broad and it can be difficult to reproduce the pain with resisted activation. Proximal olecranon enthesophytes can be seen, but can also be an incidental finding. A distal tendon or muscle belly can encroach upon the lateral or medial retrocondylar groove and can snap over the epicondyles with resisted elbow extension. Dynamic ultrasound can be useful to delineate such cases. **Olecranon bursitis** presents as swelling over the proximal ulna and can arise after an impact or chronic pressure on the area. It is frequently associated with skin reddening that is often treated as cellulitis. Elastic compression bandages are sometimes used to encourage fluid resorption. Aspiration carries a risk of recurrence, infection, or a chronic draining sinus.[42]

*Anterior*: **Distal biceps tendonitis** pain can typically be reproduced near the site of its insertion on the proximal radius with resisted supination. When injection is considered, it is typically done under ultrasound guidance from a posterolateral approach to avoid anterior neurovascular structures but is often deferred due to risk of subsequent rupture. **Distal biceps tendon ruptures** require surgical evaluation as soon as possible, because the chance of a successful repair diminishes after about 2 weeks, leading to profound forearm supination weakness and partial elbow flexion weakness.[43]

## Shoulder Pathology

Most cases of anterolateral shoulder pain are attributed to **rotator cuff dysfunction**, primarily involving the supraspinatus tendon. Pain commonly radiates down the lateral arm. Pain is typically aggravated by overhead, lateral, or posterior reach, or with direct pressure (i.e., lying on the affected side).[44] On examination, localizing the pain to the shoulder and specifically the rotator cuff can be accomplished through the use of impingement maneuvers, including, but not limited to, Neer, Empty Can, and Hawkins tests. Imaging can be helpful when considering differential diagnoses, but as with lateral epicondylitis, a range of findings can be seen, and unless a large tear is accompanied by severe clinical pain and inability to raise the shoulder in abduction, nonoperative management is typically warranted. The differential diagnosis includes primary **glenohumeral arthritis** (unlikely in patients <50 years of age), which can cause pain and crepitus with both abducted and nonabducted maneuvers, including external and internal rotation (as opposed to abduction only, seen in rotator cuff conditions),[45] and **adhesive capsulitis**,[46] which can cause restricted and painful motion in both abduction and external rotation with a normal appearing glenohumeral joint on X-ray. Adhesive capsulitis can be idiopathic or associated with diabetes mellitus or rotator cuff pathology. Primary **acromioclavicular joint** arthritic pain is less commonly seen in isolation but is characterized by focal AC joint pain and tenderness aggravated by crossed shoulder adduction. **Proximal biceps tendonitis** typically occurs in conjunction with rotator cuff pathology, rather than alone, and is characterized by focal bicipital groove pain and tenderness, sometimes radiating into the biceps muscle. Pain in the **scapular region** is often nonspecific and attributed to myofascial pathology or radiation from the neck. Scapular motion should be observed for subtle dyskinesis, during elevation (shoulder shrug), depression, protraction (reaching the entire arm forward by serratus anterior activation via the long thoracic nerve), retraction (pinching the shoulder blades together during a rowing motion), rotation (during "snow angel" motion), and tilt. Scapular pain commonly occurs in association with primary shoulder conditions placing greater demands on scapular motion or in conjunction with **cervical myofascial pain syndromes.**[47] Neurologic causes of shoulder pain are discussed below.

## Upper Extremity Neurological Disorders Affecting Musicians

Numbness in the hand and fingers is a common presenting symptom. Painful numbness and tingling in the palmar aspect of the thumb, index, middle, and/or ring fingers is characteristic of **carpal tunnel syndrome,**[48,49] although variations exist in the way people experience the distribution of symptoms, such as inclusion of the small finger or absence of thumb symptoms. However, palmar wrist pain in the absence of numbness or tingling is not characteristic. More advanced cases can lead to atrophy of thenar muscles with loss of thumb abduction and opposition, a particular concern for musicians. Opposition can be tested clinically by bringing the entire base of the thumb toward the base of the small finger, as occurs when pinching the thumb against the small finger. Diagnosis is primarily clinical, with support from electrodiagnostic and/or ultrasound studies in less straightforward cases. Treatment for many patients will eventually become surgical, but symptoms can be reduced or even temporarily eliminated with the use of nocturnal neutral wrist splinting or steroid injections.[49,50]

Numbness exclusively in the ulnar aspect of the hand, usually the small and ring fingers (and occasionally the middle finger), can usually be attributed to **ulnar nerve** irritation at the medial elbow, less commonly at the wrist. In some patients, the numbness will be painless, and, in some cases, weakness of ulnar-innervated hand intrinsic muscles develops. This is particularly pertinent to musicians since the interossei and lumbricals all contribute to metacarpophalangeal joint flexion and interphalangeal joint extension, as required to form a fingerboard-type position, maintain a bow hold, or depress woodwind keys. Finger abduction and adduction would also be affected with the exception of thumb abduction and opposition. Electromyography has limited sensitivity for mild cases and is most useful to assess for concomitant carpal tunnel syndrome in atypical cases. Ultrasound of the ulnar nerve can be a useful adjunct for diagnosis but is not always definitive.[51-53] Treatment consists of activity modification, including avoiding direct pressure on the medial elbow, avoiding >90 degrees elbow flexion (which at night may require an elbow extension splint or sleeve), and, for some cases, avoiding forceful repetitive gripping and twisting. Recalcitrant cases may require ulnar nerve surgical decompression, which is increasingly performed in situ, although some cases require subcutaneous or submuscular transposition.[54]

Some cases of paresthesias in the hand or fingers may represent other etiologies. Dorsal thumb and first–second web space numbness may occur with **cheiralgia paresthetica** or irritation of the superficial radial sensory nerve, which sometimes accompanies severe de Quervain tenosynovitis or use of a tight watch or bracelet. **Symptomatic thoracic outlet syndrome** is a frequently cited but difficult to prove and controversial entity[55] (as opposed to the rare, severe, objectively verifiable compressive forms) found by some to be common among musicians.[56] If present, it would typically involve the lower portion of the brachial plexus, inducing upper extremity pain accompanied by numbness or paresthesias in the small and ring fingers and medial forearm. Report of exacerbation with shoulder/arm position is an important distinguishing feature, but the classic physical exam maneuvers for thoracic outlet syndrome are notoriously unreliable. Lederman reported the most success attempting to reproduce symptoms (not pulse obliteration) with shoulder hyperabduction or shoulder downward traction in an internally rotated position. Ulnar neuropathy and cervical radiculopathy should not be overlooked as alternative or concomitant diagnoses, keeping in mind that mild cases cannot be excluded by electrodiagnostic testing. Once other diagnoses have been considered, there is generally little harm in pursuing physical therapy directed presumptively at this condition, which can also address concomitant myofascial symptoms and should focus on restoring appropriate shoulder and neck posture. Surgery is invasive, carries risks, and should generally be reserved only for severe demonstrable cases unresponsive to conservative management.[56] **Cervical radiculopathy** can cause paresthesias or numbness to the thumb, index, and middle fingers and dorsal forearm (C6-7 roots) or much less commonly mimic ulnar nerve distribution (C8 root).[57] It can also mimic or accompany shoulder or elbow pathology with higher root involvement (C4-5, also rare). Distinguishing characteristics of cervical radiculopathy include the presence of radiating ipsilateral neck pain extending down the arm and often down the forearm into the hand, with extremity symptoms aggravated by neck position. **Electromyography (EMG)** has limited sensitivity for mild cases and is most useful to look for alternative diagnoses or rule out severe involvement. MRI is sensitive to look for potential nerve root compression, but has limited specificity given the prevalence of disc protrusions among the general population. **Neuralgic amyotrophy** (also known as brachial neuritis or Parsonage-Turner syndrome) is often characterized by relatively sudden onset of severe pain in the shoulder or periscapular region that at least partially resolves over 1–2 weeks, with the subsequent development of weakness in one or more nerve distributions involving the brachial plexus, nerve roots, or peripheral nerves.[58] When the diagnosis is in question, EMG can be useful for localization at least 3 weeks after initial symptoms, MRI of the cervical spine can help to rule out compressive cervical radiculopathy as a competing diagnosis, and, at some institutions, highly specialized MR neurography can identify abnormalities in the affected nerves. In most cases, expectant, symptomatic, and rehabilitative management are the norm. Secondary musculoskeletal and myofascial conditions can develop as a result of ongoing weakness and suboptimal mechanics, usually affecting the shoulder and scapula. Weakness resolves substantially for most patients within 1–2 years, but physical therapy is important for optimizing mechanics during the period of weakness and for regaining strength later in the course. Many advocate for an early short oral steroid course for pain relief and with the goal of improving outcomes, but its efficacy has not been established.

**Focal task specific dystonia** is a neurological condition affecting 1%–2% of professional musicians,[59] characterized by loss of fine motor control due to involuntary muscle contraction during a particular repetitive task.[60] Common manifestations involve ring and small finger flexion in a pianist's or guitarist's right hand or a violinist's left hand; middle and ring finger interphalangeal joint extension in a woodwind player; or thumb and index finger flexion in a banjo player or pianist.[61] The condition itself is painless but can induce compensatory musculoskeletal pain. Research has implicated maladaptive sensorimotor plasticity, impaired inhibition, and motor network abnormalities including cortical, subcortical, and cerebellar regions.[62,63] Musicians are at a higher risk than the general population due to early and intensive repetition of idiosyncratic fine motor tasks. Instruments tending toward fast repetitive fine motions seem to predominate, such as violin, piano, and guitar, while cello and bass are cited as more rare.[64] Possible risk factors also include perfectionist traits or anxiety,[65] among others. Diagnosis is clinical, particularly by history, as it can be difficult to recreate the dystonic movements in clinic. Patients may be asked to bring in videos of the dysfunctional movements or asked to play their instruments in clinic. The natural history is progression over a period of months to a few years, sometimes with involvement of nonmusical activities, and then long-standing stability. Prolonged absence from playing is unhelpful. Treatment is challenging, particularly for the goal of returning to play at a high level. Options include oral medications (limited by side effects and poor efficacy), selective botulinum toxin administration (limited by the potential induction of excessive temporary muscle weakness and/or spread to adjacent muscles[66]), and sensorimotor retraining. Recently, there have been promising preliminary studies of transcranial direct current stimulation and more invasive neurosurgical techniques, including stereotactic ventro-oral thalamotomy and deep brain stimulation, although more studies and follow-up are needed.[67,68]

## INSTRUMENT-SPECIFIC INJURIES AND TECHNICAL CONSIDERATIONS

Studies have shown that musicians have similar rates of symptoms/injury among the various instrument families.[9] Although some risk factors seem to be inherent in music making, instrument ergonomics associated with specific instruments also play an important role. Therefore, it is beneficial for the performing arts provider to be familiar with each instrument's specific challenges. What follows is a sampling of instrument-specific technical considerations, as an exhaustive listing is beyond the scope of this chapter.

### Problems by Instrument
#### Piano
**Piano** is one of the most widely played musical instruments. The seated position invites a relatively static posture during practice. The wrist has been found to be the most common site of injury, followed by the fingers, with the most common complaints consisting of pain, stiffness, weakness, and cramping.[69] Advanced repertoire requires the ability of the hand to span at least an octave, and some studies suggest that hand size may be a significant risk factor in the development of playing-related injury. Measurements of keyboard span on older instruments have shown that the average key width increased

in the late 1800s.[70] This is significant in that much of the standard piano repertoire was composed on narrower keyboards. It has been suggested that the use of slightly narrower piano keyboards for those with smaller hands may result in a lower prevalence of injury.[71] One study of pianists with hand pain showed that regular practice using wide-reaching techniques, such as octaves and certain chords, increased the risk of experiencing pain.[72] A case series of pianists in a hand surgeon's practice found muscle strain of the hands and extrinsic flexors and extensors of the fingers and wrists, trigger finger, de Quervain tenosynovitis, shoulder rotator cuff impingement, elbow epicondylitis, carpal tunnel syndrome, and focal dystonia of the fingers.[69]

### Upper Strings

Several studies have shown that pain is the most common complaint among violinists and violists.[73] There also exists a small number of reports of primary bowing tremor as a distinct entity.[74,75] It is suggested that the most common sites of pain include the little finger, inner elbow, wrist, and shoulder with a higher prevalence of left-sided pain.[15,73,76] Common issues among violinists and violists include excessive flexion of the radiocarpal joint during bowing, excessive pressure exerted on the chin rest or strings, and poor posture.[22,24,77] Playing asymmetrically held instruments such as the violin or viola often promotes lateral deviation of the neck that may lead to neck and back pain.[78] Ideally, the instrument should be played with a relaxed and balanced posture wherein the musician can maximize the use of body weight and gravity and assume the most neutral position of the spine and head. The posture should support efficient movements, allowing for freedom of musical expression. Suboptimal postures lead to unnecessary muscle activation to support the weight of the instrument and increase the risk of injury.[79] Adjustments in the positioning of chair, music stand, and instrument can be made to optimize comfort and ergonomics. One study found that weight was more evenly distributed for violinists standing or sitting to the left of a music stand and allowed for less restricted movements of the bowing arm.[80] Other relatively easy sites of adjustment are the chin rest and shoulder rest. Adjusting the height of one or both can help to optimize head and neck position and relieve excessive left shoulder tension and pressure on the chin rest.[81,82]

### Lower Strings

Cellists and bassists were found in one study to have a high prevalence of right upper extremity symptoms and back problems with neuropathic symptoms.[15] Although cellists perform in a seated position, bassists often alternate between standing and sitting on a high stool. Most cellists and bassists use chairs or stools without lumbar support, and this may contribute to back pain. Bassists playing from a seated position often lean forward toward their instrument, which could also contribute to poor ergonomics.

One study has shown that the presence of scapulo-humeral dysrhythmia, scapular winging, and differences in resting shoulder height to be significant risk factors of PRMDs in cellists.[83] The prolonged shoulder flexion and abduction required of the cellist's bow arm may contribute to shoulder injuries such as rotator cuff tendinopathy.[84] Several studies have shown that female cellists are more likely to suffer injury than male cellists, and although the sample size for female bassists has been considerably small to make statistically significant conclusions, it is reasonable to surmise that the risk of injury among women may increase with the size of the instrument.[7,84]

### Guitar

Guitar is one of the most commonly played musical instruments in the United States.[85]

Playing-related injury is most common among classical guitarists but is also prevalent among musicians playing popular music on the acoustic guitar, electric guitar or electric bass, and banjo. Several studies have shown a proclivity for left-sided pain and injury, including muscle strains distal to the elbow, tenosynovitis of the wrist or fingers, carpal tunnel syndrome, focal dystonia wrist ganglia,[85,86] and index finger radial neuropathies.[76] Banjoists have been shown to also commonly develop problems in the right wrist, left shoulder, and back.[85] Brandfonbrenner recommended avoiding excessive wrist flexion or deviation in favor of a neutral position of the wrist and suggested that the hyperflexion is responsible for many musculoskeletal problems.[23]

### Woodwinds

The main instruments of the woodwind family include the flute, oboe, clarinet, English horn, saxophone, bassoon, and recorder. Among these, only the flute is held asymmetrically (although the bassoon is held across the front of the body at an angle). To maintain a neutral position of the head and neck, a flutist must lift the flute nearly perpendicular to the floor. Flutists, such as other musicians using an elevated arm position such as violinists, violists, and trumpeters, are prone to neck and shoulder pain.[87,88] The National Flute

Association reported that the most common sites of pain among flutists are neck, upper back, fingers, wrists, and shoulders.[89] Due to the sustained extension required of the left wrist, flutists often experience wrist and tendon problems.[90] In addition, flutists can be susceptible to digital neuropathy at the radial aspect of the left index finger, where the weight of the instrument is borne.[76,91] Ergonomic adjustments are particularly important in the prevention and treatment of flute-related pain and injury.

Among oboists and clarinetists, musculoskeletal problems are most common on the right side of the body. For both these instruments, the right thumb is responsible for holding and stabilizing the instrument, placing significant strain on the right thumb, hand, and wrist. Unsurprisingly, the most common site of complaint among these instrumentalists is the right thumb.[20] Common problems include muscle and tendon pain as well as interphalangeal and metacarpophalangeal joint pain.[92−94] Modifications of the thumb rest are sometimes helpful, as are the use of a neck strap or post among clarinetists and endpin for English horn players.[92]

Other common PRMDs include muscle strain distal to the elbow, intrinsic strains, extrinsic flexor group involvement, extrinsic extensor problems, and neuropathic symptoms of the elbow and wrist.[15,95]

Different from the oboe or clarinet, the weight of the saxophone and bassoon are often at least partially supported by a neck or shoulder sling and sometimes by a floor peg or seat strap for the bassoon. The majority of problems for these instrumentalists are left-sided. One study reported a 49.3% occurrence of left wrist pain and a 38.0% occurrence of left hand pain among bassoonists.[93]

## Brass

Brass instruments include the trumpet, French horn, trombone, and tuba. Brass instrumentalists show a high prevalence of neuropathic symptoms of the mouth, involuntary facial muscle movements, and embouchure dystonia, although facial problems will not be discussed at length here.[15] Both the trumpet and trombone require an elevated arm posture, predisposing these instrumentalists to neck and shoulder problems.[88] For trumpet players, the right hand works the valves, and both right and left arms support the weight of the trumpet. The sites of common injuries for trumpet players include left-hand fingers, right elbow, left shoulder, and lower back.[96]

French horn and trombone players have been found to have a high prevalence of left-sided problems. This is unsurprising given that the left hand and arm are used to support and stabilize the instruments while the right hand remains relatively relaxed. The highest rates of playing-related problems for trombonists include the left shoulder, left hand, and left wrist, with the most severe pain caused by left wrist cramping. Activation of the anterior deltoid muscle required to support the weight of the instrument may contribute to the high prevalence of left shoulder pain. Female trombonists have been found to have a higher rate of PRMDs than males, which may be related to smaller hand and arm size.[96,97]

Dynamic splinting and the use of harnesses, support bars, or left-hand braces may be useful in the treatment of these symptoms.[97,98] Tuba players have been found to have a high prevalence of right wrist problems. The right hand and arm support the weight of the instrument, manipulate the valves, and provide pressure against the embouchure.[96]

## Harp

With 7 foot pedals and 47 strings, the concert harp is demanding for the entire body. Playing requires balancing the approximately 80-lb instrument on the right shoulder in a manner that allows for freedom of movement of both arms and legs. This makes adjusting the positioning of the instrument to the body, rather than the body to the instrument, of particular importance. Surveys indicate that major sites of pain for harpist are back, neck, and shoulders.[99] Common injuries include flexor and extensor tenosynovitis of thumbs, extensor carpi radialis tendinitis, and medial epicondylitis. Some harp methods require that the shoulders be abducted to approximately 90 degrees. This position may be problematic for the shoulder and result in hyperextension of the wrist. Kondanassis recommends avoiding resting the wrists against the sounding board or curling in the little finger while playing to reduce tension in the hand.[100] In addition to playing-related injuries, moving the harp can present challenges of its own, and care should be taken to avoid lifting it with suboptimal mechanics.

## Percussion

Percussionists produce tone by striking the instrument, usually with a stick or mallet. The percussion family of instruments varies widely, but most require repetitive striking movements of the wrist, hand, and arm. Musculoskeletal problems frequently affect the shoulder and regions of the arm below the elbow involving extensor muscles of the forearm, muscles of the hands, and ligaments of the wrist and thumb.[101,102] Overuse pathologies, including rotator cuff tears, calcium deposits, and bursitis, are also well documented among percussionists.[103,104]

Treatment may include adjusting the height of the instrument, practicing with softer mallets or on softer surfaces, or the use of a rubber practice pad.[103,104]

## GENERAL TREATMENT PRINCIPLES

Although the treatment of musician injuries should be customized to a particular diagnosis whenever possible, general treatment principles exist to guide recovery and rehabilitation in the majority of cases. These are largely supported by case reports and series, as high quality randomized controlled trials are lacking. Additionally, there is some disagreement as to the role of such basic principles as rest and exercises, although most practitioners would agree that some degree of initial rest followed by activity modification is appropriate. In the absence of evidence to the contrary, what follows is a practical and multifaceted approach based on available evidence, expert opinion, and experience.

First, an **accurate diagnosis** should be pinpointed where possible, and definitively treatable causes should be addressed. Occasionally, an obvious technical or ergonomic correction is all that is needed. Instrument modifications, when available and accepted by the patient, can mitigate problematic positions. Some diagnoses, such as trigger finger and carpal tunnel syndrome, have specific treatment parameters and can be quickly addressed and often cured.[44,105] Localized tendonitis or muscle strain can be easy to diagnose when confined to one or two areas. For cases in which a specific, focal diagnosis is elusive, **regional musculoskeletal use-related pain** (variably related to the terms overuse, repetitive strain, and cumulative trauma) often serves as the working diagnosis,[20] with the assumption that the restorative capacity of the tissue has been exceeded.[106] The degree and duration of initial **rest** correlates with the severity of the injury or symptoms.[20] Moderate-to-severe pain, pain with rapid recurrence while playing, or pain affecting activities of daily living probably warrant a temporary, dramatic reduction in playing time and intensity,[106] unless quickly alleviated by fixing a correctable technical error. Absolute or prolonged rest is considered by many to be counterproductive due to concerns about lack of increased benefit beyond a certain level of rest and concerns about muscle atrophy and/or loss of learned neuromuscular coordination. Much of the related research is focused on comparing early mobilization with prolonged immobilization for acute injuries, such as ligament ruptures, tendon tears

and ruptures, joint dislocations, and certain nondisplaced fractures, within a theoretical framework of the inflammatory, proliferative, and maturation/remodeling phases of acute injuries, not on repetitive use injuries.[107,108] Despite the above concerns, failing to respond to use-related injuries with a timely adjustment in activities may risk increasing the degree of impact and chronicity. Anecdotal experience and common sense would suggest that activity that worsens the pain should be modified or reduced to a degree. When pain with daily activities or low levels of playing has subsided, a gradual return to regular levels of playing should be undertaken. More research and perhaps even new theoretical frameworks are needed to better understand these principles and objectively investigate the efficacy of current practices or alternative strategies.[106]

**Physical and occupational therapists** experienced in treating musicians provide essential resources including evaluating mechanics and technique, guiding exercise programs, discussing activity modification strategies, providing manual therapies and modalities, and spending valuable one-on-one time and attention with the patient. I will not attempt here to describe the wide-ranging expertise, approach, and techniques of skilled performing arts therapists. However, their skills and treatment complement those of physicians and contribute to a team-based approach to care, In addition to therapists, a somatic/body awareness program can be a helpful resource, and in some regions, instrument modification specialists are available for custom adjustments.

A graduated **return-to-play program** focuses first on rest from aggravating activities, followed by a disciplined schedule of short playing periods interspersed with frequent breaks, similar to a return-to-run program.[106] If the patient starts worsening, the patient returns to a prior point on the schedule or institutes another short period in the rest phase. Intensity as well as duration of playing must be considered. Alternative forms of practicing should be incorporated into the schedule to continue forward momentum, including active listening, visualization, and transcription.[109] Failure to apply some methodology to the return-to-play schedule may result in stagnation in the rest phase. Set-backs should be anticipated, and patients should be prepared with strategies for navigating them.[110] In addition, in moderate-to-severe cases, patients should be educated that it can take many months and in some cases years to recover from playing-related injuries, even when the diagnosis is straightforward.

The **total daily load** on the limb includes not just playing, but also activities of daily living, not the least of which is computer and handheld technology use. When a musician reduces playing time, care should be taken not to simply replace that time with other repetitive activities (including smartphone apps and video games). The patient should undertake an inventory of all upper limb activities and determine which can be avoided or reduced (seeking or hiring help where possible), which can be modified or replaced with assistive hands-free or mechanized devices (i.e., voice-to-text, alternative mouse, food processor), and which activities the patient is unable or unwilling to modify or reduce. Simply "doing nothing" with your time is not possible, and the patient should plan ahead how to employ the time and energy previously spent on aggravating activities.

**Psychosocial factors** are essential considerations for a successful treatment plan. Most patients indicate that their injury creates stress and anxiety about the future. Recurrent overuse pain can at times be unpredictable, showing an inconsistent relationship with the amount or timing of activities. The resultant stress simply adds to the cumulative adverse effect on quality of life. Additionally, an unsettled mind may render the patient susceptible to impulsive decisions, such as indulging in hours of intense practice after feeling better for a single day. **Mindfulness** or cognitive behavioral strategies can be taught to help the patient become aware of thoughts that shift into worries about the future ("will I ever get better?") or regrets about the past ("why did this happen to me?"). As practitioners we may not always be able to eliminate physical pain, but we can help patients learn to understand, accept, cope with, and manage their lives amidst the pain.[111]

Corticosteroid or other **injections** should be applied sparingly, in conjunction with a multifaceted treatment program, and only when a specific diagnosis or localization has been identified. The adverse effects of steroid injection include initial pain flare that could affect playing for several days or even a week, cutaneous discoloration, and tissue weakening or atrophy with repeated injections. Steroid injection does not consistently produce relief of symptoms, and relief may be transient. In addition, immediate pain relief may promote a precipitous return to activity and/or lack of incentive to engage in the broader treatment program. Exceptions to this are certain conditions that are perhaps more amenable to steroid injection and have an effective follow-up surgery available, including trigger finger, de Quervain tenosynovitis, and carpal tunnel syndrome, or nontendinous conditions, such as thumb CMC arthritis.

Surgical authors who treat musicians have generally advocated a sparing approach to **surgery**,[112] and only when a specific diagnosis has been identified that has a predicable surgical result. It has been stated that there is no role for exploratory or empiric surgery in musicians.[113] Musicians tend to be averse to invasive procedures, including injections and surgery,[114] perhaps out of fear of damaging their valuable, highly trained hands. In some cases, avoiding procedures may be wise; however, avoidance of appropriate, predictable surgeries may delay needed care, sometimes leading to prolongation of symptoms and a poorer long-term outcome.[114] For instance, moderate-to-severe nerve entrapments (such as carpal tunnel syndrome, ulnar neuropathy at the elbow, and cervical radiculopathy or myelopathy) with progressive neurologic deficit despite nonoperative treatment can lead to irreversible neurological injury if not addressed in a timely fashion. Surgeons operating on musicians should keep in mind their unique functional demands and consider that mild residual deficits or postoperative complications that would allow a satisfactory outcome for a nonmusician may be devastating to the fine control necessary for high-level musical performance. Surgeons should evaluate the patient with instrument in hand[113] (or have the patient bring in a video demonstration) and consider the anticipated postoperative positioning, range of motion, and forces needed for playing. In some cases, return-to-play time can influence the choice of surgical options and timing.[115] Musicians who play in wrist and finger flexion may need additional postoperative reminders to avoid such positioning in the first 10−12 days after carpal tunnel release, to reduce the risk of bowstringing (encroachment of the tendons through the divided ligament).[116]

Other specific surgical modifications have been advocated including fingertip skin grafting rather than open healing, restoration of distal tissue loss, avoidance of bone shortening,[117] lower threshold for distal replantation or single digit proximal replantation, avoiding incisions in critical contact areas, higher standards for fracture alignment including rotation, lower threshold for digital nerve repair in traditionally "unimportant locations," lower angle threshold for Dupuytren intervention, lower threshold for Darrach procedure (with sparing modifications) to restore pronation and supination, avoidance of A1 pulley release in guitarists due to concern for subtle functional bowstringing and using FDS ulnar slip resection instead, first dorsal compartment release along dorsal rim of retinaculum at insertion on radius, and utilization of silastic implant with LRTI for thumb CMC arthritis in pianists to preserve length.[116,118,119]

Fry wrote insightfully years ago regarding an uncontrolled observational series of 379 musicians (out of 900 musicians examined) from six symphony orchestras, nine music schools, and other referral sources with mostly chronic "overuse syndrome," in which he felt no focal traditional diagnosis of tendonitis could be applied, postulating a tissue overload mechanism. He described a treatment program of radical rest from all pain-inducing activities for severe cases, and activity modification, ergonomics, and body awareness for mild-to-moderate cases. Although this was not a particularly quantitative analysis, one could argue that Fry's insights and treatment strategies remain relevant well into the 21st century.[120]

## PREVENTION

When possible, the best treatment for musicians' injuries is avoidance of initial injury. It is considerably harder to get symptoms under control and prevent recurrence once significant problems have begun. Thus, a key step between primary and secondary prevention involves **early identification** of developing symptoms or at-risk situations and instituting treatment strategies early.[121] This is a reflection of the considerable overlap between prevention and treatment, as much of treatment consists of preventing further aggravation of symptoms and preventing recurrence.

For starters, healthy practice habits should be taught and encouraged. Mechanically sound technique, relaxed/optimized posture, sensible instrument and seating ergonomics with frequent reprieves from static positions, moderation in duration and intensity of playing with frequent breaks, body awareness including tension levels, and a relaxed rather than forced mental approach have all been identified as optimal principles.[15,122,123] Recording one's practice and performance with video can increase awareness of tension. It should be noted that external pressures can at times conflict with these goals, and planning ahead can be critical to avoid being faced with a sudden high-intensity, high-duration, and high-stress situation, such as a last-minute entry into a challenging audition process. Systemic and environmental factors are difficult for the individual musician to control and should be addressed at the organizational level.

A broader approach also includes **optimizing general health**, including general fitness, healthy sleep and dietary patterns, and psychological/emotional health.[124,125] It has been noted that musicians tend to be more sedentary than athletes, and recently many have advocated for the adoption of sports medicine practices in music, including warm-up routines, stretching, and targeted muscular strengthening of activity-related and proximal muscle groups.[23,125,126]

## CONCLUSION

Musicians perform a tremendous service to society and tend to be passionate about their art. They are at risk for musculoskeletal injury that can dramatically affect their playing and, in turn, their lives and psychological/emotional health. Although efforts have increased to educate musicians regarding prevention strategies, many are **caught off-guard** by injury. It can be challenging to find local providers with awareness of their unique needs, and delays in engagement with a treatment plan can lead to unnecessary prolongation of symptoms. On the other hand, most playing-related injuries in musicians improve with appropriate management, allowing a return to playing.[127] A combination of healthy playing habits, attention to general physical and mental health, early recognition and treatment of injury, a sound diagnosis, affirmation of patient concerns, and adequate patient education can alleviate the trauma of injury and provide each patient with the best chance for returning to play. Further research is essential to better elucidate the pathophysiology and mechanisms of use-related injury, optimal strategies for prevention and rehabilitation, and novel treatments capable of restoring chronically relapsing patients to their prior level of resilience. Less-studied populations, such as freelance jazz, rock, and folk musicians, merit increased attention. Ongoing education and system-level strategies are critical to the prevention of injury, particularly in less populated regions where performing arts medicine providers may be less available.

A special thanks to Michael Charness, MD for his assistance with content review.

## REFERENCES

1. Ackermann BJ. How much training is too much? *Med Probl Perform Art.* 2017;32(1):61–62.
2. Bragge P, Bialocerkowski A, McMeeken J. Understanding playing-related musculoskeletal disorders in elite pianists: a grounded theory study. *Med Probl Perform Art.* 2006;21(2):71–79.
3. Ciurana Monino MR, Rosset-Llobet J, Cibanal Juan L, Garcia Manzanares MD, Ramos-Pichardo JD. Musculoskeletal problems in pianists and their influence on professional activity. *Med Probl Perform Art.* 2017;32(2): 118–122.

4. Furuya S, Nakahara H, Aoki T, Kinoshita H. Prevalence and causal factors of playing-related musculoskeletal disorders of the upper extremity and trunk among Japanese pianists and piano students. *Med Probl Perform Art.* 2006; 21(3):112−117.

5. Kochem FB, Silva JG. Prevalence and associated factors of playing-related musculoskeletal disorders in Brazilian violin players. *Med Probl Perform Art.* 2017;32(1):27−32.

6. Cayea D, Manchester RA. Instrument-specific rates of upper-extremity injuries in music students. *Med Probl Perform Art.* 1998;13(1):19−25.

7. Middlestadt SE, Fishbein M. The prevalence of severe musculoskeletal problems among male and female symphony orchestra string players. *Med Probl Perform Art.* 1989;4(1):41−48.

8. Park A, Guptill C, Sumsion T. Why music majors pursue music despite the risk of playing-related injuries. *Med Probl Perform Art.* 2007;22(3):89−96.

9. Roset-Llobet J, Rosines-Cubells D, Salo-Orfila JM. Identification of risk factors for musicians in Catalonia (Spain). *Med Probl Perform Art.* 2000;15(4):167−174.

10. Lockwood AH. Medical problems of musicians. *N Engl J Med.* 1989;320(4):221−227.

11. Bird HA. Overuse syndrome in musicians. *Clin Rheumatol.* 2013;32(4):475−479.

12. Newmark J, Lederman RJ. Practice doesn't necessarily make perfect: incidence of overuse syndromes in amateur instrumentalists. *Med Probl Perform Art.* 1987;2(4): 142−144.

13. Hulin BT, Gabbett TJ, Lawson DW, Caputi P, Sampson JA. The acute:chronic workload ratio predicts injury: high chronic workload may decrease injury risk in elite rugby league players. *Br J Sports Med.* 2016; 50(4):231−236.

14. Rodriguez-Romero B, Perez-Valino C, Ageitos-Alonso B, Pertega-Diaz S. Prevalence and associated factors for musculoskeletal pain and disability among Spanish music conservatory students. *Med Probl Perform Art.* 2016; 31(4):193−200.

15. Abréu-Ramos AM, Micheo WF. Lifetime prevalence of upper-body musculoskeletal problems in a professional-level symphony orchestra: age, gender, and instrument-specific results. *Med Probl Perform Art.* 2007; 22(3):97−104.

16. Zaza C, Farewell V. Musicians' playing-related musculoskeletal disorders: an examination of risk factors. *Am J Ind Med.* 1997;32(3):292−300.

17. Hoppmann RA, Reid RR. Musculoskeletal problems of performing artists. *Curr Opin Rheumatol.* 1995;7(2): 147−150.

18. Patrone NA, Hoppman RA, Whaley J, Chauncey B. Benign hypermobility in a flutist: a case study. *Therapy.* 1988:159.

19. Brandfonbrener AG. Joint laxity and arm pain in a large clinical sample of musicians. *Med Probl Perform Art.* 2002;17(3):113−115.

20. Lederman RJ. Neuromuscular problems in musicians. *Neurologist.* 2002;8(3):163−174.

21. Graffman G. Doctor, can you lend an ear. *Med Probl Perform Art.* 1986;1(1):3.

22. Davies J, Mangion S. Predictors of pain and other musculoskeletal symptoms among professional instrumental musicians: elucidating specific effects. *Med Probl Perform Art.* 2002;17(4):155−168.

23. Brandfonbrener A. The Etiologies of Medical Problems in Performing Artists in Performing Arts Medicine. In: Sataloff RT, Brandfonbrener A, Lederman RJ, eds. San Diego, CA: Singular Publishing Group, Inc.; 1998.

24. Kruta De Araújo NC, Gatto Cárdia MC, Soares Másculo F, Gomes Lucena NM. Analysis of the frequency of postural flaws during violin performance. *Med Probl Perform Art.* 2009;24(3):108−112.

25. Aulisa L, Tamburrelli F, Padua R, Romanini E, Lo Monaco M, Padua L. Carpal tunnel syndrome: indication for surgical treatment based on electrophysiologic study. *J Hand Surg.* 1998;23(4):687−691.

26. McDermott JD, Ilyas AM, Nazarian LN, Leinberry CF. Ultrasound-guided injections for de Quervain's tenosynovitis. *Clin Orthop Relat Res.* 2012;470(7): 1925−1931.

27. Sawaizumi T, Nanno M, Ito H. De Quervain's disease: efficacy of intra-sheath triamcinolone injection. *Int Orthop.* 2007;31(2):265.

28. Amirfeyz R, McNinch R, Watts A, et al. Evidence-based management of adult trigger digits. *J Hand Surg Eur Vol.* 2017;42(5):473−480.

29. Makkouk AH, Oetgen ME, Swigart CR, Dodds SD. Trigger finger: etiology, evaluation, and treatment. *Curr Rev Musculoskelet Med.* 2008;1(2):92−96.

30. Peelman J, Markiewitz A, Kiefhaber T, Stern P. Splintage in the treatment of sagittal band incompetence and extensor tendon subluxation. *J Hand Surg Eur Vol.* 2015; 40(3):287−290.

31. Khashan M, Smitham PJ, Khan WS, Goddard NJ. Suppl 2: Dupuytren's disease: review of the current literature. *Open Orthop J.* 2011;5:283.

32. Fox PM, Chang J. Treating the proximal interphalangeal joint in swan neck and boutonniere deformities. *Hand Clin.* 2018;34(2):167−176.

33. Van Der Giesen F, Van Lankveld W, Kremers-Selten C, et al. Effectiveness of two finger splints for swan neck deformity in patients with rheumatoid arthritis: a randomized, crossover trial. *Arthritis Care Res.* 2009;61(8): 1025−1031.

34. Boyer MI, Gelberman RH. Operative correction of swan-neck and boutonniere deformities in the rheumatoid hand. *J Am Acad Orthop Surg.* 1999;7(2): 92−100.

35. Gude W, Morelli V. Ganglion cysts of the wrist: pathophysiology, clinical picture, and management. *Curr Rev Musculoskelet Med.* 2008;1(3−4):205−211.

36. Peterson B, Szabo RM. Carpal osteoarthrosis. *Hand Clin.* 2006;22(4):517−528 (abstract vii).

37. Faro F, Wolf JM. Lateral epicondylitis: review and current concepts. *J Hand Surg.* 2007;32(8):1271−1279.

38. Trudel D, Duley J, Zastrow I, Kerr EW, Davidson R, MacDermid JC. Rehabilitation for patients with lateral epicondylitis: a systematic review. *J Hand Ther.* 2004; 17(2):243−266.

39. Tarpada SP, Morris MT, Lian J, Rashidi S. Current advances in the treatment of medial and lateral epicondylitis. *J Orthop.* 2018;15(1):107−110.

40. Rosenbaum R. Disputed radial tunnel syndrome. *Muscle Nerve.* 1999;22(7):960−967.

41. Myburgh C, Larsen AH, Hartvigsen J. A systematic, critical review of manual palpation for identifying myofascial trigger points: evidence and clinical significance. *Arch Phys Med Rehabil.* 2008;89(6):1169−1176.

42. Kim JY, Chung SW, Kim JH, et al. A randomized trial among compression plus nonsteroidal antiinflammatory drugs, aspiration, and aspiration with steroid injection for nonseptic olecranon bursitis. *Clin Orthop Relat Res.* 2016;474(3):776−783.

43. Strauch RJ. Biceps and triceps injuries of the elbow. *Orthop Clin.* 1999;30(1):95−107.

44. Hubbard MJ, Hildebrand BA, Battafarano MM, Battafarano DF. Common Soft tissue musculoskeletal pain disorders. *Prim Care.* 2018;45(2):289−303.

45. Macías-Hernández SI, Morones-Alba JD, Miranda-Duarte A, et al. Glenohumeral osteoarthritis: overview, therapy, and rehabilitation. *Disabil Rehabil.* 2017; 39(16):1674−1682.

46. Le HV, Lee SJ, Nazarian A, Rodriguez EK. Adhesive capsulitis of the shoulder: review of pathophysiology and current clinical treatments. *Shoulder & Elbow.* 2017;9(2): 75−84.

47. Giamberardino MA, Affaitati G, Fabrizio A, Costantini R. Myofascial pain syndromes and their evaluation. *Best Pract Res Clin Rheumatol.* 2011;25(2):185−198.

48. Palmer KT, Harris EC, Coggon D. Carpal tunnel syndrome and its relation to occupation: a systematic literature review. *Occup Med.* 2007;57(1):57−66.

49. Ibrahim I, Khan W, Goddard N, Smitham P. Suppl 1: Carpal tunnel syndrome: a review of the recent literature. *Open Orthop J.* 2012;6:69.

50. Weng C, Dong H, Chu H, Lu Z. Clinical and electrophysiological evaluation of neutral wrist nocturnal splinting in patients with carpal tunnel syndrome. *J Phys Ther Sci.* 2016;28(8):2274−2278.

51. Chang KV, Wu WT, Han DS, Ozcakar L. Ulnar nerve cross-sectional area for the diagnosis of Cubital tunnel syndrome: a meta-analysis of ultrasonographic measurements. *Arch Phys Med Rehabil.* 2018;99(4): 743−757.

52. Yoon JS, Walker FO, Cartwright MS. Ultrasonographic swelling ratio in the diagnosis of ulnar neuropathy at the elbow. *Muscle Nerve.* 2008;38(4):1231−1235.

53. Beekman R, Visser LH, Verhagen WI. Ultrasonography in ulnar neuropathy at the elbow: a critical review. *Muscle Nerve.* 2011;43(5):627−635.

54. Staples JR, Calfee R. Cubital tunnel syndrome: current concepts. *J Am Acad Orthop Surg.* 2017;25(10): e215−e224.

55. Franklin GM. Work-related neurogenic thoracic outlet syndrome: diagnosis and treatment. *Phys Med Rehabil Clin.* 2015;26(3):551−561.

56. Lederman RJ. Thoracic outlet syndromes. *Med Probl Perform Art.* 1987;2(3):87.

57. Dillin W, Booth R, Cuckler J, Balderston R, Simeone F, Rothman R. Cervical radiculopathy. A review. *Spine.* 1986;11(10):988−991.

58. Torres MO, Mesfin FB. *Brachial Plexitis (Parsonage Turner Syndrome, Brachial Neuropathy, Brachial Radiculitis).* 2017.

59. Altenmüller E. Focal dystonia in musicians: phenomenology, pathophysiology, triggering factors, and treatment. *Med Probl Perform Art.* 2010;25(1):3−9.

60. Altenmüller E, Jabusch H-C. Focal hand dystonia in musicians: phenomenology, etiology, and psychological trigger factors. *J Hand Ther.* 2009;22(2):144−155.

61. Newmark J, Hochberg FH. Isolated painless manual incoordination in 57 musicians. *J Neurol Neurosurg Psychiatry.* 1987;50(3):291−295.

62. Furuya S, Hanakawa T. The curse of motor expertise: use-dependent focal dystonia as a manifestation of maladaptive changes in body representation. *Neurosci Res.* 2016; 104:112−119.

63. Stahl CM, Frucht SJ. Focal task specific dystonia: a review and update. *J Neurol.* 2017;264(7):1536−1541.

64. Conti AM, Pullman S, Frucht SJ. The hand that has forgotten its cunning—lessons from musicians' hand dystonia. *Mov Disord.* 2008;23(10):1398−1406.

65. Enders L, Spector JT, Altenmüller E, Schmidt A, Klein C, Jabusch HC. Musician's dystonia and comorbid anxiety: two sides of one coin? *Mov Disord.* 2011;26(3): 539−542.

66. Ross MH, Charness ME, Sudarsky L, Logigian EL. Treatment of occupational cramp with botulinum toxin: diffusion of toxin to adjacent noninjected muscles. *Muscle Nerve.* 1997;20(5):593−598.

67. Charness ME. Brain surgery for musician's dystonia. *Ann Neurol.* 2013;74(5):627−629.

68. Horisawa S, Taira T, Goto S, Ochiai T, Nakajima T. Long-term improvement of musician's dystonia after stereotactic ventro-oral thalamotomy. *Ann Neurol.* 2013;74(5): 648−654.

69. Dawson WJ. Upper-extremity problems caused by playing specific instruments. *Med Probl Perform Art.* 2002; 17(3):135−140.

70. Sakai N. Keyboard Span in old musical instruments: concerning hand span and overuse problems in pianists. *Med Probl Perform Art.* 2008;23(4):169−171.

71. Manchester RA. The keyboard instruments. *Med Probl Perform Art.* 2014;29(2):55.

72. Sakai N. Hand pain related to keyboard techniques in pianists. *Med Probl Perform Art.* 1992;7(2):63−65.

73. Hiner SL, Brandt KD, Katz BP, French R, Beczkiewicz TJ. Performance-related medical problems among premier violinists. *Med Probl Perform Art.* 1987;2(2):67−71.

74. Lederman RJ. Primary bowing tremor. *Med Probl Perform Art.* 2012;27(4):219−223.

75. Lee A, Altenmüller E. Primary task-specific bowing tremor: an entity of its own? *Med Probl Perform Art.* 2012;27:224—226.

76. Lederman RJ. Neuromuscular and musculoskeletal problems in instrumental musicians. *Muscle Nerve.* 2003; 27(5):549—561.

77. Ramella M, Fronte F, Converti RM. Postural disorders in conservatory students: the Diesis project. *Med Probl Perform Art.* 2014;29(1):19—22.

78. Park KN, Kwon OY, Ha SM, Kim SJ, Choi HJ, Weon JH. Comparison of electromyographic activity and range of neck motion in violin students with and without neck pain during playing. *Med Probl Perform Art.* 2012;27(4): 188—192.

79. Chan C, Ackermann B. Evidence-informed physical therapy management of performance-related musculoskeletal disorders in musicians. *Front Psychol.* 2014;5:706.

80. Spahn C, Wasmer C, Eickhoff F, Nusseck M. Comparing violinists' body movements while standing, sitting, and in sitting orientations to the right or left of a music stand. *Med Probl Perform Art.* 2014;29(2):86—93.

81. Rabuffetti M, Converti RM, Boccardi S, Ferrarin M. Tuning of the violin-performer interface: an experimental study about the effects of shoulder rest variations on playing kinematics. *Med Probl Perform Art.* 2007;22(2): 58—66.

82. Okner MAO, Kernozek T, Wade MG. Chin rest pressure in violin players: musical repertoire, chin rests, and shoulder pads as possible mediators. *Med Probl Perform Art.* 1997;12(4):112—121.

83. Rickert D, Barrett M, Halaki M, Driscoll T, Ackermann B. A study of right shoulder injury in collegiate and professional orchestral cellists: an investigation using questionnaires and physical assessment. *Med Probl Perform Art.* 2012;27(2):65—73.

84. Hopper L, Chan C, Wijsman S, Ackland T, Visentin P, Alderson J. Torso and bowing arm three-dimensional joint kinematics of elite cellists. *Med Probl Perform Art.* 2017;32(2):85—93.

85. Fjellman-Wiklund A, Chesky K. Musculoskeletal and general health problems of acoustic guitar, electric guitar, electric bass, and banjo players. *Med Probl Perform Art.* 2006;21(4):169—176.

86. Rigg JL, Marrinan R, Thomas MA. Playing-related injury in guitarists playing popular music. *Med Probl Perform Art.* 2003;18(4):150—152.

87. Wahlström Edling C, Fjellman-Wiklund A. Musculoskeletal disorders and asymmetric playing postures of the upper extremity and back in music teachers: a pilot study. *Med Probl Perform Art.* 2009;24(3):113—118.

88. Nyman T, Wiktorin C, Mulder M, Johansson YL. Work postures and neck-shoulder pain among orchestra musicians. *Am J Ind Med.* 2007;50(5):370—376.

89. Lonsdale K, Laakso EL, Tomlinson V. Contributing factors, prevention, and management of playing-related musculoskeletal disorders among flute players internationally. *Med Probl Perform Art.* 2014;29(3): 155—162.

90. Nemoto K, Arino H. Hand and upper extremity problems in wind instrument players in military bands. *Med Probl Perform Art.* 2007;22(2):67—69.

91. Cynamon K. Flutist's neuropathy. *N Engl J Med.* 1981; 305(16):961.

92. Smutz WP, Bishop A, Niblock H, Drexler M, An K-N. Load on the right thumb of the oboist. *Med Probl Perform Art.* 1995;10:94—99.

93. Thrasher M, Chesky KS. Prevalence of medical problems among double reed performers. *Med Probl Perform Art.* 2001;16(4):157—160.

94. Banzhoff S, Del Mar Ropero M, Menzel G, Salmen T, Gross M, Caffier PP. Medical issues in playing the oboe: a literature review. *Med Probl Perform Art.* 2017;32(4): 235—246.

95. Dawson WJ. Common problems of wind instrumentalists. *Med Probl Perform Art.* 1997;12(4): 107—111.

96. Chesky K, Devroop K, Ford IJ. Medical problems of brass instrumentalists: prevalence rates for trumpet, trombone, French horn, and low brass. *Med Probl Perform Art.* 2002; 17(2):93—98.

97. Wallace E, Klinge D, Chesky K. Musculoskeletal pain in trombonists: results from the UNT trombone health survey. *Med Probl Perform Art.* 2016;31(2):87—95.

98. Quarrier NF, Norris RN. Adaptations for trombone performance: ergonomic interventions. *Med Probl Perform Art.* 2001;16(2):77—80.

99. Semmler CJ. Harp aches. *Med Probl Perform Art.* 1998; 13(1):35—39.

100. Kondonassis Y. *On Playing the Harp.* Carl Fischer, LLC; 2006.

101. Sandell C, Frykman M, Chesky K, Fjellman-Wiklund A. Playing-related musculoskeletal disorders and stress-related health problems among percussionists. *Med Probl Perform Art.* 2009;24(4):175—180.

102. Papandreou M, Vervainioti A. Work-related musculoskeletal disorders among percussionists in Greece: a pilot study. *Med Probl Perform Art.* 2010;25(3):116—119.

103. Judkins J. The impact of impact: the percussionist's shoulder. *Med Probl Perform Art.* 1991;6:69—70.

104. Judkins J. A performance application for rehabilitating the rotator cuff in the percussionist. *Med Probl Perform Art.* 1992;7:83—86.

105. Zamborsky R, Kokavec M, Simko L, Bohac M. Carpal tunnel syndrome: symptoms, causes and treatment options. Literature reviev. *Ortop Traumatol Rehabil.* 2017;19(1): 1—8.

106. Lederman RJ, Calabrese LH. Overuse syndromes in instrumentalists. *Med Probl Perform Art.* 1986;1(1): 7—11.

107. Kannus P, Parkkari J, Järvinen TL, Järvinen TA, Järvinen M. Basic science and clinical studies coincide: active treatment approach is needed after a sports injury. *Scand J Med Sci Sports.* 2003;13(3):150—154.

108. Nash CE, Mickan SM, Del Mar CB, Glasziou PP. Resting injured limbs delays recovery: a systematic review. *J Fam Pract.* 2004;53(9):706—712.

109. Freymuth M. Mental practice for musicians: theory and application. *Med Probl Perform Art*. 1993;8(4):141.

110. Norris RN. Return to play after injury: strategies to support a musician's recovery. *Work*. 1996;7(2):89–93.

111. Wong SY-S, Chan FW-K, Wong RL-P, et al. Comparing the effectiveness of mindfulness-based stress reduction and multidisciplinary intervention programs for chronic pain: a randomized comparative trial. *Clin J Pain*. 2011; 27(8):724–734.

112. Winspur I, Parry CBW. Musicians' hands: a surgeon's perspective. *Med Probl Perform Art*. 2000;15(1):31–35.

113. Amadio PC. Surgical assessment of musicians. *Hand Clin*. 2003;19(2):241–245. vi.

114. Eaton R, Nolan W. *Diagnosis and Surgical Treatment of the Hand*. In: *Textbook of Performing Arts Medicine*. New York: Raven Press; 1991:205–227.

115. Sheibani-Rad S, Wolfe S, Jupiter J. Hand disorders in musicians: the orthopaedic surgeon's role. *Bone Joint J*. 2013; 95-b(2):146–150.

116. Winspur I, Warrington J. The instrumentalist's arm and hand: surgery and rehabilitation. *Perform Arts Med*. 2010;3:229–245.

117. Dumontier C. Distal replantation, nail bed, and nail problems in musicians. *Hand Clin*. 2003;19(2): 259–272.

118. Ragoowansi R. Solutions to two difficult surgical problems in musicians: modified surgical techniques for basal thumb arthritis and trigger finger. *Med Probl Perform Art*. 2008;23(1):16–19.

119. Rosenbaum AJ, Vanderzanden J, Morse AS, Uhl RL. Injuries complicating musical practice and performance: the hand surgeon's approach to the musician-patient. *J Hand Surg*. 2012;37(6):1269–1272.

120. Fry H. The treatment of overuse syndrome in musicians. Results in 175 patients. *J R Soc Med*. 1988;81(10):572.

121. Shafer-Crane GA. Repetitive stress and strain injuries: preventive exercises for the musician. *Phys Med Rehabil Clin*. 2006;17(4):827–842.

122. Storm SA. Assessing the instrumentalist interface: modifications, ergonomics and maintenance of play. *Phys Med Rehabil Clin N Am*. 2006;17(4):893–903.

123. Ackermann BJ, Adams RD. Perceptions of causes of performance-related injuries by music health experts and injured violinists. *Percept Mot Skills*. 2004;99(2):669–678.

124. Barton R. Effectiveness of an educational program in health promotion and injury prevention for freshman music majors. *Med Probl Perform Art*. 2008;23(2):47–53.

125. López TM, Martínez JF. Strategies to promote health and prevent musculoskeletal injuries in students from the high conservatory of music of Salamanca, Spain. *Med Probl Perform Art*. 2013;28(2):100–106.

126. Chan C, Driscoll T, Ackermann BJ. Effect of a musicians' exercise intervention on performance-related musculoskeletal disorders [AGB award 2014]. *Med Probl Perform Art*. 2014;29(4):181.

127. Knishkowy B, Lederman RJ. Instrumental musicians with upper extremity disorders. *Med Probl Perform Art*. 1986; 1(3):85–89.

## CHAPTER 5

# Musicians' Health Problems: A Psychophysiological Approach

JOHN P. CHONG, MD, FRCPC

The Performing Arts Medicine Association, dedicated to improving the well-being of performing artists, began in the 1983 and now has grown as an international multidisciplinary organization including physicians, audiologists, psychologists, therapists, performers, educators, researchers, and administrators. The chapters in this book on Hearing Health, Neuromusculoskeletal and Vocal Health, and Psychological Health lay the basic groundwork for clinical assessment of common health problems among musicians.

Doidge,[1] in his book "the Brain that Changes Itself", made popular the concept of neuroplasticity, that the nervous system is changeable, malleable, or modifiable. He has recently further explored this concept in "the Brain's Way of Healing."[2] However, when confronted by the extraordinary rates of injury among musicians as published by Ackermann,[3] psychological as well as physical risk factors urgently need to be targeted for risk reduction strategies especially early in musical training. For example, in professional orchestras, there is an 84% lifetime prevalence and 50/50 chance of playing hurt. With the refinement of neural imaging and other technology, a growing body of evidence can lead to a greater understanding of the risks to health and interventions to treat or prevent adverse health outcomes. The Musicians' Clinics of Canada was created in 1986 at the request of the Organization of Canadian Symphony Musicians to address the unmet health care needs of musicians in Canada. Chong[4] reviewed this experience. The Artists' Psychophysiology and Ergonomic Laboratory (APELab) has been constructed to evaluate treatment interventions in ongoing $n$-of-1 clinical trials.

Many neurological aspects of music making and listening have been outlined in the writings of Jourdain,[5] Levitin,[6] and Sacks[7] exploring the underlying biological structures involved in the neural processing of music. Schlaug[8] has studied the effect of musical training on the auditory-motor tract called the arcuate fasciculus and shows that the musician has a larger tract in both hemispheres than in the nonmusician. Zatorre's group (2009)[9] studied the effects of music on the dopamine binding in the caudate and ventral striatum demonstrating anticipation and experience temporal responses implicated in movement and pleasure. Altenmuller,[10] however, describes the dark side of the increasing specialization and prolonged training in musicians that could result in loss of control and degradation of skilled movement known as focal dystonia. Musical performance continues to be studied, for example, how the activation of the brain networks involved in reward, emotion, and motivation mediates powerful effects on neuroplasticity. Understanding how psychological factors such as anxiety and perfectionist tendencies are implicated in the development of motor control problems is a prioritized area of research. An excellent example of these concepts can be seen in the documentary "Two Hands" where Leon Fleisher[11] describes in intimate detail the stress of the life of a concert pianist and then his struggles with focal dystonia.

Coyle,[12] in the Talent Code, identifies three key elements to develop optimal performance—deep practice, ignition, and master coaching by the myelination of neural networks increasing speed and accuracy of movements and thoughts. He describes three rules of deep practice—Rule One: Chunk It Up; Rule Two: Repeat It; and Rule Three: Learn to Feel It. Wolff[13] stated that the body will adapt to demands or shed, the "use it or lose it" principle. Hebb[14] stated that "when an axon of cell A is near enough to cell B and repeatedly or persistently takes part in firing it, some growth process or metabolic change takes place in one or both cells such that A's efficiency, as one of the cells firing B, is increased" or more simply stated "cells that fire together, get wired together". But then the phenomenon called "mirror neurons" was accidently discovered while studying the grasping movement of a monkey, which has led researchers such as Iacoboni[15] to explore this in social environments and culture. Theorell[16] in a systematic review of 59 studies evaluating work and

Performing Arts Medicine. https://doi.org/10.1016/B978-0-323-58182-0.00005-5

depressive symptoms found that there was moderately strong evidence for high psychological demands, low decision latitude, and bullying as having significant impact on the development of depressive symptoms. Lesser evidence was shown for psychological demands, effort reward imbalance, low support, unfavorable social climate, lack of work justice, conflicts, limited skill discretion, job insecurity, and long working hours. The juxtaposition of this evidence creates a construct upon which health care professionals and educators can develop clinical and pedagogical environments that foster musical performance excellence or the contrary, high-risk environments for injury and illness.

Mate[17] in "When the Body Says No—the Cost of Hidden Stress" comes to the following conclusions: (1) Who gets ill and who does not are not random acts of fate, but very much related to our social and emotional lives; (2) Contrary to mainstream medical practice, both ancient wisdom and modern science tell us the mind and body cannot be separated nor can individual humans be separated from their psychological and social relationships; (3) Understanding these unities helps us to maintain or to regain health; and (4) Authentic self-expression is the key—including but not limited to artistic self-expression. Stress is a major factor in the onset of all chronic illness having its origins in emotions resulting in measurable physical events in the body involving the brain, hormone, immune, and other physiological systems. The cumulative experience of adverse childhood, educational, occupational, and personal events creates a chronic stress response that may lead to health effects such as heart disease, stroke, diabetes, cancer, arthritis, multiple sclerosis, and dementia.

Felitti[18] found that the number of Adverse Childhood Experiences (ACEs) in a study of over 17,000 individuals was strongly associated with adulthood high-risk health behaviors such as smoking, alcohol and drug abuse, promiscuity, and severe obesity, and correlated with ill-health including depression, heart disease, cancer, chronic lung disease, and shortened lifespan. Compared to an ACE score of zero, having four adverse childhood experiences was associated with a sevenfold increase in alcoholism, a doubling of risk of being diagnosed with cancer, and a fourfold increase in emphysema; an ACE score above six was associated with a 30-fold increase in attempted suicide. What neurobiological mechanisms could explain such a strong dose response relationship.

Selye[19] was the first to demonstrate the existence of biological stress building upon the ideas of Bernard and Cannon's "homeostasis" into the "general adaptation syndrome" whereby the body copes with stress by activating the hypothalamic—pituitary—adrenal axis (HPA axis) system and then recovers. McEwen[20] went further to show that in the face of stressful situations and stimuli, activation of neural, neuroendocrine, and neuroendocrine-immune mechanisms occurred. This adaptation has been called "allostasis" or maintaining stability through change through hormonal mediators of the stress response, cortisol, and epinephrine or adrenaline. However, when the stress is chronic over a long-time period the resulting "allostatic overload" accelerates disease processes by chemical imbalances in the autonomic nervous system, central nervous system, neuroendocrine, and immune systems. Four conditions that lead to allostatic overload are: (1) Repeated frequency of stress responses to multiple novel stressors; (2) Failure to habituate to repeated stressors of the same kind; (3) Failure to turn off each stress response in a timely manner due to delayed shut down; and (4) Inadequate response that leads to compensatory hyperactivity of other mediators. Sapolsky[21] in the documentary "Stress—Portrait of a Killer" elegantly reviews the effects of allostatic overload and implications for long-term health from prolonged exposure to the stress hormone cortisol where inequalities of rank exist in hierarchical social and environmental structures.

Porges[22] explores in the "Polyvagal Theory" the regulation of the autonomic nervous system. This theory outlines the structure and function of the two distinct branches of the vagus nerve that originates in the medulla, both of which are inhibitory in nature via the parasympathetic nervous system (PNS). The vagal system is in opposition to the sympathetic-adrenal "fight or flight" system, which is involved in mobilization of the defense survival response. The dorsal branch of the vagus originates in the dorsal motor nucleus and is considered the older branch. This branch is also known as the "vegetative vagus" because it is associated with primal survival strategies such as freezing when threatened, conserving metabolic resources. The dorsal vagal complex (DVC) provides primary control of sub-diaphragmatic visceral organs and maintains regulation of the digestive processes. The ventral vagal complex (VVC) or social engagement system is more sophisticated to modulate behavioral and affective responses to increasingly stressful environments. This branch is also known as the "smart vagus" because it is associated with the regulation of sympathetic nervous system or "fight or flight" system. This VVC regulates the defense survival circuits and provides primary control of supra-diaphragmatic visceral organs, such as the esophagus, bronchi, pharynx, and larynx and the heart. When vagal tone to the heart is high the vagus acts as a restraint or brake limiting heart rate however when vagal tone is low there is less inhibition to the mobilization of the "fight or flight" response. As the vagus plays such an integral role in the PNS by the regulation of heart rate, the amplitude of respiratory sinus arrhythmia (RSA) is a good index of PNS activity to see how the vagus modulates heart rate activity in response to stress. This creates psychophysiological intervention strategies that could have an enormous potential to protect musicians from the effects of chronic stress.

The high rates of injuries among musicians have been largely documented by measures of playing-related musculoskeletal disorders (PRMDs) as described in the systematic review of incidence and prevalence by Zaza[23] leading to the widely held belief that ergonomic interventions such as postural correction and modification of technique could reduce the risk of injury. However, Gevirtz[24] proposed that sympathetic nervous system (SNS) innervated muscle spindles connects musculoskeletal system to the story of defense survival "fight or flight" responses resulting in myofascial pain and muscle tension. The possibility that there are more than biomechanical risk factors involved in the mechanism of injuries must be considered to provide a comprehensive model for diagnosis, treatment, and prevention.

Miller[25] reviewed the role of inflammation on psychological health problems such as depression (MDD) and as a common mechanism of disease with elevation of inflammatory cytokine production. This elevated production has been linked back to the excito-toxicity of the chronic stress hormone cortisol on the glial cells that are the "glue" of the nervous system responsible for support of the neural networks, process of myelination, and neuro-regulation of the immune system. There are three types of glial cells: (1) astrocytes; (2) oligodendrocytes; and (3) microglia, the latter most responsible for regulation of immune function. Under chronic stress activation the psychopathological process leads to major adverse health consequences and most importantly chronic pain as reviewed by Milligan.[26] Loggia[27] demonstrated the elevation of a marker of glial activation in patients with chronic low back pain compared to controls that herald a new era in the study of the pathophysiology and treatment of pain and depression.

Kenny[28] found a complex relationship between severity of PRMD and depression in the Australian professional orchestra study. In three groups, there was an association between pain and depression; however, the fourth group denied depression but had the most severe

pain suggesting somatization of their psychological distress. There was also a strong relationship between PRMD severity and music performance anxiety (MPA). These findings are indeed profound and highlight the need to reduce the stress of musical performance, beginning as early as possible in the rehabilitation process. In addition, this evidence points to new treatment targets to ameliorate the effects of chronic stress.

Slavich[29] proposes a "social signal transduction theory" of depression whereby situations involving social threat are represented in the central nervous system such as the anterior insula and dorsal anterior cingulate cortex (dACC) that process experiences of negative affect and distress. These connect to lower level subcortical structures such as the hypothalamus and brainstem that influence systemic inflammation by modulating the activity of the HPA axis and SNS increasing production of proinflammatory cytokines and inflammatory responses. Major life stressors especially involving interpersonal stress and social rejection are among the strongest risk factors for depression that elicit profound changes in behavior including depressive symptoms such as sad mood, anhedonia, fatigue, psychomotor retardation, and socio-behavioral withdrawal. The risk to health from adverse cortisol effects from psychologically traumatic events is 22 times, equivalent to the health risks from tobacco and asbestos.

Lanius[30] in the text "The Impact of Early Life Trauma on Health and Disease—The Hidden Epidemic" comprehensively examines various aspects of the issue. The connection of parental verbal anger and peer verbal bullying is associated with cortical and subcortical structural abnormalities in the arcuate fasciculus, cingulate, fornix, insula, and superior temporal gyrus shown by diffusion tensor imaging. Offord[31] constructed the Ontario Child Health Study, which has yielded epidemiological evidence significantly influencing healthcare systems and policy makers. The American Academy of Pediatrics[32] issued a policy statement stating that psychological maltreatment is as harmful as physical assault and includes spurning, terrorizing, isolating, exploiting, corrupting, denying emotional responsiveness, and mental health/medical/educational neglect. The film Whiplash[33] written and produced by Damien Chazelle portrays a first-year university jazz drumming student subjected to traumatic stress and abuse by the conductor and teacher. This film graphically illustrates the connection to the above evidence in the music industry and the need to establish policies on healthy boundaries. More recently awareness has increased due to the uncovering of widespread physical, psychological, and sexual abuse in high profile cases.

Epel[34] studied the effect of chronic stress in a group of mothers of handicapped children and found that psychological elements such as (1) seeing red; (2) rumination; (3) threat to ego; and (4) negative mind wandering, shortened telomere length; 1 year of chronic stress equaled 6 years of biological aging. Telomere length, a measure of cellular aging, is regulated by the enzyme telomerase, and Blackburn[35] received the Nobel Prize in Medicine for this research on telomeres. Ornish[36] found that comprehensive lifestyle changes such as diet, exercise, stress management, and social support increased telomere length in a group of men with early prostate cancer. The same intervention program has been effective at reversing heart disease. Now much interest in the emerging field of integrative medicine has focused on the evaluation of antiinflammatory diets, development of exercise programs to increase core stability and cardiovascular fitness, the widespread acceptance of mindfulness-based meditation and yoga, and attention to healthy boundaries in interpersonal relationships. If these types of integrative medicine programs with an increased awareness on health and wellness were implemented on a large-scale basis in rehabilitation and music education, a significant positive health impact could be achieved.

Solovitch,[37] in a heartfelt account of her story "Playing Scared" as a gifted pianist struggling with MPA, underscores the need to recognize and treat musician health problems early to prevent dropping out of music education and to suffer a lifelong loss of the pleasure to perform music in public. LeDoux,[38] one of the foremost researchers in psychological health has put forward the premise that fear and anxiety are not innate states waiting to be unleashed from the brain in response to threatening stimuli but instead experiences that are assembled cognitively from the psychophysiological responses of the body. This has enormous implications for treatment and prevention in that interventions must address both conscious and underlying unconscious processes of anxiety and harness the powers of neuroplasticity. He posits that feelings and working memory are made from a soup of ingredients including (1) executive function such as attention, monitoring, labeling, and attributing; (2) memory including sematic, episodic, autobiographical, and implicit; (3) body response feedback including behavioral and physiological; (4) brain arousal; (5) survival circuit activity; and (6) sensory processing. The driving force of defensive responses and supporting physiological responses in the brain and body is the amygdala; which accelerates the response. The ventromedial prefrontal cortex (VMPFC) is the brake on these responses. By understanding the neural circuitry of threat memories involving the VMPFC, hippocampus and amygdala, the conditioning and extinction of defense survival responses becomes possible. The development of extinction techniques to enhance exposure therapy effectiveness will become useful in reducing the chronic stress from musical performance and traumatic events that may occur during music education and competition. How music students at risk from chronic stress will be identified early for these interventions will be an enormous challenge for clinicians and music educators.

Van der Kolk[39] in the most comprehensive text to date "The Body Keeps the Score" reviews some of the neurobiological evidence in treating trauma survivors from combat veterans, victims of accidents and crimes, those touched by the hidden toll of sexual and family violence, and communities and schools devastated by abuse, neglect, and addiction. Crucial in the healing from trauma is the presence of safe and secure attachments mediated by oxytocin and the provision of treatments based on restoring the capacity of the body and mind to self-regulate. Interventions such as cognitive behavioral therapy (CBT) and eye movement desensitization and reprogramming (EMDR) are proposed interventions. Yoga shows enormous promise as a treatment as well as a modality to prevent the deleterious effects of chronic stress and to improve resilience. It is possible that biofeedback interventions including surface electromyography (sEMG), heart rate variability, and neurofeedback will form the foundation for trauma treatment in the future. Ogden[40] similarly reviews the neurobiological evidence upon which to design a treatment approach based on sensorimotor techniques to down regulate defensive survival responses and to upregulate neural networks to create safety and integration of somatic stabilization with self and attuned relationships. Siegel[41] has been enormously influential in creating "interpersonal neurobiology", a framework for maintaining mental health and well-being by promoting secure attachment, mindfulness meditation, and effective psychotherapy. Ongoing trials of various forms of meditation as described by Epel[42] may provide evidence of slowing the rate of cellular aging. Given that effective treatments are available based on these neurobiological mechanisms the challenge for the music industry and educators is to design referral systems to identify musicians at risk and provide access to interventions for healing.

Williamon[43] in "Musical Excellence" reviews some ground rules for achieving musical excellence, examines effective and efficient practice methods, and then introduces methods for enhancing musical achievement.

Although the goal of musical training is to optimize strategies to maximize performance, reducing the risks of illness and injury is of paramount importance. Some of the techniques such as physical fitness, Alexander technique, biofeedback and neurofeedback, mental skills training, and cognitive feedback may have some benefit to enhance resilience of the musician under chronic stress; however, more needs to be done to identify those at risk and to make treatment accessible. Kenny[44] comprehensively examines MPA with various conceptualizations of the problem and continues to examine various treatment approaches. Although there may be effective treatments for MPA, those students at risk must be identified early and have access to effective and efficient treatment modalities.

Morton[45] in "The Authentic Performer—Wearing a Mask and the Effect on Health" examines the connection between authenticity and health, being an authentic performer, perseverance or abuse in training, and the relationship between body language and creating balance with authenticity, which are germane to creating a safe environment in the performing arts industry education as well as pursuing artistic excellence. The US Preventive Services Task Force[46] has released recommendations on the benefits and harms of screening for depression. Screening should be implemented with adequate systems in place to ensure accurate diagnosis, effective treatment, and appropriate follow-up. Tuning the music industry and educational environment to listen for both physical and psychological health problems will require the education of musicians in these issues and will create a conversation of what methodology could be implemented to address the early recognition of musicians at risk.

This body of evidence can now be utilized to create a psychophysiological approach for treatment in musician rehabilitation and prevention utilizing quantitative measurement technology. Although Performing Arts Medicine is a relatively new field of endeavour compared to Sports Medicine, the medical problems of performing artists are alarming common and career threatening. Medical problems of performing artists require specialized clinical and educational interventions targeted at populations exposed to highly stressful activities and environments. Since 1986 the Musicians' Clinics of Canada has treated over 10,000 musicians with muscle fatigue, anxiety, depression, nerve entrapments, and various stress-related medical conditions. The acronym MADNESS—muscle fatigue, anxiety, depression, nerve entrapments, and stress syndromes—encompasses the spectra of observed medical phenomenon and creates the possibility for targeted treatment interventions.[47] In Canada healthcare services are universal, accessible, and portable across the provinces, except Quebec, allowing the performing artist to seek medical consultations and obtain treatment interventions for their occupational health problems.[48]

Specific risk factors that have been identified[49] are as follows:
- Long practice sessions
- Insufficient rest
- Excess muscle tension
- Poor posture
- Muscle fatigue
- Sudden increase in playing
- Repertoire scheduling
- Stress
- Lack of fitness
- Insufficient warm-up

The focus of the earlier versions of the Musicians' Clinics of Canada from 1990 to 1996 were ergonomic interventions such as posture, tension, force, support, duration, repetition, technique, recovery, strength, fitness, and size. These concepts are common in occupational and sports medicine however do not on their own explain the extremely high injury rates and extent of impairment and disability of performing artists.

In 1996 the clinic expanded to include assessment of psychophysiology and explored techniques to reduce the effects of chronic stress following ABCDEFG paradigm:
- ALIGNMENT
- BREATHING
- COORDINATION
- DIET
- EXERCISE
- FOCUS
- GOALS

The following elements were added as quantitative measurement technology was developed and evidence-based interventions were refined for clinical practice. A detailed review of each of these methods is beyond the scope of this chapter[50] but briefly are summarized as follows:

**Surface Electromyography** measures electrical signals generated by neuromuscular recruitment of muscles with wireless sensors to assess fatigue, power spectrum, and power output during musical performance. This allows the modification of ergonomic factors that relate to excessive force, duration, repetition, and technique.

**Motion Analysis** examines postural alignment and dynamic movements during musical performance objectively measuring factors that may create excessive biomechanical loads on anatomically vulnerable structures.

**Audio/video Feedback** is crucial during the process of synchronizing the musical performance to muscle and movement data recorded in real time and available for playback analysis.

**Heart Rate Variability (HRV) Analysis** before, during, and after musical performance can examine the balance of the sympathetic and parasympathetic nervous system.

**Neurofeedback Analysis** measures the frequency of brain waves from very low to high frequencies to tune the mind–body connection into the zone of calm focus.

**Psychotherapy Techniques** such as mindfulness based stress reduction (MBSR), CBT, and psychodynamic therapy (PT) form the building blocks to down-regulate the effects of chronic stress related to performance and the artistic lifestyle.

**Acupuncture Techniques** can deactivate trigger points that are created by excessive stimulation from the sympathetic nervous system and ergonomic biomechanical imbalances.

**Medications** can be prescribed to modify or regulate neurotransmitter and hormonal regulation problems created by chronic stress.

Specific psychophysiological and ergonomic parameters can be measured with state-of-the-art biofeedback technology to allow the performing artist and clinician to collaborate in a problem-solving methodology. By seeing and feeling how these objective measurements relate to performance health problems, awareness of risk factors such as alignment, breathing, and coordination create possibilities for restoration of autonomic regulation and homeostasis. Lifestyle modifications related to diet, exercise, focus, and goals are integral to reverse the effects of biological aging and to increase multisystem resilience outcomes. In 2015 the creation of the APELab allows an *N*-of-1 strategy[51] to evaluate performance-related health problems and interventions that increase an individual's resilience.

The following case example illustrates the integrative approach to management and prevention:

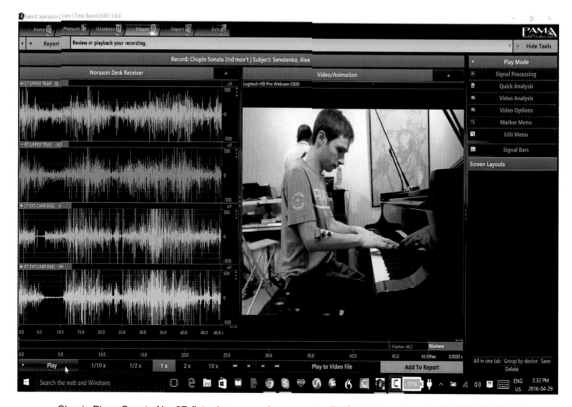

Chopin Piano Sonata No. 2B flat minor second movement sEMG video/audio analysis APELab MC2.

Alex "the Gr88!" Seredenko, concert pianist graduate of the Artist Diploma Program Glenn Gould School, was referred at age 21 in 2008 to MC2 for playing-related pain in the neck, back, and upper extremities. He was born in Moscow, started playing piano at age 3, and settled in North Toronto. He has been under intense family pressure to make it and live up to the legacy of the great Russian pianists. Quantitative analysis of neuromuscular function utilizing sEMG techniques showed dramatic fatigue response in the left greater than right forearms. Psychological assessment was consistent with a diagnosis of musician performance anxiety with major depression and posttraumatic stress disorder (PTSD).

The initial treatment plan included a noninflammatory diet, moderate aerobic exercise, learning multimodal stress reduction techniques, enhanced restorative sleep, mindfulness-based cognitive psychotherapy, and the medication pregabalin 75 mg at bedtime. Further medications were added to control the pain and depressive symptoms: nabilone 0.5 mg at bedtime and duloxetine 30 mg in the morning with an increase in pregabalin to 150 mg at bedtime.

A psychodynamic approach to rewrite the trauma narrative of ACEs emphasizing interpersonal boundaries, safe attachments, and trauma desensitization techniques was used. A nonjudgmental harm reduction approach to substance use of alcohol, tetrahydrocannabinol (THC), stimulants, and opiates was taken. Psychotherapy sessions addressed multiple stressors including financial instability, relationship breakups, and music competition anxiety. In depth, reflections on the life of Glenn Gould and an exploration of the history of great Russian pianists were undertaken to address the intense peer competition and parental pressure to succeed. Very strict monitoring of practice routine behavior using an iPad app revealed a cumulative piano performance load approximately 22,000 h.

With control of the PRMD, MPA, and major depressive disorder/PTSD symptoms, he was able to win the Canadian Chopin competition and prestigious Rebanks Scholarship at the Glenn Gould School with numerous international competitions lined up. Follow-up treatment included monthly sessions in APELab to prevent relapse, create resilience under performance pressure, and taper the medications as necessary. Diversification of career goals was necessary due to the scarcity of funding and performance opportunities for young Canadian performing artists.[52]

In 2009 the Dean of the Glenn Gould School at the Royal Conservatory in Toronto made a request to create the "Performance Awareness" course, which is mandatory for all Performance Diploma and Artist Diploma students. Basic mechanisms of performance-related stress on health are covered in detail followed by interactive demonstrations of techniques to measure and reduce specific risk factors related to performance related injury and illness. The application of targeted psychophysiological interventions is formulated and evaluated with objective outcomes for each student. Long-term outcomes of the course are being evaluated. Moreover, further educational collaboration with the National Youth Orchestra of Canada and Toronto Summer Music Festival is ongoing during the summer months to continue the effort of injury prevention on a national basis. University Faculties of Music are now starting similar courses to address this urgent need.

Other organizations interested in performing arts medicine began working with PAMA with an international initiative called PAMAForte with the following goals:

- Promoting the highest quality of care to all performing artists and bringing to that care an appreciation of the special needs of performing artists.
- Developing educational programs designed to enhance the understanding and prevention of medical problems related to the performing arts.
- Promoting communication among all those involved in the healthcare and well-being of performing artists.
- Fostering research into the etiology, prevention, treatment, and rehabilitation of medical problems of performing artists.

Progress thus far includes the following: international leadership and collaboration, social media development and sharing, development of more regional meetings, highlighting the annual symposium with the Aspen Music Festival and School, partnerships with the International Association of Dance Medicine and Science, American College of Sports Medicine, National Association of Schools of Music, Music Teachers National Association, National Athletic Trainers Association, and others. This culminated in the first International Congress in Performing Arts Medicine in New York City in 2016. A Task Force on Psychological Health published a series of State of the Art Reviews that are available on the PAMA website at artsmed.org.[53]

This chapter on the psychophysiological approach to musicians' health problems provides strong evidence for clinicians and music educators to implement (1) primary prevention strategies to educate musicians and the music industry about psychophysiological health risks and implement mandatory stress reduction interventions; (2) secondary prevention strategies to create systems for early detection such as screening for psychophysiological health problems among musicians, especially those at risk; and (3) tertiary prevention strategies to provide access to effective and efficient treatment of psychophysiological health problems among musicians. The collective contributions by authors of this book will further elucidate issues of key importance and provide more relevant evidence to effect change and to protect the psychophysiological health of musicians.

## REFERENCES

1. Doidge N. *The Brain that Changes Itself*. London: Penguin Books; 2007. ISBN 978-0-14-311310-2.
2. Doidge N. *The Brain's Way of Healing*. New York: Viking; 2015. ISBN 978-0-670-02550-3.
3. Ackermann B, Driscoll T, Kenny DT. Musculoskeletal pain and injury in professional orchestral musicians in Australia. *Med Probl Perform Art*. 2012;27(4):181–187.
4. Chong J. *Playing Healthy Staying Healthy: Creating the Resilient Performer*. Vol. 64. American Music Teacher; 2015:25–27.
5. Jourdain R. *Music, the Brain, and Ecstasy*. New York: William Morrow and Co.; 1997. ISBN:0-688-14236-2.
6. Levitin DJ. *This Is Your Brain on Music*. New York: Dutton; 2006. ISBN:0-525-94969-0.
7. Sacks O. *Musicophilia*. New York: Knopf; 2007. ISBN 978-0-676-97978-7.
8. Schlaug G, Chi C. The Brain of Musicians. [book auth.] Zatorre RJ, Peretz I. *The Biological Foundations of Music*. Vol. 930. New York: Ann. N.Y Acad. Sci; 2001:281–299.
9. Salimpoor V, et al. Anatomically distinct dopamine release during anticipation and experience of peak emotion to music. *Nat Neurosci*. 2011;14:257–264.
10. Altenmuller E, Jabusch H-C. Focal dystonia in musicians. *Med Probl Perform Art*. 2010;25:3–9.
11. Kahn N. *Two Hands: The Leon Fleisher Story*. Crazy Boat Pictures; 2006.
12. Coyle D. *The Talent Code*. New York: Bantam Dell; 2009. ISBN 978-0-553-80684-7.
13. Wolff J. *The Law of Bone Remodelling*. Berlin: Springer; 1892.
14. Hebb DO. *The Organization of Behaviour: A Neuropsychological Theory*. New York: Wiley and Sons; 1949. ISBN 978-0-47136727-7.
15. Iacoboni M. *Mirroring People*. New York: Farrar, Straus and Giroux; 2008. ISBN 978-0-374-21017-5.
16. Theorell T, Hammarstrom A, Aronsson G, et al. A systematic review including meta-analysis of work environment and depressive symptoms. *BMC Public Health*. 2015;15:738–748.
17. Mate G. *When the Body Says No: The Cost of Hidden Stress*. Toronto: Alfred A. Knopf; 2003. ISBN:0-676-97311-6.
18. Felitti VJ, Anda RF, Nordenberg D, et al. Relationship of childhood abuse and household dysfunction to many leading causes of death in adults: the adverse childhood experiences (ACE) study. *Am J Prev Med*. 1998;14:245–258.
19. Selye H. *The Stress of Life*. New York: McGraw-Hill; 1956. ISBN 978-0-070-56212-7.
20. McEwen BS. Protective and damaging effects of stress mediators. *New Eng J Med*. 1998;338:171–179.
21. Sapolsky R. *Stress – Portrait of a Killer*. National Geographic; 2008.
22. Porges SW. *The Polyvagal Theory: Neurophysiological Foundations of Emotions, Attachment, Communication, and Self-regulation*. New York: W. W. Norton and Company; 2011. ISBN 978-0-393-70700-7.
23. Zaza C. Playing-related musculoskeletal disorders in musicians: a systematic review of incidence and prevalence. *CMAJ*. 1998;158(8):1019–1025.
24. Gevirtz R. The muscle spindle trigger point model of chronic pain. *Biofeedback*. 2006;34(2):53–57.
25. Miller AH, Maletic V, Raison CL. Inflammation and its discontents: the role of cytokines in the pathophysiology of major depression. *Biol Psychiatry*. 2009;65(9):732–741.
26. Milligan ED, Watkins LR. Pathological and protective roles of glia in chronic pain. *Nat Rev Neurosci*. 2009;10(1):23–36.
27. Loggia ML, Chonde DB, Akeju O, et al. Evidence for brain glial activation in chronic pain patients. *Brain*. 2015;138(Pt 3):604–615.
28. Kenny D, Ackermann B. Performance-related musculoskeletal pain, depression and music performance anxiety in professional orchestral musicians: a population study. *Psychol Music*. 2015;43(1):43–60.
29. Slavich GM, Irwin MR. From stress to inflammation and major depressive disorder: a social signal transduction theory of depression. *Psychol Bull*. 2014;140(3):774–815.
30. Lanius RA, Vermetten E, Pain C. *The Impact of Early Life Trauma on Health and Disease: The Hidden Epidemic*. Cambridge: Cambridge University Press; 2010. ISBN 978-0-521-88026-8.
31. Offord DR, Boyle MH, Fleming JE, et al. Ontario child health study: summary of selected results. *Can J Psychiatry*. 1989;34(6):483–491.
32. Hibbard R, Barlow J, MacMillan H. Psychological maltreatment. *Pediatrics*. 2012;130:372–378.
33. Chazelle D. *Whiplash*. Sony; 2014.
34. Epel ES, et al. Accelerated telomere shortening in response to life stress. *Proc Natl Acad Sci*. 2004;101(49):17312–17315.
35. Blackburn EH. *Telomeres and Telomerase: The Means to the End*. Nobel Lecture; December 7, 2009.
36. Ornish D, et al. Effect of comprehensive lifestyle changes on telomerase activity and telomere length in men with biopsy proven low-risk prostate cancer. *Lancet Oncol*. 2013;14:1112–1120.
37. Solovitch S. *Playing Scared: A History and Memoir of Stage Fright*. New York: Bloomsbury; 2015. ISBN: 978-I-62040-091-3.
38. LeDoux J. *Anxious: Using the Brain to Understand and Treat Fear and Anxiety*. New York: Viking; 2015. ISBN 978-0-670-01533-7.
39. Van der Kolk BA. *The Body Keeps the Score: Brain, Mind and Body in the Healing of Trauma*. New York: Viking; 2014. ISBN 978-0-670-78593-3.

40. Ogden P, Minton K, Pain C. *Trauma and the Body: A Sensorimotor Approach to Psychotherapy*. New York: W. W. Norton and Company; 2006. ISBN:978-0-393-0457-0.

41. Siegel DJ. *The Mindful Brain: Reflection and Attunement in the Cultivation of Well-being*. New York: W. W. Norton and Company; 2007. ISBN 978-0-393-70470-9.

42. Epel E, et al. Can meditation slow rate of cellular aging? Cognitive stress, mindfulness, and telomeres. *Ann NY Acad Sci*. 2009;1172:34−53.

43. Williamon A. *Musical Excellence: Strategies and Techniques to Enhance Performance*. Oxford: Oxford University Press; 2004. ISBN 978-0-19-852535-6.

44. Kenny DT. *The Psychology of Music Performance Anxiety*. Oxford: Oxford University Press; 2011. ISBN: 978-0-9-958614-1.

45. Morton J. *The Authentic Performer − Wearing a Mask and the Effect on Health*. Oxford: Compton Publishing Ltd.; 2015. ISBN 978-1-909082-47-2.

46. Siu AL, USPSTF. Screening for depression in adults: US preventive services Task force recommendation. *JAMA*. 2016; 315(4):380−387.

47. Chong J, Lynden M, Harvey D, Peebles M. Occupational health problems of musicians. *Can Fam Physician*. 1989; 35:2341−2348.

48. Chong J, Zaza C, Smith F. *Med Problems Perform Artists*. 1991;6(1):8.

49. Ackermann BJ, Kenny DT, Driscoll T, O'Brien I. *Sound Practice Health Handbook for Orchestral Musicians*; 2015. http://www.australiacouncil.gov.au/research/wp-content/uploads/2017/06/SoundPractice-WHS-handbook-orchestral-musicians.pdf.

50. Peper E, Tylova H, Gibney KH, Harvey R, Combatalade D. *Biofeedback Mastery − an Experiential Teaching and Self-training Manual*. Association for Applied Psychophysiology and Biofeedback. 2008. ISBN 978-0-9842979-0-0.

51. Guyatt G, Sackett D, Taylor DW, Chong J, Roberts R, Pugsley S. Determining optimal therapy−randomized trials in individual patients. *N Engl J Med*. 1986;314(14): 889−892.

52. van den Eynde J, Fisher A. *Working in the Australian Entertainment Industry: Final Report*; 2016. https://static1.squarespace.com/static/584a0c86cd0f68ddbfffdcea/t/587ed93e3e00be6f0d145fe0/1486006488652/Working+in+the+Australian+Entertainment+Industry_Final+Report_Oct16.pdf.

53. Chong JP, et al. *Psychological Health in Schools of Music: State of the Art Reviews*; 2017. http://www.artsmed.org/sites/default/files/files/stars-nasm-pama-psychological-health_v2.pdf.

Respectfully submitted,

Prof Nim Chimpsky

John Chong MD BASc MSc DOHS FRCPC FACPM CGPP ARCT

Medical Director, Musicians' Clinics of Canada, Hamilton, Ontario

Assistant Professor, Department of Family Medicine

Faculty of Health Sciences, McMaster University, Hamilton, Ontario

Adjunct Professor, Music and Health Research Collaboratory

Faculty of Music, University of Toronto, Toronto, Ontario

Performance Awareness, Glenn Gould School, Royal Conservatory, Toronto, Ontario

Past President and Treasurer, Performing Arts Medicine Association

Governor General Diamond Jubilee Medal

Musicians' Clinics of Canada

565 Sanatorium Road, Suite 201

Hamilton, Ontario, Canada, L9C 7N4 Office: (905)-574-5444 Fax: (905)-574-1119 E-mail: john.chong@sympatico.ca

Performing Arts Medicine Association
Website: artsmed.org

## CHAPTER 6

# Managing Auditory Symptoms in Musicians

MARSHALL CHASIN, MSC, AUD

## INTRODUCTION

Hearing loss is frequently referred to as the invisible handicap. Different from many other injuries in the performing arts field, hearing loss is slow and gradual, without pain that may only manifest itself after many years of music exposure. It is generally the family and friends who may notice the hearing loss long before the musician may notice it. The need for hearing loss prevention is something that has only become explicitly realized by musicians over the last generation.

There are a number of parallels between the study of noise exposure and that of music exposure. Both are based on a combination of laboratory studies that examine the effects on permanent threshold shift (PTS) in mammals such as the chinchilla and guinea pig and studies on the effects of humans with a temporary threshold shift (TTS) paradigm. In a TTS paradigm a worker's or musician's hearing status is measured prior to an exposure and then immediately after—the difference being a measure of TTS in decibels (dB). In addition, there are considerable large-scale surveys resulting in models of hearing loss for industrial workers who have been exposed to noise from industry.

## PERMANENT THRESHOLD SHIFT

As the name suggests, PTS is the permanent loss of sensitivity to certain sounds as a result of exposure to noise and/or music. The vast majority of cases concern a long-term exposure that has the effect of damaging cochlear hair cells resulting in apoptosis or cell death. In some rare cases, single traumatic insults such as an explosion or a feedback squeal can also cause PTS but the pathophysiology is less well defined, most likely being related to a combination of apoptosis, necrosis, and a mechanical breakage of some of the inner ear structures.

Between 1968 and 1973 there were six important studies on the relationship between industrial noise exposure and PTS as a function of duration and sound exposure level.[1-6]

The first five studies formed the basis for the 1973 United States Environmental Protection Agency Criteria Document[7] and noted among other things that there was minimal measureable PTS for exposures less than 85 decibels A-weighted (dBA) if the individual was exposed for 8 h a day over 40 years. The "A-weighting" (in dBA) is a special filter that is applied to a sound level meter where the results relate to the human ear's sensitivity. In these studies, PTS was measured as the average hearing loss for 500, 1000, and 2000 Hz, which is considered to have a low-frequency bias by today's view, because noise- (and music)-induced hearing loss manifests itself in the 3000−6000 Hz region. There was good agreement between the five studies for these lower frequency regions. There was poor agreement however for PTS for higher frequencies such as 4000 Hz, especially at higher noise exposure levels. Although the EPA document is still in effect, the United States defunded many of the EPA activities in the 1980s.

The sixth study[6] formed the basis of the National Institute for Occupational Safety and Health (NIOSH) model.[8] This model was in agreement with the five other studies for PTS at lower exposure levels but predicted a greater PTS at higher exposure levels.

A more recent model of PTS that is currently considered to have high validity for prediction of a group hearing loss as a function of duration and of exposure level is the International Standard Organization (ISO) 1990 Standard R-1999.[9] This model is considered accurate enough for use by regulators and

Performing Arts Medicine. https://doi.org/10.1016/B978-0-323-58182-0.00006-7

administrators to make policy suggestions for workers[10] but "group results cannot and should not be used at any time when an individual is considered" (p. 54).[11] (Table 6.1)

## 3 AND 5 DB EXCHANGE RATE

In 1966 the Committee on Hearing and Bioacoustics (CHABA) attempted to develop a model that would relate exposure level to duration of exposure in an attempt to develop damage risk contours (DRC). For example, can we relate an exposure of 85 dB for 20 h a week to the potential risk for someone who is exposed to 90 dB for 18 h a week? Such a relationship is called an "exchange rate" or "trading relationship."

The 3 dB exchange rate is based on the "equal energy hypothesis" that the effects of noise (or music) exposure that is summed over time adds up to a well-defined exposure energy that is independent of being steady state or intermittent. In this scenario an exposure to 90 dBA for 40 h a week is identical to 93 dBA for 20 h a week (…96 dBA for 10 h a week, 99 dBA for 5 h a week, and so on). This "3 dB exchange rate" is the policy of NIOSH[8,12] in the United States and most other jurisdictions around the world.[13]

The 5 dB exchange rate is predicated on the assumption that equal amounts of temporary threshold shift (TTS) are equally damaging. In this scenario, an exposure of 90 dBA for 40 h a week is identical to 95 dBA for 20 h a week (… 100 dBA for 10 h a week, 105 dBA for 5 h a week, and so on). There is very little theoretical research to support this view since PTS is not correlated to TTS. Subsequently this "5 dB exchange rate" is not found commonly in policies around the world but the Occupational Safety and Health Administration (OSHA)[14] in the United States and a few jurisdictions in Canada do subscribe to this view.

Embleton, in reporting on results of an International Institute of Noise Control Engineering Working Party paper, concluded that "the scientific evidence is that 3 dB is probably the most reasonable exchange rate

for daily noise exposure. Statistically it is also a good approximation for the results of many epidemiological studies relating to intermittent exposures, even though these show considerable spread about any mean curve" (p. 18).[15]

## TEMPORARY THRESHOLD SHIFT

As the name suggests, TTS is a temporary loss in sensitivity to certain sounds for a period following an exposure to noise or music. The pathophysiology is not well understood but appears to be in part related to the temporary disarticulation between the outer hair cells and the tectorial membrane in the cochlea (which re-establishes itself after 16—18 h) and glutamate levels that become ototoxic, where the levels return to a normal (lower) level after 16—18 h. This may be noted by the individual as a feeling of fullness or numbness after a loud event with or without tinnitus. The tinnitus may continue for several days after the event. TTS, being a "threshold" change, assesses cochlear pathology and indeed other measures of cochlear function such as otoacoustic emission (OAE) testing would also show a temporary reduction in cochlear sensory function for a period after an exposure to noise or music. OAEs assess the function of the outer hair cells (efferently innervated) in the cochlea, so TTS is considered to be a cochlear sensory (rather than neural) dysfunction.

## TTS HAS TO BE DISCUSSED IN TWO TIME PERIODS

Prior to the year 2000, TTS was considered to be a benign feature of exposure to noise or music resolving in 16—18 h—a temporary cochlear phenomenon. Because TTS was "temporary," it was a paradigm commonly used to assess whether a person was subjected to an overly high level of noise or music. Academic research review boards had little concern with approving such studies. Much of the research revolved

| TABLE 6.1 | | | | | |
|-----------|---|---|---|---|---|
| **Predicted PTS for a Range of Exposure Levels (in dBA) for a Number of Studies** | | | | | |
| **Sound Level (dBA)** | **Passchier-Vermeer (1971)** | **Robinson (1968)** | **Baughn (1973)** | **NIOSH (1973)** | **ISO R-1999 (1990)** |
| 85 | 8 | 6 | 9 | 5 | 6 |
| 90 | 15 | 12 | 14 | 11 | 11 |
| 95 | 23 | 18 | 17 | 20 | 21 |

around whether a measure of TTS could be used to predict future PTS; however, no research has shown that TTS (or the pattern of recovery from TTS) can be used as a predictor of future PTS.

After the year 2000, a number of studies have demonstrated that despite hearing thresholds returning to the pre-exposure level (i.e., no measureable TTS), there can be some permanent neural deficits that may not be immediately detectable. That is, despite a return to normal cochlear function (with a normal audiogram), there can be neural deficits that remain. Specifically, the synapse from the cochlear inner hair cells (afferently innervated) to the VIII auditory nerve can be permanently altered with a reduced amplitude on the Wave I on a traditional Audiometric Brain Response (ABR) evoked audiometry paradigm. This has been referred to as "cochlear synaptopathy."[16–19] There are currently no accurate measures of cochlear synaptopathy, and its prevalence is not well defined.

Although prevalence estimates of cochlear synaptopathy in animal models are found in the literature, it would be erroneous to relate this to humans. There is very little data, but there has been some research on human temporal bones. Viana et al.[20] counted the number of synapses in five temporal bones. As a function of age, there were fewer synaptic connections at the time of death. Another study by Makary et al.[21] showed that again, as a function of age in 100 human temporal bones, there was a marked decrease in cochlear spiral ganglion cells, despite having intact cochlear sensory cell populations at the time of death.

Cochlear synaptopathy has colloquially been referred to in the media as "hidden hearing loss" and while that can grab headlines, at this point in time, little is known about how this can manifest itself in humans, how this can be reliably measured, and what the prevalence actually is.

## MUSIC AND NOISE

Music is noise. Both music and noise have many features in common. They are both time-varying sources of vibration in air that have peaks and valleys in their amplitudes. Both music and noise can be "intermittent" or "steady state." Occupational noise can have sustained levels in excess of 100 dBA, and many forms of music can have sustained levels in excess of 100 dBA. Having said this, industrial noise sources tend to have more energy in the lower frequency regions whereas music can have significant mid and high frequency energy, although even this gross generalization can be simplistic. Moreover, the audiometric configuration of long-term noise exposure is even similar to that

of long-term music exposure (see Fig. 6.1). It is frequently difficult to differentiate a noise-induced hearing loss from a music-induced hearing loss purely on audiometric data. A thorough case history is required as the differentiating element.

It is therefore not surprising that many of the research results using noise as a stimulus can apply (or have been applied) to music in many national and international regulations and policies.

## MUSIC SOUND LEVELS

Because of the physics of musical instruments, room acoustics, and even electronic sound re-enforcement, music can be played at a number of different levels. Table 6.2, adapted from Chasin,[22] shows typical sound levels in dBA from over 1000 musicians measured at a distance of 3 m when music is played at an "average" or mezzo forte level. The top and bottom quartiles were removed from these data. In the vast majority of instruments (except for acoustic piano and singing), sound levels far exceeded 85 dBA. These data are from solo performances. In real life performances of bands or orchestras, the overall levels would be much greater.

There are dedicated sound level meters that can be used to measure the sound level. There are also many Smartphone apps that are available on both the OS and Android platforms that can perform this function as well. Although there are limitations with many of these apps, they can be accurate for mid-level sounds. Unfortunately (unless otherwise designed), Smartphones typically use a form of "compression" that can lower the measured sound levels, especially for high-level sound sources, providing erroneous results. In addition, Smartphone apps can rely on more than one microphone source (within the Smartphone) imparting a directional bias, thereby further reducing the measured sound level from off-axis sources. Subsequently, caution should be exercised when concluding whether any music source is potentially damaging, especially when based on only several measurements.[23]

## MUSIC AND DOSE

A result that stems from the use of exchange rates is that there is a "maximum dose" that can be measured such as "100% dose of music exposure." If one assumes that an exposure of 85 dBA for 40 h each week is "100% dose" then 88 dBA (85 dBA + 3 dB) for 40 h each week would be "200% dose" and 85 dBA for only 20 h each week would be "50% dose." This above

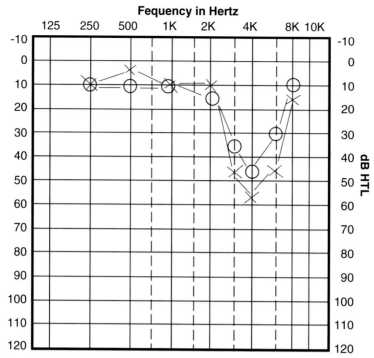

FIG. 6.1 Audiogram of a musician with a music-induced hearing loss showing poorer sensitivity in the 3000–6000 Hz region. "O" represents the right ear and "X" represents the left ear. (From the Musicians' Clinics of Canada; with permission.)

dose calculation assumes a 3 dB exchange rate. If the dose calculation would have used the 5 dB exchange rate, then the 88 dBA exposure for 40 h each week would have been closer to a 150% dosage. The 5 dB exchange rate is more conservative than the 3 dB exchange rate.

| TABLE 6.2 | |
|---|---|
| **Typical Ranges of Some Sound Levels of Music From 3** | |
| **Musical Instrument at 3 m** | **Sound Level (dBA)** |
| Normal piano practice | 60–90 |
| Cello | 80–104 |
| Flute | 98–114 |
| Trumpet | 88–108 |
| Amplified guitar | 105–112 |
| Vocalist | 70–85 |
| Saxophone | 75–110 |

Adapted from Chasin M. Sound levels for musical instruments. *Hear Rev* 2006;13(3):34–41; with permission.

The result of research into the effects of noise (and music) demonstrates that it is not just the sound level (in dBA) but the sound level over a period of time that can potentially damage one's hearing. There is nothing wrong with going to a rock concert on Friday night as long as you do not mow your lawn on Saturday. It is the dose that we try to keep below "100%."

There are many dedicated dosimeters that can be used (where a light may flash red when 100% dose is achieved), and recently some Smartphone-based dosimeters have become available. The Smartphone-based apps do suffer from the same microphone and compression issues mentioned with sound level meter apps, but again, can be used as a first estimate in any hearing conservation program. Fig. 6.2

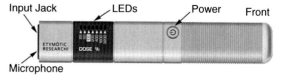

FIG. 6.2 Hand held dosimeter showing the percentage of dose of noise or music exposure. (From Etymotic Research; with permission.)

shows a commercially available dosimeter that many musicians use.

## HEARING PROTECTION

Because of the laws of physics where high frequency sounds acoustically "see" any obstruction better than lower frequencies, conventional industrial hearing protection tends to provide only about 20–25 dB of protection for the lower frequency sounds but up to 35–40 dB for the higher frequency sounds. Because sound energy can enter the skull directly to the cochlea (in the 2000 Hz region), the maximum limit of attenuation on any hearing protector is 40 dB.[24]

The musicians' earplug utilizes an acoustic network (either Holmholtz or wavelength based) to reestablish much of the mid- and high-frequency sound energy; the result being a flat or uniform hearing protector. Having a uniform attenuation hearing protector allows the musician to hear the proper balance between the lower frequency fundamental (or tonic) energy and the higher frequency harmonic energy. All acoustic energy in the music is reduced identically from a potentially damaging to a nondamaging sound level. Various manufactures of the musicians' earplugs have different strategies to accomplish this but most provide approximately 15 dB of sound attenuation. Although 15 dB does not sound like a lot, every 3 dB reduction effectively cuts the dose of exposure in half. A musician wearing a 15 dB uniform hearing protector can then be in a musical environment for 32 times as long as without hearing protection—more is not necessarily better.

What the physician treating musicians need to know:

- What are some factors that can affect hearing loss? The two main factors are the sound level of the music or noise, and how long one has been exposed to it. We know from research that prolonged exposure to 85 dBA or greater, over time will cause a permanent hearing loss. The "A-weighting" (in dBA) is a special filter that is applied to a sound level meter where the results relate to the human ear's sensitivity. A level of 85 dBA is not particularly loud—a dial tone on a telephone is about that! Even though it is not loud, the sound level is enough to be damaging. However, it also depends on how long you are exposed to it. Research has found that the maximum exposure each week should be less than 85 dBA for 40 h. This is identical to 88 dB for only 20 h. That is, for each increase of 3 dB, you can only be exposed for half as long. Saying it differently, for every 3 dB increase, your

exposure doubles. Other less significant factors are general health, environmental concerns, and hereditary factors.

- Can a single, short duration sound cause permanent hearing damage? If so at what level?
This is called "acoustic trauma" and is quite rare. Different from most types of hearing loss from loud noise or music that is gradual and happens over many years, a single intense blast can create a sudden permanent hearing loss at exactly the frequency of the insulting sound. A common example is a feedback squeal from a loud speaker—a permanent hearing loss can occur and will occur at exactly the frequency of the feedback squeal (e.g., 1500 Hz). This example is not a typically frequency tested one by an audiologist, so care should be taken to assess as many frequencies as possible during testing to eliminate this.
  - This is a common concern for sax and clarinet players—instruments where the top teeth touch the mouthpiece. Sound can be generated from the instrument, through the teeth and by way of bone conduction, go directly to the ear. There are no studies that I know of about the exact sound level, but indirect evidence suggests that the sound can be quite intense. One can minimize the potential effect by ensuring that the earplug does not "trap" the sound in the ear. This is called the occlusion effect. As a sax player, unless the band is VERY loud, you should not be wearing an ER-25. At most, the ER-15 would be sufficient. I am a clarinet player and I use the vented/tuned earplugs. These use a small hole that would let the bone conducted sound out of my ear.
- Which are more damaging: low or high frequencies? Actually, this is an important question. A few research studies concluded that some frequencies are "slightly" more damaging than others, but in reality, all frequencies are equally damaging. The reason we have our worst hearing in the 3000–6000 Hz region (around the top note of the piano keyboard) has more to do with the way our ear is made up, rather than the sound(s) that cause the hearing loss. For this reason, a flute and a bass player would have similar hearing losses.
- I have had tinnitus for 2 years. Is my drumming career over?
Tinnitus is almost always associated with some hearing loss. Treating the hearing loss may result in "treating the tinnitus." Most people find that some external noise (either from a hearing aid or from a

"tinnitus masker") tends to block out the tinnitus. That is why many people with tinnitus do not find that it is as bothersome when there is background noise. Many musicians find that external noise allows them to play and enjoy their music. In fact, there is a type of tinnitus therapy called tinnitus retraining therapy (TRT) that has been shown to be successful for many musicians.

- So what is Tinnitus Retraining Therapy?

  Tinnitus is actually created in the brain—not the ear. The hearing loss (from too much loud music) causes the nerve endings in the ear to become damaged. The brain cells that receive the impulses from these nerve endings say "where is the sound?" These cells become "lonely" and start to generate their own sound. TRT is a method that involves counselling and the use of a noise generator (or masker). The cells in the brain say "Oh! Here is the sound" and gradually (after a year or so) stop producing their own noise. The tinnitus is reduced (or at least becomes less bothersome and noticeable). Many audiologists offer this type of tinnitus therapy but there are other tinnitus reduction therapies as well.

- What can be done if I do have tinnitus that would not go away?

  Do not panic—this is rather uncommon, but it does occur on occasion. There is almost always a hearing loss associated with the tinnitus. Using hearing aids (and there are some that fit invisibly into the ear canal) not only will help you hear better, but will tend to mask or reduce the tinnitus in the majority of people. Being overly concerned about it is another problem. The last thing someone should do is become stressed as this may make the tinnitus more noticeable. There are therapy programs that serve to retrain the brain to ignore tinnitus and these can be very successful. Contact your local audiologist or doctor if this becomes a problem.

- What else can happen as my hearing gets worse?

  In some sense, hearing loss is the least of your worries. After all, hearing loss is very gradual, and only affects the very high pitched sounds... so you may not notice it for years to come. However, with hearing loss comes two other things that can be very annoying—or if you are a musician—can be career ending. They are pitch perception problems and permanent tinnitus. Pitch perception problems, as the name suggests, means that a person with a significant hearing loss may hear one note as another (and have limited understanding for speech). Moreover, can you imagine having a constant hum

or whistle in your head day and night? So, ... prevention of hearing loss is where it is at.

- If my tinnitus goes away after 16 h, is it safe to go to another concert after?

  The short answer is "yes" and "no." It is true that the ear recovers after about 16 h and can take on new challenges of loud music, but TTS is a warning signal of being exposed to too much music. If you go to a rock concert on Friday night, do not mow your lawn until Sunday (or better yet, get someone else to do it!) However, once you have a music related (or noise induced) hearing loss, it is permanent, so do whatever it takes to prevent it. Certainly, moderation is one idea. Enjoy that loud song, but when it is over, turn down the volume a bit to give your ears a rest.

- Well, ... thank you for that, but what is TTS?

  TTS stands for temporary threshold shift. This is a fancy way of saying temporary hearing loss. After a loud concert, or a day in the factory, your hearing is temporarily reduced. After about 16−18 h, this hearing loss resolves and your hearing should return to the level it was before (hopefully normal). When the hearing is reduced, there is frequently tinnitus, which is especially noticeable in quiet places such as when you are trying to sleep. The tinnitus and hearing loss (sometimes felt as a numbness in your ears) should completely resolve after 16 h. However, it turns out that TTS may not be just a benign characteristic of too much noise or music. Recent research indicates that while the hearing loss (as measured with puretones on a hearing test or audiogram) can return to normal, that there can still be permanent neural damage.

- What is hyperacusis?

  Hyperacusis is an awful sounding word meaning an "abnormal sensitivity to loud sound." People may complain that "medium sounds are OK but loud sounds that don't bother most people, seem to bother me!" This is actually an early warning sign of hearing loss. That is, not only does sound have to be a bit louder to hear, but also the tolerance to loud sounds is reduced. Most modern hearing aids are specially designed to not only amplify softer sounds but make louder sounds softer. Most people with hyperacusis have some hearing loss. On rare occasions, some people with normal hearing have hyperacusis as well. It also turns out that the part of the brain that lights up with a functional MRI scan for people that have hyperacusis is also the same part of the brain that shows hyperactivity for those who have tinnitus. Many strategies to reduce tinnitus can be quite useful for those people complaining of hyperacusis.

- Could low-frequency hearing loss be caused by music?

  NO. All music (and noise exposure) manifests itself in the higher frequency region (with the greatest hearing loss being near the top note on the piano keyboard—being between 3000 and 6000 Hz). If someone has a low frequency hearing loss it is either related to the outer and middle ears (e.g., wax, ear infection, or a stiffening of the bones in the middle ear) or by an unusual condition of the inner ear. In all cases, you should seek out the medical opinion of an ear, nose, and throat doctor (an otolaryngologist). Depending on where you live, you may require a referral from your primary care physician.

- Can my hearing loss be treated with medicine or surgery?

  Only hearing losses that are from the middle ear (where kids get ear infections) or from the outer ear (such as wax occlusion) can be treated. Rarely, can a hearing loss be treated if it is from the inner ear. The inner ear is actually in the brain, so inner ear surgery is brain surgery! Having said all this, researchers are working on a "vaccination" that can be given to reverse inner ear hearing loss but this is still years away.

- What are some other causes of permanent hearing loss?

  Other than hearing loss associated with aging (called presbycusis), the single greatest cause is working around noise or music. The ear does not know the difference between loud noise and loud music. To the ear, noise and music are just vibrations in the air. Rarely, a person may suffer a permanent hearing loss from a virus or even a brain tumor. These usually have a sudden onset and may be accompanied by dizziness. Hearing loss from noise or music tends to be gradual in nature with no dizziness. If one experiences dizziness or a sudden hearing loss, one should immediately contact their primary care physician.

- Can headphones damage hearing?

  Headphones are no more damaging than listening to music from a loudspeaker. One will always adjust the volume to a comfortable listening level, and the ear does not know whether the music is coming from headphones (3 cm from the ear) or a loudspeaker (3 m from the ear). The potential danger is when headphones are used in conjunction with "portable" music such as an MP3 player. Listening to music in a noisy environment can be damaging, because one tends to turn up the volume over the background noise.

- So what volumes are safe when I listen to my MP3 player?

  There is a good rule of thumb called the "80/90 rule." This stands for "80% volume on your MP3 player for 90 minutes a day." This exposure "dose" will provide one half of your daily exposure. If your favorite song comes on, turn up the volume and enjoy it; but turn down the volume after.

- Are noise cancelling earbuds/headphones better for your hearing?

  Portable or recreational music exposure such as those from MP3 players can be potentially damaging simply because people listen in noisy everyday environments. The tendency is to turn up the volume over the background noise, and this is where the danger lays. Using either noise cancelling headphones or "isolation" earphones that lessen the environmental noise means that you do not need to turn up the volume as much. So, yes, these earphones can be very useful. However, beware of not being as able to hear a car coming up behind you!

- I teach music in a high school and the room is awful. Is there anything I can do to improve it? P.S. I do not have much money.

  Actually there are several things you can do that are easy to accomplish and inexpensive. You can place the trumpet players on risers as this will allow the higher pitched harmonics of the trumpet to literally go over the heads of the other musicians "downwind." You can put up some drapes over the blackboard behind you while you are conducting to dampen the unwanted reflections. These drapes can be pulled aside when you want to use the blackboard. Finally, get the Art Department to make some 3-D relief art that can be placed on the side walls. This will also help to lessen the unwanted reflections. High school band teachers, because of the number of hours each week that they must be in a band room should consider musicians' earplugs. Teachers are at risk of hearing loss and have successfully won cases with some Worker's Compensation Boards, or their equivalent, in the past.

- When I go to a concert in a large venue, the band is set back from the edge of the stage. Is this to protect them from the fans?

  How observant you are! It may be to protect them, but there is an acoustic reason as well. The lip of the stage in front of the band or orchestra acts as an acoustic mirror. That is, the higher pitched sounds of the band not only come off the stage to the audience but also reflect off the lip of the stage, thereby enhancing the higher pitched sounds. The band members do not have to play as loud up on stage for the people in the audience to hear it better. Not only are the musicians performing at a safer level, but the potential for arm and wrist injuries are lessened.

- Can this be helped by diet and lifestyle?

Diet is obviously critical to maintaining optimal health. Drinking plenty of fluids and eating healthy (vegetarian) meals can do alot to extend your musical career, especially if you are on the road. Many 24-h supermarkets stock easy to prepare frozen foods that can be heated up in the night-club's microwave. Try to keep caffeine and alcohol to an acceptable minimum—having two beers and not four. (And of course no beer if you are under age!)

- What are some causes of music-related injuries?

Most music-related health problems come from the interaction between the musician and their instrument or the musician and the environment. Too much force, too many repetitions, and too much force or volume can all result in injury. Musicians tend to be stuck in one position and repetitive strain injuries can occur. Faulty technique can also contribute to problems.

I understand that rock music can be damaging to my hearing, but I cannot believe that Mozart or Beethoven can be bad for me.

Believe it or not, but Classical music—or specifically playing classical music—can be more damaging than rock music. Research has shown that about 37% of rock musicians have a hearing loss, and about 52% of classical musicians suffer from this problem. The main difference is that classical musicians rehearse, perform, and teach more hours each week than typical rock musicians. Moreover, classical musicians tend to be clustered closer together than rock musicians. So even though the peak sound levels in a rock band may be higher than in an orchestra, the total weekly dosage of a classical musician is greater.

- Can I do anything with my loudspeakers to hear the music better and to protect myself from further hearing loss?

Loudspeakers do not send all sounds out equally. Typically the low pitched bass notes emanate from all parts of the loudspeaker—bass notes are equally loud from the back, front, top, and sides. However, the higher pitched notes come out almost like a

laser beam—in a straight line. If the loudspeakers can be tilted to aim toward your ears, you will hear a flatter "truer" sound. Moreover, importantly, if the loudspeaker is aimed at your ears, the overall volume control level will be lower. In this manner, even though the music will sound as loud, it will be at a lower sound level. That means it will be less damaging. Sound level is what causes hearing loss, whereas loudness is simply your impression of the sound. Some researchers suggest elevating the loudspeakers, and this can be useful, but be careful. Some loudspeakers are designed to be left on the floor. Check with the manufacturer before you elevate loudspeakers to see if this would be a problem.

- I have also seen some baffles hooked onto the back of some seats at the symphony. What are these used for?

These are typically used on the seats of violinists and viola players. In many cases, these musicians need to sit in front of the brass or percussion sections, and the baffles serve to lessen the energy from these louder instruments. The only problem with a seat baffle is that it has to be within 7 inches (18 cm) of the violinist's ear. If it is further away, there is minimal benefit because of the reflections off the floor, ceiling, and music stands.

- I have seen some clear plastic shields up on stage in front of the drummer. What are these used for and do they work?

These are called baffles and are usually made of Plexiglas or Lucite. All baffles, because of the laws of physics, attenuate (or lessen) the higher pitched sounds more than the lower bass notes. These baffles are designed to lessen the energy for those high pitched high hat cymbals, and rim shot hits that a drummer may make. This protects the other musicians and helps to improve the balance of the music. Note that the low bass thumping sounds from the bass drum is not really affected. The only "trick" with baffles is that they should not extend up above the drummer's ear. The last thing anyone would want is to cause more hearing loss in the drummer by being forced to hear his music, not once, but twice (the initial sound and the reflection off the back of the baffle).

- I have seen musicians on TV wearing what look like hearing aids connected to small wires. What are these?

These are called in-the-ear monitors, and they are a form of a modified hearing aid. Musicians use them as their own monitoring system instead of the small "wedge" monitors on the floor of the stage. The wires are connected to the sound amplification system either directly or through a wireless transmitter. The musician can then hear their own music as well as that of the other musicians, but at a safer level. When musicians use in-the-ear monitors, the overall sound level on stage is typically much less than if they were using conventional wedge monitors.

## REFERENCES

1. Passchier-Vermeer W. *Hearing Loss Due to Exposure to Steady-state Broadband Noise (Rep. No. 35)*. The Netherlands: Institute for Public Health Engineering; 1968.
2. Passchier-Vermeer W. Steady-state and fluctuating noise: its effects on the hearing of people. In: Robinson DW, ed. *Occupational Hearing Loss*. New York: Academic Press; 1971.
3. Robinson DW. The relationship between hearing loss and noise exposure. In: *National Physical Laboratory Aero Report Ae32*. London, England: National Physical Laboratory; 1968.
4. Robinson DW. Estimating the risk of hearing loss due to continuous noise. In: Robinson DW, ed. *Occupational Hearing Loss*. New York: Academic Press; 1971.
5. Baughn WL. *Relation Between Daily Noise Exposure and Hearing Loss as Based on the Evaluation of 6835 Industrial Noise Exposure Cases*. Dayton, Ohio: Aerospace Medical Research Laboratory, Wright-Patterson Air Force Base; 1973. TR-AMRL-TR-73-53 (AD767 204).
6. Lempert BL, Henderson TL. *NIOSH Survey of Occupational Noise and Hearing: 1968 to 1972*. Washington, DC: US Department of Health, Education and Welfare, National Institute for Occupational Safety and Health, TR 86; 1973.
7. Environmental Protection Agency. *Public Health and Welfare Criteria for Noise. (EPA Rep. No. 550/9-73-002)*. Washington, DC: Author; 1973.
8. NIOSH. *Occupational Noise and Hearing 1968-1972. HSM 73-11001*. Washington, DC: NIOSH; 1973.
9. International Organization for Standardization. *Acoustics-Determination of Occupational Noise Exposure and Estimation of Noise-induced Hearing Impairment*. 2nd ed. Geneva, Switzerland: Author; 1990. International Standard ISO 1999.
10. Johnson DL. Field studies: industrial exposures. *J Acoust Soc Am*. 1991;90:170−174.
11. Glorig A, Linthicum FE. The relations of noise-induced hearing loss and presbycusis. *J Occup Hear Loss*. 1998;1:51−60.
12. NIOSH. *Criteria for a Recommended Standard, Occupational Noise Exposure, DHHS (NIOSH), Publication No. 98-126*. Washington, DC: NIOSH; 1998.
13. Suter AH. Development of standards and regulations for occupational noise. In: Crocker M, ed. *Handbook of Noise and Vibration Control*. Hoboken: John Wiley and Sons, Inc.; 2007:377−382.
14. OSHA. Occupational noise exposure: hearing conservation amendment; Final Rule, effective 8 March 1983. 29 CFR 1910.95; 1983.
15. Embleton T. Upper limits on noise in the workplace. Report by the international Institute of noise control Engineering working party. *Can Acoust*. 1995;23(2):11−20.
16. Kujawa SG, Liberman MC. Adding insult to injury: cochlear nerve degeneration after "temporary" noise-induced hearing loss. *J Neurosci*. 2009;29:14077−14085.
17. Kujawa SG. Putting the 'neural' back in sensorineural: primary cochlear neurodegeneration in noise and aging. *Hear J*. 2014;67:8.
18. Kujawa SG, Liberman MC. Synaptopathy in the noise-exposed and aging cochlea: primary neural degeneration in acquired sensorineural hearing loss. *Hear Res*. 2015;330:191−199.
19. Liberman MC, Kujawa SG. Cochlear synaptopathy in acquired sensorineural hearing loss: Manifestations and mechanisms. *Hear Res*. 2017;349:138−147.
20. Viana LM, O'Malley JT, Burgess BT, et al. Cochlear neuropathy in human presbycusis: Confocal analysis of hidden hearing loss in post-mortem tissue. *Hear Res*. 2015;327:78−88.
21. Makary CA, Shin J, Kujawa SG, Liberman MC, Merchant SN. Age-related primary cochlear neuronal degeneration in human temporal bones. *J Acad Res Otolaryngol*. 2011;12:711−717.
22. Chasin M. Sound levels for musical instruments. *Hear Rev*. 2006;13(3):34−41.
23. Chasin M. Smartphones and microphones. *Hear Rev*. 2017;24(12):10.
24. Berger EH. Methods of measuring the attenuation of hearing protection devices. *J Acoust Soc Am*. 1986;79:1655−1687.

## CHAPTER 7

# Care of the Marching Musician

STEVEN ROCK, MD • SERENA WEREN, DMA

The marching arts encompass activities such as marching band, drum corps, and amusement park performers. The physical demands of participation in the marching arts can vary greatly, depending on the performance (i.e., competition performance vs. parade), the instrument being played, the fitness of the participant, the type of music being performed, and the style of marching. Despite the large numbers of participants, there has been little research done on these activities and their participants.

## BACKGROUND

Across the country, many individuals are involved in high school and collegiate marching band. Most marching bands have all musicians participating on the field during rehearsals and performances and include various combinations of percussion (referred to as the drumline), woodwinds, brass, color guard, dancers, twirlers, and drum majors. A subset of percussionists, often referred to as the front ensemble or pit, play from the front of the field but do not march. The dynamics of the activity can vary between marching bands. Some units may have limited marching when playing, whereas other groups may incorporate highly choreographed moves at high intensities while playing instruments with precision. Some high school marching bands perform only at halftime of sporting events or parades. Other high school marching bands enter band competitions throughout the fall in addition to the halftime performances and parades. The competitive marching bands will typically perform a single show throughout the season, making modifications to improve the show as the season progresses. The bands that only perform at halftimes may learn a new show each week of the football season, which is common among collegiate marching bands. Additionally, marching bands at all levels often participate in parades throughout the year, and while not as technical as a competitive show, often require continuous marching and playing for many miles with little rest. Each of these

situations creates a different set of demands on the marching athletes. Marching bands that perform the same show for the entire season can be at risk for overuse or repetitive use injuries, due to the number of repetitions of movements they are required to practice and perform. Those bands learning a new show each week can be at greater risk of acute injury with the changes in timing and patterns of movement.

Drum corps is a competitive summertime activity with marching ensembles consisting of brass instruments, drumline, color guard, drum major(s), and a front ensemble. Similar to competitive high school marching bands, drum corps work to perfect a 12-min show over the span of the summer competitive season. For each of these activities, individuals audition for a position with a particular corps. In Drum Corps International (DCI), world class corps are considered to be the elite level. World class corps are active 10−14 h a day, often rehearsing during the day, competing in the evening, traveling by bus during the night, and sleeping the remainder of the night on gym floors. The world class corps comprised high school and college aged individuals up to age 22. Open class corps have a less demanding competition and travel schedule. Typically, members are younger, ranging in age from 9 to 22 years old. The open class rehearsals can be nearly as long, but the performance itself is less technically and physically demanding. Drum Corps Associates (DCA) corps do not have an upper age limit, but typically compete on weekends and have a less intense rehearsal schedule.

SoundSport is another predominantly summertime marching activity similar to DCI and DCA, but is performed on a much smaller field allowing for more choice in performance venues both indoor and outdoor. Other related marching activities include competitive winter guard, winter drumline, and winter winds. Although there are fewer participants and groups, these activities are often the source of inspiration for competitive high school marching band performances. The majority of drum corps athletes are also involved in high school or collegiate marching band.[1] A subset of these

Performing Arts Medicine. https://doi.org/10.1016/B978-0-323-58182-0.00007-9

individuals will participate in summer, fall, and winter marching arts activities, making them a year-round marching athlete. These individuals have little time for rest and recovery from injury and are at high risk for overuse.

Instrument weights and shapes differ considerably (Table 7.1). High school and collegiate marching bands often utilize woodwind instruments, which weigh as little as 1 pound. At the other end of the spectrum, low brass instrument weights are often 25 pounds or greater and tenor drums can weigh nearly 35 pounds. This can be particularly significant for younger musicians where the instrument is a greater percentage of their body weight and their relative strength and endurance are less. Most instruments are not designed with optimal ergonomics in mind for playing while seated, let alone while marching. The instruments may shift the center of gravity in front of the musician, causing them to lean backward, increasing stress on the shoulders, upper back, and lower back. Color guards utilize flags, rifles, sabres, and other props with varying weights and resistances to create a visual effect.

Published estimates of workload in the marching arts are 4.5–6 METs, which are derived from a single study of treadmill marching at a steady rate and parade marching.[2] This equates the marching arts with activities such as archery and shooting baskets.[3] Another study demonstrated heart rates between 120 and 200 while comparing different marching techniques.[4] Unpublished data from a study of drum corps athletes demonstrated similar heart rate ranges and total daily caloric expenditures of over 5000 kcal/day. The intensity of the activity during the 8–10 h a day of drum corps rehearsal varies greatly, from standing and rehearsing music, to full drill (rehearsing parts of or the full show). When rehearsing full drill, step rates may briefly be over 200 steps per minute, with an average of 120–140 steps per minute. During the active portions of rehearsals and performances, workloads can approach 10 METs, as demonstrated in a quad drummer who was monitored during a rehearsal. His heart rate was reported to average 180 bpm and his VO2 during the rehearsal reached 40 mL/kg per minute, which approximates 9–10 METs.[5,6] This level of activity compares to vigorous calisthenics and vigorous circuit training.[3] Particularly with drum corps and competitive marching bands, this higher estimate likely is more reflective of the demands of the marching arts as they have evolved and deserves further study.

## MARCHING STYLES AND TECHNIQUE

Participation in the marching arts across all performance and age levels predominantly fall into two marching style categories: corps style and traditional style. Although both styles have many similarities, the purpose, music, and marching techniques are very often different and therefore, the demands on the marching athlete vary. Marching techniques for each style are developed to create a more cohesive visual and musical presentation, but are often highly repetitive, unnatural, or physically demanding to perform well. The foundational marching techniques of each style are emphasized heavily in rehearsals that create a risk factor for overuse and repetitive strain musculoskeletal injuries. Unsurprisingly, a majority of these musculoskeletal injuries affect the lower extremities.[7,8] The following is a brief overview of the major marching techniques within each style.

Corps style marching is the most common and is the standard for competitive marching activities from the high school level through DCI. The most common foundational marching technique utilized across this style consists of variations on the glide step. The forward-moving glide step, or roll step, is performed by moving one leg forward leading with the ankle dorsiflexed 90°, allowing the heel to hit the ground first,

| TABLE 7.1 Marching Instrument Approximate Weights | |
|---|---|
| **Instrument** | **Approximate Weights** |
| Flute | 1 lb |
| Clarinet | 1.5 lbs |
| Alto saxophone | 4.6–5 lbs |
| Tenor saxophone | 6.5–7.5 lbs |
| Baritone saxophone | 11–15 lbs |
| Trumpet | 2.5–3 lbs |
| Mellophone | 3.5–4 lbs |
| Trombone | 4–5 lbs |
| Baritone | 5.5–6 lbs |
| Euphonium | 7–8 lbs |
| Tuba/contrabass | 20–28 lbs |
| Sousaphone | 25–50 lbs |
| Cymbals | 7.2–15 lbs |
| Snare drum (without carrier) | 13.2–25 lbs |
| Tenor drums (without carrier) | 20–34 lbs |
| Bass drum (without carrier) | 13–30 lbs |

and then rolling smoothly through the foot. The upper body remains as upright and still as possible throughout the step, giving the impression of gliding. The purpose of this step is to allow for a very visually fluid motion across the field at all tempos and control over the upper body that does not impede the consistent airflow needed to produce a sustained sound on a wind instrument. Variations in the glide step are dependent upon how straight the knee remains throughout the marching motion and range from bent knee to straight leg marching. Drum corps, as well as some high schools and university bands, utilize straight leg marching where the knee must remain almost completely straight throughout the movement. The marcher's weight is shifted to the ball of the foot and used to push the marcher forward. This gait creates the cleanest visual on the field, but is difficult, physically demanding, and unnatural to produce. If not performed correctly or without necessary physical conditioning, straight leg marching can result in lower extremity musculoskeletal injuries. Those marching bands—not able to commit the time to train straight leg marching—bend the knee, which is more comparable to a natural gait.

When moving backwards, marchers maintain the straight leg of the glide step, but remain on the balls of their feet without the heels touching the ground. As they move backward, they drag their toes on the ground that helps to provide the same visually fluid motion as moving forward. Similar to the variation in the forward glide step, another backward marching technique bends the knee and rolls the foot from the toe through the heel. When moving in lateral directions, or sliding, these marching techniques continue to be used; however, the toes will point or drag in the direction of motion and the upper body will twist from the hips to keep the shoulders parallel to the front of the field regardless of the direction of motion. Quick changes in direction, especially at high tempos, are a common source of acute injury.

The drumline has a unique technique called the crab step that is used when moving laterally. It visually allows the drums to stay parallel to the front of the field, but it also presents unique injury risks in this population. The crab step involves crossing the trailing leg in front of the leading leg while keeping the upper body and hips parallel to the front of the field. For example, when moving laterally to the right, the left leg will always cross in front with the foot rolling from the outside edge to the inside. This is similar to a carioca run done in sport warm-ups although it does not alternate legs front and back.

Other marching techniques that are commonly used in corps style include flanks and other types of turns. A flank is a sharp 90° turn with the entire body. The step is produced by either planting the heel or the toe pointing toward the new direction and then making the sharp turn with the next step. Turns of various degrees can be produced using this technique. The sharpness with which performers may be asked to create these turns and the marching surface upon which the heel or ball of the foot rotates can lead to possible knee and ankle injuries.

The color guard and other dance units may utilize the techniques outlined above, but they are often required to move further than the instrumentalists in the same amount of time to create the visual displays appropriate within their function on the field. Much of the choreography for the color guard is influenced by different dance styles and utilizes the jazz run as a basic movement technique. As with the glide step, the upper body remains still and upright so that it still appears to glide, but in the jazz run, the body is lowered by bending the knees and each step is a controlled lunge led with a pointed toe and the leg externally rotated. This technique is used by instrumentalist when they must quickly cover large distances, but is sparingly used while playing.

Corps style has evolved significantly over the past 20 years, which has increased the technical and physical demands placed upon the marching athlete. The movement techniques have grown to include extremely complex and varied motions including interactions with large and small props on the field. Although they create a very engaging performance for the audience, they require more training and physical conditioning to perform safely. These demands are exemplified by the DCI world class corps. Many high school marching bands emulate the movements and show concepts of these corps, but often do not have access to the same number of trained staff; in addition, participants have a wider range of fitness levels, with less time to learn and develop compared with DCI.

Traditional style marching bands, also known as show bands, are more regionally or culturally situated and are mainly for entertainment, not competition. These bands use marching techniques unique to their cultural traditions and can vary greatly. An example of a show band style is that used by historically black colleges and university (HBCU) marching bands. HBCU marching bands often use highly choreographed movements and an ankle knee step. The ankle knee step is produced by lifting the ankle to the height of the opposite knee. Opposite of the glide step, the toe is the last part of the foot to leave the ground and the first to return to the ground. HBCU show band style also often includes more dance, exaggerated motion, and significant rhythmic movement of the instruments and upper bodies while marching.

Another common example of a traditional style band is that used by many of the Big Ten university bands. Instead of the ankle knee step, these bands often use the chair step, which is similar except the elevated leg forms right angles at the hip and knee with the toe pointed down creating a chair shape in profile. Due to the physical demands of performing this step for prolonged periods, some bands only lift the leg to a 45° angle in extended performances such as parades. Both the chair and ankle knee step may use stop action, which requires a momentary stop in motion at the peak of each step. This increases the physical demands on the performer to control each step.

At the university level, it is not uncommon to have a mixture of styles. For example, the pregame show may feature a traditional style and the halftime show may be more corps style. It is also not uncommon for corps style bands to use tradition style movements as effects within a show. There are also other types of marching bands such as military bands, fife & drum corps, and scatter bands. Participation in these styles is less common and draws upon many similar marching techniques described above. A detailed discussion is beyond the scope of this chapter, but as with all of these techniques, they can be described and demonstrated by a marching athlete patient. Numerous videos and written resources are also available on the marching arts that may be helpful.

## INJURIES

Musculoskeletal injuries in the marching arts are largely overuse injuries. Detailed discussion of injury treatment in the marching arts is beyond the scope of this chapter. The approach to treatment of chronic and acute injuries in the marching arts does not differ from the sport athlete. Relative rest, limited participation, and gradual progression back to activity can be challenging. Depending on the situation, the marching athlete may be worried about losing their dot, or spot on the field, to a reserve member or letting their teammates in the band down by leaving an empty spot on the field during performances or competition. Just as the sports medicine team should meet with athletic coaches in the preseason, the medical team should meet with the directors of the marching arts group to develop policies and procedures regarding injuries and return to play,

develop, and rehearse emergency action plans, and advocate for the health and safety of the marching athlete. Unfortunately, many high school and some university marching bands are separated from the athletic infrastructure and do not have any or easy access to athletic trainers or other medical staff, guidelines for healthy and safe participation, and are led by music educators with minimal training in these issues. Many marching athletes have an expectation that they will go back to activity unrestricted after injury. To create a functional progression within the activity, the author has found it helpful to recommend a gradual increase in the number of repetitions of segments of the show during rehearsal. For example, the returning member can be instructed to start with 1 rep out of 5 and increase gradually as long as their symptoms do not recur.

The marching athlete should be encouraged to bring in their instrument to clinic appointments, if possible. This will help the clinician to understand the physical demands of holding and playing the instrument. Having video of the performance/rehearsals and a copy of the rehearsal/competition schedule can be helpful with planning for treatment and rehabilitation of injuries and ultimately progression back to full participation.

## LOWER EXTREMITY INJURIES

Injuries in the marching arts most often involve the lower extremities and are largely overuse injuries. In surveys of collegiate marching bands, 25% of respondents reported a musculoskeletal injury, of which 88.7% involved the lower extremity.[7,8] Injuries are more common early in the season, often during band camp and in the first month of the season, when rehearsals are longer and more intense.[7,8] Shin splints, patellofemoral stress syndrome, stress fractures, and ankle sprains are common issues. Based on experience with this activity, most drum corps have more than one member with a stress fracture per season, some of which may not be reported or detected until after the season. In the marching arts, the performance surface can be uneven, particularly with natural grass fields and can lead to ankle sprains and fractures. Poor biomechanics can result in patellofemoral pain, patellar dislocation, or anterior cruciate ligament tear due to landing with valgus alignment at the knee. Depending on the marching technique, individuals can be at risk for tibialis anterior tendonitis/tenosynovitis. The straight leg marching technique requires a deliberate foot roll, from heel strike with the ankle held at 90°, through toe off, creating an excessive eccentric load on the ankle dorsiflexors.

Members of the drumline experience lower extremity issues less commonly seen in other sections. The crab step, or lateral marching by continuously crossing the trailing leg in front of the leading leg while keeping the upper body and hips parallel to the front of the field, is a heavily used movement by drumlines. Based on the author's experience, high volumes of crab stepping during practices and performances can lead to adductor injuries, trochanteric bursitis, iliotibial band syndrome, and iliopsoas snapping hip/bursitis. The carrier harnesses used in the marching percussion can put pressure on the lateral femoral cutaneous nerve, causing meralgia paresthetica. This can be alleviated by adding padding beneath the harness to dissipate the pressure over the nerve or by flipping the carrier plate.

## UPPER EXTREMITY INJURIES
Shoulder pain is common, particularly for marching athletes carrying brass instruments. The posture of holding the instrument stresses the shoulders and can lead to a decompensated posture. Decompensated posture can cause a forward positioning of the shoulder complex, resulting in scapulothoracic dyskinesis and secondary impingement syndrome. At a minimum, decompensated posture can result in significant muscle soreness and tightness in the scapular stabilizers. The asymmetric posture required to hold some instruments (i.e., flute, trombone, contrabass) can lead to altered posture while playing, leading to shoulder impingement and other upper extremity pain.[9]

The cymbal player is at risk for shoulder injury, as the playing technique involves holding a 4 kg disc in each hand with the elbows nearly fully extended. The shoulder is held between 70 and 90° of forward flexion. The cymbals are flipped and spun for visual effect, stressing the entire shoulder complex.[10]

Forearm and wrist pain are most commonly encountered in the color guard, marching percussion, and front ensemble. Prolonged and/or repetitive flag and rifle work in the color guard and hours of percussion activity lead to overuse issues. In the authors' experience, tears of the triangular fibrocartilage complex or radial styloid tenosynovitis are common sources of persistent wrist pain. These same activities can lead to trigger point formation in the forearm as well as medial and lateral epicondylitis. Metacarpal fractures can occur, most often with a missed catch of a rifle or sabre.

Pain in the wrist and digits, mainly thumb, is reported by woodwind players, likely due to the asymmetric posture involved with playing their instruments.[11] Some of the weight of a woodwind instrument is borne by the thumb, and the wrists can spend prolonged time in an unnatural position. Some possible conditions that may be observed are de Quervain's tenosynovitis, carpal tunnel syndrome, tendonitis, and entrapment of the median or ulnar nerve. The use of proper woodwind instrument harnesses can relive some of the pressure on the digits and wrists and improve overall posture.

## LUMBOSACRAL INJURIES
Low back and sacroiliac joint problems are common, particularly in the color guard.[12] Their activity on the field combines elements of dance with the use of flags, rifles, sabres, and other props. The repetitive and prolonged jumping and landing on uneven ground along with lumbar flexion, extension, and rotating to throw and catch their props lead to both acute and overuse injuries in the lumbosacral spine. For the instrumentalists, the addition of the carried weight of the instrument shifts the center of gravity cephalad and forward, leading to a tendency to hyperextend the lumbar spine in a compensatory manner. A recent report of spondylolysis in nonelite athletes identified marching band as having the second highest prevalence of symptomatic spondylolysis in females.[13]

## CONCUSSION
The marching arts athlete with a concussion requires additional consideration with return to activity. Concussions can be sustained in the marching arts as a result of being struck by a rifle or flag in color guard, collisions on the field, or due to trauma while loading or unloading the equipment. Marching artists and musicians also may have sustained a concussion outside of their marching arts activity. The marching arts athlete who is suspected of having a concussion, like all athletes, should be removed from practice and play (performance) until cleared by a provider trained in the diagnosis and management of concussion.[14] The progression back to activity needs to incorporate the additional factors of significant sound exposure, instrument playing technique, marching while playing the instrument, and the dynamics of the individual marching band. Dizziness, slowed cognition, and impaired dual task gait can negatively impact performance and place the musician at higher risk of repeat injury.[15] No studies currently exist that have evaluated concussions in the marching arts or return to activity in musicians postconcussion. Nevertheless, participation in the arts should be included in the planning for return to learn and return to activity progressions.

## PREVENTION

Preseason conditioning programs should be encouraged for all marching arts athletes. At a minimum, a general fitness program should be recommended for preparation for band camp and the marching season. More specific programs can be designed to address strength and endurance for holding the instrument and aerobic conditioning to aid in quicker recovery during performances and allow for better respiratory control while playing and marching.

Footwear for the marching arts should be selected with respect to the activity requiring rapid movements from side to side as well as forward and backward. Based on expert recommendation, the optimal shoe type is a cross trainer or trail shoe. Both shoe types afford the multidirectional support needed, as compared to popular minimalist shoes and running shoes, which are designed for straight ahead activity. A study of collegiate marching band injuries from the 1993–94 season noted that a majority of the injuries occurred in those wearing other types of shoes (running shoes, tennis shoes, walking shoes, etc.).[8] In those who were wearing the recommended cross trainers when they were injured, the shoes were found to be in poor condition.[8] Individuals in collegiate and high school marching bands typically will need one pair of shoes per season. Drum corps athletes will need *at least* two pairs of shoes for each season. Because of the lengthy rehearsals and dynamics of the activity, each pair of shoes will wear out within 4–6 weeks of use.

Hearing loss and hearing protection have been covered in Chapter 6. It is important to understand that the outdoor environment does not confer a safe hearing environment. Research done on a drum corps found that, despite practicing outdoors, sound exposure levels exceeded safe limits each day of rehearsal.[16,17] Even with the use of musician's earplugs, some members of the drum line would have exceeded safe limits daily and are at risk for noise induced hearing loss.[16] Marching musicians should be educated about noise induced hearing loss and encouraged to wear appropriate hearing protection.

## ENVIRONMENTAL ISSUES

Environmental stressors, including heat, cold, and severe weather exposure of the marching athlete, are relatively unique issues in the performing arts world. The marching athletes are often expected to practice and perform in weather extremes. In general, weather guidelines for athletic activities should be followed for the marching arts. Although state high school athletic associations often mandate weather guidelines for sport, some states leave the development and implementation of weather guidelines for marching band to band directors.

Heat illness is a particular concern for drum corps, high school, and collegiate marching bands. Preseason band camps for high school and collegiate marching bands occur in August, and some are scheduled to take place over 5–7 days, lasting 8–10 h each day. Many of the participants in marching band do not have the opportunity or guidance to undertake appropriate heat acclimatization practices. Whereas there have been guidelines and rules in place for heat acclimatization of athletes,[18] these rules and guidelines may not be followed for marching bands. In addition, performance attire is not always designed for prolonged wear in the heat. Rehearsals and pregame/precompetition warm ups may take place in less than ideal locations, such as parking lots, turf fields, or grass fields with no possibility of shade.

Marching artists should acclimatize to heat, just as other athletes preparing for late summer and fall athletic activities.[18,19] Music educators should be trained to recognize the signs and symptoms of heat illness and respond appropriately. Practice scheduling should follow the same recommendations and accommodations for extreme heat and humidity as other sports. Marching athletes should be allowed to hydrate frequently, and rehearsal environments should be selected to reduce heat exposure[20] (i.e., rehearsing on a grass field vs. a parking lot, seeking shaded areas for parts of rehearsal). When possible, marching uniforms should be adaptable for performances in the heat and, when applicable, the extreme cold.

In the North, football games are rarely cancelled due to the cold. Bands will be present for these contests. Hypothermia and frostbite may occur. Some woodwind instruments must be played with exposed fingertips. For many schools, the same uniform is worn throughout the season. Having the ability to layer clothing under the uniform is essential as well as considering appropriate outerwear while in the stands during the game.[21]

Planning for weather extremes should include contingencies for when the marching arts group should be permitted to leave the performance venue. Examples include modifying or cancelling the performance (or rehearsal) in the event of extreme heat, extreme cold, or snow. Thunderstorm and severe weather guidelines should be followed for marching groups as they would for all other athletic activities. Ideally, these would be written guidelines prepared before the season begins.

Each marching arts group should develop an emergency action plan (EAP) to prepare for the season.[22,23] The emergency action plan should be developed with the input of appropriate health care personnel along with the leadership of the marching arts organization. The EAP should include venue specific information for each practice and performance site. Specific roles and responsibilities of individuals should be listed. A one-page EAP should be available for each venue used, with a more detailed EAP for different medical emergencies (allergic reaction, cardiac arrest, heat illness, etc.), severe weather guidelines, etc.

Online resources are available for development of an EAP. The National Athletic Trainers Association and the National Federation of High Schools have resources available for developing an EAP on their respective websites. Many athletic departments and school systems already have an EAP developed for other activities, and these could be adapted for the marching arts activities.

Marching athletes with allergies and asthma, like other athletes, should be encouraged to participate. For their safety, directors and staff should be informed of the allergy and how to respond in case of an exposure. Appropriate medications should be kept nearby, ideally with the allergic individual. The response to an allergic exposure should be rehearsed, particularly for severe allergies.[24]

## PREPARTICIPATION PHYSICAL EXAMS

Preparticipation exams should be encouraged for all marching arts participants. The goals of the PPE, as discussed in the Preparticipation Physical Exam monograph, are divided into the primary objectives of (1) screening for conditions that may be life threatening or disabling and (2) screening for conditions that may predispose to illness or injury. The secondary objectives are (1) determining general health, (2) serving as an entry point into the health care system for adolescents, and (3) providing an opportunity to initiate discussion on health-related topics.[25] The endorsing organizations of the Preparticipation Physical Examination monograph recommend the PPE to become an integral part of the health-screening exam for all active individuals.

## CONCLUSION

The marching arts are a widespread activity, which is significantly understudied. The marching arts have evolved into a highly dynamic physical activity that deserves further research to develop evidence-based recommendations for preseason conditioning, injury prevention, and injury treatment. Current sports medicine principles can guide the evaluation and treatment of the marching musician, but as research progresses in the marching arts, guidelines can be developed for the marching arts athlete.

## REFERENCES

1. Drum Corps International. DCI Parents: About Drum Corps. https://www.dci.org/news/dci-parents-about-drum-corps. Accessed 18.8.8.
2. Erdmann LD, Graham RE, Radlo SJ, Knepler PL. Adolescents' energy cost in marching band. *Percept Mot Skills*. 2003;97(2):639−646.
3. Compendium of Physical Activities. Activity Categories. https://sites.google.com/site/compendiumofphysicalactivities/Activity-Categories. Accessed 18.8.8.
4. Lauhon P, Walsh R, Binoniemi B, et al. The cost of performance: a study on the effect of marching style and tempo on energy expenditure during marching. Proceedings of the 2015 Industrial and Systems Engineering Research Conference. June 2015.
5. DCI Athletes. https://www.youtube.com/watch?v=6WWmM1jpM8I. Accessed 18.8.8.
6. Metabolic Equivalents. http://www.globalrph.com/metabolic_equivalents.htm. Accessed 18.8.8.
7. Beckett S, Seidelman L, Hanney WJ, Liu X, Rothschild CE. Prevalence of musculoskeletal injury among collegiate marching band and color guard members. *Med Probl Perform Art*. 2015;30(2):106−110.
8. Mehler AS, Brink DS, Eickmeier KM, Hesse DF, McGuire JW. Marching band injuries. A one-season survey of the University of Michigan marching band. *J Am Podiatr Med Assoc*. 1996;86(9):407−413.
9. Sataloff RT, Brandfonbrenner AG, Lederman RJ, eds. *Performing Arts Medicine*. 3rd ed. Narberth, PA: Science & Medicine, Inc.; 2010.
10. Oregon Crusaders Cymbal Technique Packet. http://oregoncrusaders.org/wp-content/uploads/2015/02/OCP-Cymbal-Technique-Book-20151.pdf; 2015.
11. Arino H, Nemoto K. Hand and upper extremity problems in wind instrument players in military bands. *Med Probl Perform Art*. 2007;22(2):67−69.
12. Harman SE. Medical problems of marching musicians. *Med Probl Perform Art*. 1993;8(4):132.
13. Selhorst M, Fischer A, MacDonald J. Prevalence of spondylolysis in symptomatic adolescent athletes: an assessment of sport risk in nonelite athletes. *Clin J Sport Med*. 2017:1−5. https://doi.org/10.1097/JSM.0000000000000546.
14. McCrory P, Meeuwisse W, Dvořák J, et al. Consensus statement on concussion in sport—the 5th international conference on concussion in sport held in Berlin, October 2016. *Br J Sports Med*. 2017;51:838−847.
15. Grants L, Powell B, Gessel C, Hiser F, Hassen A. Gait deficits under dual-task conditions in the concussed adolescent and young athlete population: a systematic review. *Int J Sports Phys Ther*. 2017;12(7):1011−1022.

16. Neumann S, Bondurant L, Smaldino J. Hearing conservation programs for drum and bugle corps: implications for educational audiologists. *J Educ Audiol.* 2013;19: 25−37.

17. Su-Hyun J, Nelson PB, Schlauch RS, Carney E. Hearing conservation program for marching band members: a risk for noise-induced hearing loss? *J Educ Audiol.* 2013; 22:26−39.

18. National Athletic Trainers Association Consensus Statement. Preseason heat acclimatization guidelines for secondary school athletics. *J Athl Train.* 2009;44(3): 332−333.

19. American College of Sports Medicine. Position stand: exertional heat illness during training and competition. *Med Sci Sports Exerc.* 2007;39(3):556−572.

20. American College of Sports Medicine. Position stand: exercise and fluid replacement. *Med Sci Sports Exerc.* 2007; 39(2):377−390.

21. American College of Sports Medicine. Position Stand: prevention of cold injuries during exercise. *Med Sci Sports Exerc.* 2006;38(11):2012−2029.

22. National Athletic Trainers Association position statement: emergency planning in athletics. *J Athl Train.* 2002;37(1): 99−104.

23. Lemak L, Unruh B. Athletic Departments Must Design and Practice Emergency Action Plan. Oct 2015. https://www. nfhs.org/articles/athletic-departments-must-design-and-practice-emergency-action-plan/. Accessed 18.8.8.

24. Athletes With Allergies, Asthma Can Play It Safe. June 2011. http://acaai.org/news/athletes-allergies-asthma-can-play-it-safe. Accessed 18.1.14.

25. *PPE Preparticipation Physical Evaluation.* 4th ed. American Academy of Pediatrics; 2010.

## FURTHER READING

1. Inter-association consensus statement on best practices for sports medicine management for secondary schools and colleges. *J Athl Train.* 2014;49(1):128−137.

2. National Athletic Trainers Association position statement: lightning safety for athletics and recreation. *J Athl Train.* 2013;48(2):258−270.

## CHAPTER 8

# Foot and Ankle Injuries in Dancers: Guidance for Examination, Diagnosis, and Treatment

NANCY KADEL, MD

## INTRODUCTION

Dance as an art form requires intense training from an early age for those who aspire to perform at an elite level. The dancer's foot and ankle complex are subjected to high forces, often at the extremes of joint range of motion, particularly ankle plantar flexion.[1−3] The foot and ankle complex functions as a base of support, a lever to propel the dancer in dynamic maneuvers, and a shock absorber. Unlike most other sports, in dance the foot is essential for expressing the artistic (aesthetic) line of the leg, regardless of the dance style being performed. Dance footwear is rarely shock absorbing nor does it allow for orthotics.[4]

Reports on professional dancers show a high prevalence of injury in ballet, modern, and Irish dancers.[5−11]. In one Swedish study of a professional ballet company, 95% of the dancers sustained at least one injury during a one-year study period.[12] An international cross-sectional study looking at self-reported injuries in 260 professional modern and ballet dancers found a point prevalence of 46.3% and 54.8%, respectively. In addition, more than 15% of the surveyed injured professional dancers had failed to report their injury.[13] The foot and ankle together are the most frequently injured areas in dancers (14%−77% of all injuries reported in dancers), with significantly higher rates reported in female ballet dancers.[9,14] The sur les pointes position requires maximal ankle, hindfoot, and midfoot plantar flexion, while placing high forces across those joints.[1−3] Dance injuries may be the result of acute trauma, such as landing from a leap or turn or more commonly from repetitive microtrauma, often after a rapid increase in training volume and intensity. Menstrual irregularities, disordered eating, low energy availability, low vitamin D, and osteopenia may contribute to dancers' risk for injury or delayed healing.[15,16]

Epidemiologic studies in younger dancers report injury incidence rates ranging from 0.77 to 1.55 per 1000 dance hours. During adolescence, an important time of growth and maturation, the concurrent rise in training volume, and intensity for young dancers appears to increase their risk of injury.[14] Over a 2-year period Steinberg et al. found that 40%−48% of all dancers aged 8 to 18 sustained an injury, and Ekegren found a risk of injury of 76% over 1 year in preprofessional ballet students.[17,18,21] These studies both attributed the high rate of injury in large part to increased training intensity. The foot and ankle complex is reported in many studies of adolescent dancers to be the most frequently injured body part. The majority of injuries in young dancers are the result of overuse (72%−82% is some studies), which is postulated to be due to the highly specific repetitive movements practiced on a day-to-day basis.[14,17−23] By way of contrast, overuse injuries reported in elite adolescents in other sports account for only 15%−63% of injuries.[24] Training levels in elite young dancers often exceed those in other sports, including technique classes and/or rehearsals 6 days per week. This article will review some common problems involving the foot and ankle in dancers, clinical presentation, diagnostic tips, and treatment recommendations.

## ANKLE SPRAIN

Ankle sprain is the most frequent traumatic injury in dancers and may be related to the increased time

Performing Arts Medicine. https://doi.org/10.1016/B978-0-323-58182-0.00008-0

**63**

dancers spend weight-bearing in ankle plantar flexion, a highly unstable position for the ankle joint. The usual mechanism of injury includes rolling over the lateral border of the foot while on sur les pointes (Fig. 8.1) or demi-pointe (Fig. 8.2) or landing improperly from a jump. In most ankle sprains the lateral ligaments are injured, especially the anterior talofibular ligament (ATFL). The ATFL is injured when the ankle is in plantarflexion; the calcaneofibular ligament (CFL) is injured when the inversion occurs with the ankle (foot) in dorsiflexion (or neutral) position. It is well recognized that the greatest risk factor for an ankle sprain is a previous inversion injury, and those dancers with a cavus foot type and varus heel also have higher inversion injury risk.[25-30]

The dancer with an acute ankle sprain will present with pain, usually anterolateral swelling and ecchymosis of the ankle and hindfoot. Weight-bearing may be painful. Findings on physical examination include tenderness to palpation over the lateral ankle ligaments, swelling, and ecchymosis. Laxity on ankle drawer testing may be present but must be compared to the contralateral ankle. Any tenderness over the fibula, sinus tarsi, or fifth metatarsal should alert the clinician to obtain foot and ankle radiographs. Tenderness over the syndesmosis, a positive "squeeze test," or

pain with dorsiflexion/external rotation stress should alert the clinician to a high ankle sprain. Acute injury to the deltoid ligament (medial ankle sprain) is rare, but if the dancer's turnout is poorly controlled at the hip, then chronic pain may occur in this area due to excessive pronation causing a chronic strain of the deltoid ligament.

A computed tomography (CT) scan or magnetic resonance imaging (MRI) scan should be obtained to identify possible osteochondral injury to the talus or occult fracture if symptoms have not started to improve in a weeks' time. For those skilled in ultrasound, a joint effusion and ligament injury may be demonstrated. MRI of the ankle may reveal patchy marrow edema in the talus or hindfoot—a common finding noted in previous MRI studies of dancers.[31,32] The authors caution that the marrow edema may represent a normal variation in ballet dancers rather than a pathologic process such as a stress fracture. The MRI changes likely represent an overuse syndrome related to the unique stresses of weight-bearing in ankle plantar flexion (the demi-pointe or sur les pointe positions) along with the intensity of the dance training. When symptomatic, reduction of training intensity is recommended, but be cautious in limiting dance participation based solely on the presence of talar or hindfoot patchy bone marrow edema seen on MRI.

The majority of sprains resolve with conservative management. Early functional treatment of ankle sprains is recommended. Compression bandaging, briefly icing, wearing an ankle air-stirrup brace in

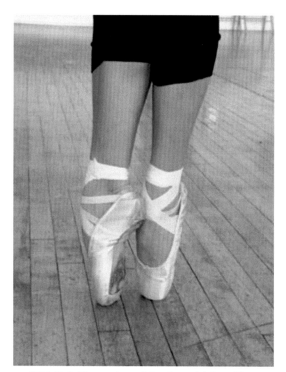

FIG. 8.1 The sur les pointes (en pointe) position.

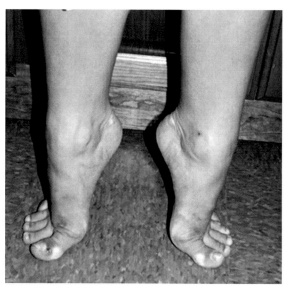

FIG. 8.2 The demi-pointe (demi-releve) position.

athletic shoes outside of class, and limiting class participation are the initial steps of treatment. Severe sprains
may require use of a removable walking boot cast for
3 weeks. The boot should be removed for icing and
range-of-motion exercises and worn for walking and
sleeping until the pain resolves (not more than
3 weeks). Dancers with high-level sprains may need to
do floor barre classes, Pilates, or Gyrotonics before
returning to class and performance. McCormack et al.
observed that dancers with generalized hypermobility
have a more prolonged recovery from soft tissue injuries
than nonhypermobile dancers.[33,34]

Attention to strengthening, edema control, range of
motion, and proprioception exercises are needed for
rehabilitation from an ankle sprain. Dancers require
full mobility of their hindfoot, midfoot, and ankle
joints to dance, especially in the demi-pointe and sur
les pointes positions. Failure to restore posterior talar
glide and full ankle dorsiflexion following an ankle
sprain may lead to posterior ankle impingement.[35]
The insufficient ATFL ligament allows the talus to
translate forward in the ankle mortise in the plantar
flexed position, resulting in impingement of bone
and/or soft tissues in the posterior ankle joint. It is
important to encourage dancers to work on attaining
full dorsiflexion at the tibiotalar joint following an
ankle sprain; therapists should be encouraged to assist
the dancer in achieving posterior talar glide and
should use manual therapy to restore subtalar joint
mobility.

Dancers often have a very flexible ankle and a
moderately or highly arched (cavus) foot. Subtle hindfoot varus may be present, increasing the prospect of
reinjury. Studies have found dancers and athletes with
previous ankle sprains have impaired dynamic postural
control (more postural sway than controls or uninjured
dancers). Even after return to full professional dance or
sport participation, and without complaints of instability, measurable differences in postural sway can be
demonstrated[25–29]

Optimization of the entire kinetic chain is crucial
for full recovery. Core strengthening, proprioception,
and proximal hip strengthening exercises should
be included in any dancer's rehabilitation from an
ankle sprain, in addition to fibularis longus and
brevis muscle strengthening. Balance tasks on unstable
surfaces or with eyes closed facilitate proprioception
retraining. Practicing elevés in parallel position with
a tennis ball held between the malleoli (the "toe
to toe" exercise) can help the injured dancer retrain
ankle strength and motion in a neutral ankle joint
position, avoiding subtle sickling during relevé[30]
(Figs. 8.3 and 8.4).

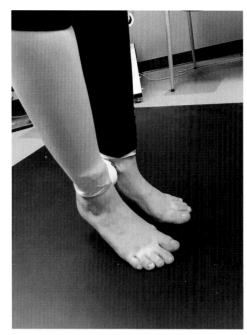

FIG. 8.3 The "toe to toe" exercise. This dancer has
not reached the complete demi-pointe position in this photo.

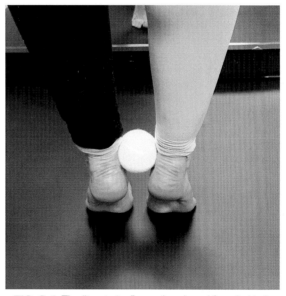

FIG. 8.4 The "toe to toe" exercise viewed from behind.

## ANKLE IMPINGEMENT SYNDROMES
### Posterior Ankle Impingement Syndrome
The term "posterior ankle impingement syndrome" or
"PAIS" is used to describe any painful condition due
to compression of soft tissues or bone between the

posterior edge of the tibia and the calcaneus, typically when the ankle is in plantar flexion. A normal ossification center is located at the posterior aspect of the talus. It usually appears at 9 to 12 years of age and fuses 1 year after its appearance. If it does not fuse with the talus, an ossicle develops, known as the os trigonum.[36] This ossicle, a fracture of the posterior lateral talar process (Sheperd's fracture), or a large posterior lateral process of the talus called a Steida process are the usual sources of bony impingement, but a prominent downsloping tibia or superior calcaneal tuberosity may also be implicated in compression of soft tissues posteriorly.[32] While it may be seen at any age, most commonly this problem presents in the adolescent dancer. Flexor hallucis longus (FHL) tenosynovitis secondary to an impinging os trigonum is also reported and should be suspected in any dancer with posterior ankle pain.[37–39] An acute fracture of the posterolateral process of the talus can also cause posterior ankle pain.[40]

Dancers with posterior ankle impingement usually describe pain in the posterolateral ankle behind the fibularis tendons, along with stiffness and limitation in plantar flexion motion. Pain is worst with plantar flexing of the ankle, as in tendu and relevé maneuvers. This condition may be mistaken for fibularis or Achilles tendonitis and may follow an ankle sprain.[35] The dancer may have difficulty achieving the full pointe position (plantar flexion) on the affected side (Fig. 8.5). Swelling and tenderness may be present behind the lateral ankle joint anterior to the Achilles tendon. Dancers with posterior ankle impingement will have a positive *plantar flexion sign*: pain with forced passive

ankle plantar flexion with the dancer's knee flexed at 90 degrees. This test will not be positive in Achilles, fibularis, or isolated FHL tendinitis.[37–39,41–46]. Those with FHL tendonitis and an os trigonum will have posteromedial ankle tenderness and pain with flexion of the great toe against resistance.

Radiographs in maximal plantar flexion, or with the dancer sur les pointes (Fig. 8.6), can demonstrate a bony block or os trigonum. MRI is useful to identify bone edema in the posterior talus, os trigonum, or calcaneus and to demonstrate fluid in the FHL tendon sheath.[31,32,40] Relief of pain with an injection of lidocaine posterior to the fibularis tendons can confirm the diagnosis.[37,38,47] Ultrasound may be useful for diagnosis and guided injections. Treatment consists initially of limitation of painful activities, including pointe work and physical therapy to strengthen and mobilize the ankle joint. The dancer should sleep with a night splint to help reduce stiffness and synovitis until symptoms resolve. Intrinsic foot strengthening exercises (especially the doming exercise) along with practice pointing the foot with a relaxed calf can reduce symptoms.[43] Surgery to remove the os trigonum and/or release the FHL tendon sheath is reserved for those dancers who fail physical therapy and

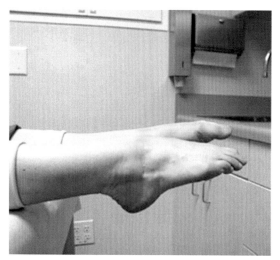

FIG. 8.5 A dancer with left posterior ankle impingement and limited plantar flexion.

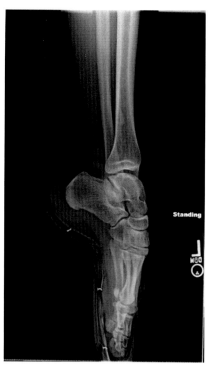

FIG. 8.6 Radiograph of a dancer en pointe in her pointe shoe.

correction of technical errors. Recovery time after surgery varies, and dancers often have some persistent symptoms for 1 year, but most return to full participation by 4−6 months (Fig. 8.7). Some dancers find benefit from changing their pointe shoe style and fit.

## Flexor Hallucis Longus Tendinitis

FHL tendinitis is common in dancers, hence the term "dancer's tendinitis." While present rarely in other athletes, it is seen most frequently in the female ballet dancer.[37,38,44−46] A biomechanical study demonstrated that the muscles crossing the metatarso-phalangeal joints (MTPJs) work 2.5 to 3 times harder than those crossing just the ankle joint in dancers rising on to full pointe position, placing these muscles and tendons (FHL and flexor digitorum longus) at risk for overuse injuries.[1] The repetitive foot transition from full plantar flexion of the en pointe position to plié with the ankle in dorsiflexion can compress the FHL tendon in its fibro-osseous tunnel along the posterome-dial talus under the sustentaculum tali, leading to inflammation.

Dancers may complain of posteromedial ankle pain, swelling, or popping. Some dancers develop triggering or locking of the great toe, the result of a nodule forming on the tendon. Crepitus can be palpated at the posteromedial ankle, and pain with resisted flexion of the hallux interphalangeal joint may be present. Functional hallux rigidus may be present, as demonstrated by a limitation of great toe dorsiflexion with the knee fully extended and the ankle in full dorsiflexion, known as the Thomasen test.[46] FHL inflammation may be present with or without an os trigonum or

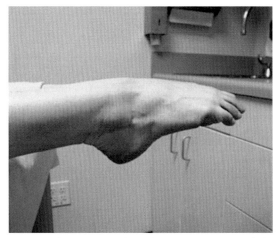

FIG. 8.7 Postsurgery this dancer has regained her flexibility.

prominent Steida process; therefore, the FHL tendon should be evaluated in any dancer suspected of posterior ankle impingement. Diagnostic ultrasound and or MRI are the recommended tests.[48]

Conservative treatment including temporary cessation of pointe work and jumps, physical therapy, and anti-inflammatory medication usually resolves the problem. Corticosteroid injection into the FHL tendon sheath is NOT recommended, as a rupture could end a dancer's career. Ultrasound-guided hydrodissection or regenerative medicine techniques may have a role. In those dancers with triggering of the hallux, a nodule on the tendon, or that fail nonoperative treatment, surgical release of the FHL sheath may be required. Open and arthroscopic procedures generally have good to excellent results in dancers, but most reports are based on retrospective studies or case series. Return to full dance participation typically is 3 to 6 months.[49−51]

## Anterior Ankle Impingement

Anterior impingement in dancers may be a consequence of hypertrophied soft tissues or osteophytes (talar neck and/or distal tibia) in the anterior ankle joint. The osteophytes are proposed to be a consequence of repeated ankle sprains or microtrauma from repetitive impact of loaded dorsiflexion.[52−54] Anterior impingement is more common in male dancers and in dancers with cavus feet. Symptoms of anterior impingement include anterior ankle joint pain with jump landings, plié, and limited ankle dorsiflexion. Some have pain when descending stairs. Swelling may or may not be present. Tenderness to palpation of the anterior ankle joint is usually found. Pain with passive ankle dorsiflexion can be present, but this may be falsely negative in anterior impingement.[52,53]

Radiographs of the ankle and an oblique view of the foot will demonstrate osteophytes. Treatment includes relative activity limitation, including avoidance of jumps and forced demi-plié, and the use of a small felt medial/lateral wedge pad under the heel to lift the lateral heel in dance and street shoes. Physical therapy to correct technical errors such as improper alignment in plié or hindfoot supination and to tape the foot to support the subtalar joint and hindfoot may help to resolve symptoms. A brief trial in a walking boot cast brace for 3 weeks and a night splint may help alleviate pain and inflammation. Judicious use of a single intra-articular corticosteroid injection may be used in select cases, followed by a walking cast brace for 3 weeks. If pain persists, surgical treatment with arthroscopic or open debridement of osteophytes and soft tissue may be required.[55–57] Postoperative care including Pilates, Gyrotonics, and pool exercises (once incisions are healed) should be initiated early, with an increase of dance activity as pain allows. Full dance participation may take as long as 3–6 months.[4,30,52]

## Achilles Tendinitis/Tendonosis

Chronic Achilles tendinopathy, retrocalcaneal bursitis, and acute tendinitis may be seen in male and female dancers. The Achilles and patellar tendons do not have synovial envelopes but instead are covered by paratenon. As such, pathologic changes at this level are referred to as paratendinopathy, acute, or chronic.[58] Comin and colleagues[59] evaluated Achilles and patellar tendons in 79 professional ballet dancers and found a 12% prevalence of sonographic abnormalities in the Achilles and patellar tendons of asymptomatic dancers. Dancers who force their turnout, leading to increased pronation in the midfoot and hindfoot, are at risk for Achilles tendon problems. Failure of the dancer to land with his or her heels on the ground while jumping can contribute to shortening of the Achilles tendon and risk for injury. The cavus foot type often favored in dance is associated with a prominent posterior-superior process of the calcaneus (Haglund deformity) and a higher risk of developing retrocalcaneal bursitis. In young dancers during periods of rapid growth, there is relative tightness and weakness of the gastrocnemius-soleus complex, placing them at risk for Achilles tendinitis and calcaneal apophysitis.[4] In a prospective study, Mahieu and colleagues[60] identified plantar flexion weakness and increased dorsiflexion excursion as significant predictors for Achilles tendon overuse injury. In the Comin study, only those dancers with hypoechoic changes seen on ultrasound later developed symptomatic Achilles tendinitis, suggesting that ultrasound in asymptomatic dancers may help identify those dancers at risk for future Achilles tendon problems.[59]

Dancers will present with pain and swelling of the Achilles tendon. Jumps, pliés, pointing the foot in tendu, and even walking may be painful. Tenderness to palpation will be present, often with fusiform swelling, thickening, crepitus, and or nodule formation.

Diagnostic ultrasound is the most advantageous imaging modality for routine clinical evaluation, although MRI is also helpful. Weight-bearing radiographs are useful if retrocalcaneal bursitis and Haglund deformity are suspected.

Tight ribbons around the ankle in ballet dancers may cause tendon irritation and can be fixed by adjusting the tension of ribbons around the ankle or the use of elastic.[19,20] Careful stretching and the use of a night splint while sleeping can alleviate most symptoms. Eccentric strengthening exercises, physical therapy with modalities such as Graston technique, ASTYM, or deep tissue massage may be beneficial. The use of a stretch box in the studio and backstage at the theater has been found to be a good preventative measure for some companies. Regenerative medicine techniques utilizing ultrasound-guided injections of whole blood and platelet-rich plasma have been shown to promote healing in Achilles tendons.[61] Corticosteroid injections should be avoided in the Achilles tendon as potential weakening of tissues could lead to rupture.

## Achilles Tendon Rupture

Rupture of the Achilles tendon is unusual in female dancers, more commonly seen in male dancers over the age of 30 as tendon elasticity and vascularity are decreased. Landing in hyperdorsiflexion or eccentric loading of the foot during push-off can result in an acute Achilles tendon rupture. It typically presents with sharp pain and the inability to rise up to demi-pointe on the affected side. The Thompson test will be positive, and when examining the patient in the prone position with the knees flexed, the relaxed resting posture of the injured leg will demonstrate more dorsiflexion than the uninjured side. A palpable defect is usually present, but acute swelling may mask this finding. Acute ruptures in dancers generally are treated with surgical repair followed by early protected motion. Any suspected rupture should be referred to an orthopedic surgeon.[47]

## Apophysitis of the Os Calcis (Sever's Disease)

Sever's disease (calcaneal apophysitis) is a traction apophysitis and should be considered in any young dancer with open physes (growth plates) who complains of heel pain. The calcaneal apophysis is located in the posterior calcaneus, oriented perpendicular to the long axis of the tuberosity. It first appears on radiographs at ages 4 to 7 years in females and 4 to 10 years in males; it does not fuse until an average age of 16 years. The Achilles tendon inserts along the posterior calcaneal tuberosity, and the plantar fascia (PF) inserts on the plantar medial tuberosity.[36,62] The diagnosis is particularly common in Irish step dancers and is seen in both males and females.[63] The dancer may complain of heel pain in the morning, pain with jumping, on heel strike when walking, and with percussive movements. Radiographs are often negative, but fragmentation or widening of the growth plate may be present. Physical examination findings include tenderness to palpation over the apophyseal calcaneal growth plate and posterior heel, pain with medial and lateral squeeze test of the calcaneus, weakness of ankle dorsiflexion, and contracture of the Achilles tendon.[64]

Treatment includes avoidance of painful activities, and in most cases use of a removable walking boot cast for 3 weeks, PF night splint for sleeping, and gentle Achilles stretches along with ankle dorsiflexion resistance band strengthening. The young dancer may need to continue the use of the night splint for sleep and wear a cushioned supportive shoe outside of class for an additional 4−6 weeks as symptoms subside. Return to dance includes relative rest, such as avoidance of jumps and other painful maneuvers, until symptoms are resolved.

## Plantar Fascia

The plantar aponeurosis is a strong band of fascia extending from the calcaneal tuberosity to attach at the plantar aspect of the proximal phalanges. The PF may be strained, partially torn, or simply inflamed (plantar fasciitis). Occasionally there is an acute injury, most often insidious in onset after increased training intensity. Walls and colleagues reported on MRI findings of the right ankles in 18 professional Irish dancers; insertional Achilles tendinopathy was observed in 14 dancers, and plantar fasciitis was seen in 7 dancers.[63]

Dancers usually present with plantar-medial arch or heel pain worse with their first few steps in the morning, which improves quickly and then worsens later with increased activity. Diagnosis is based on history and physical examination findings of tenderness over the anteromedial aspect of the heel and along the PF, worst with the foot and toes in dorsiflexion (placing the PF on stretch) and less tender with plantar flexion of the toes. This is a clinical diagnosis because radiographs are often not helpful. However, tenderness of the calcaneal wall should alert the clinician to a possible calcaneal stress fracture (or Sever's Disease in a skeletally immature dancer), and further imaging is needed.

Treatment should include relative rest (including avoidance of painful activities), dorsiflexion night splint for sleeping, and gastrocnemius, soleus, and plantar arch stretches. Use of a stiff-soled shoe for walking, such as hiking boots or clogs, can help to avoid stressing the PF by limiting extension of the MTPJs.[65] Use of the night splint and stiff-soled shoes is often needed for a minimum of 4−6 weeks. Taping the arch

of the foot can improve symptoms in many dancers. For those that fail initial conservative treatments, platelet-rich plasma injection has been found on meta-analysis to have better long-term results than corticosteroids.[66]

## Stress Fractures

Whenever loading is increased too rapidly, or there is repeated microtrauma of physiologic loads that exceed the bones' reparative capacity, a stress fracture can occur. Increased training intensity, hard floors, nutritional and hormonal factors, menstrual irregularities, low body mass index, and low energy availability have all been implicated in stress fractures. Dancing more than 5 h per day and having amenorrhea greater than 90 days have been demonstrated as risk factors for stress fractures in female dancers.[67] Metatarsal stress fractures are the most common stress fracture reported in dancers.[67,68] The fibula, tibia, spine, and hip are other potential sites for injury.

The dancer with a stress fracture will report a dull, achy pain in the injured area. Initially pain will typically occur near the end of class or with jumps. A marked increase in training intensity (such as a summer dance program) often precedes the symptoms. As symptoms progress, pain becomes more constant and may occur with walking and at night. Rarely is swelling present, and often pain is not well localized. Bony tenderness may be present. Initial radiographs are often normal. Radionuclide bone scans can be positive only a few days after the injury, but MRI is the recommended test to make the diagnosis.

Dancers are at risk for a stress fracture at the base of the second metatarsal. Running athletes typically will have a stress fracture of the midshaft or more distal aspect of the metatarsal.[68,69] In the midfoot, the second metatarsal is recessed and the second metatarsal-cuneiform joint is more proximal than the first or third metatarsal-cuneiform joints. The first and second metatarsals bear the majority of a dancer's weight whether on demi-pointe, pointe, or on landing from a jump, and those stresses are transmitted proximally to the midfoot, where the base of the second metatarsal is locked in place.[70]

Synovitis of Lisfranc's joints (the metatarsal-cuneiform joints) and a proximal second metatarsal stress fracture are difficult to distinguish with physical examination or a bone scan.[68,69,71−73] Therefore, MRI has become the preferred test in a dancer with midfoot pain, a suspected stress fracture, and negative radiographs. Healing time is prolonged for the stress fracture (6−8 weeks) compared to synovitis (3 weeks); hence, accurate diagnosis is important for managing these injuries.[71] Treatment for foot and ankle stress fractures does not usually require casting, but some dancers need a removable cast boot for pain-free walking outside of class. Bone stimulators are often used to aid healing. Attention to energy availability, calcium and vitamin D levels, and correction of any deficits is important. Conditioning can be maintained with floor barre, Pilates, pool exercises, and exercise bicycle or elliptical trainer barring pain at the fracture site with those activities. Rehabilitation includes gradual return to class with avoidance of painful activities such as pointe work, jumps, turns, and demi-pointe until healing is completed and pain resolved.

### Lisfranc Sprain/Fractures

Midfoot sprains/fractures in dancers are not common, but the physician treating dancers should have a high index of suspicion because if this injury is not recognized and treated it can be career ending. The ligaments of the tarso-metatarsal joints act to support the medial and longitudinal arches of the foot. These injuries can be easily missed as radiographic findings may be subtle, and midfoot pain can be mistaken for a possible stress fracture or synovitis. Usually these injuries have more swelling when compared to a stress fracture or isolated synovitis.

The dancer will complain of midfoot pain worse with weight-bearing, and depending on the severity of the injury, may be able to relate the exact mechanism of injury. Tenderness will be present over the dorsal midfoot (especially the first and second metatarsal-cuneiform joints). In acute cases, plantar midfoot ecchymosis may be seen, increasing the likelihood of a Lisfranc injury diagnosis. Weight-bearing AP foot radiographs may show a small diastasis between the first and second proximal metatarsal bases (comparison views of the opposite foot aid in making the diagnosis). Subtle displacement may be observed on the lateral and or oblique views. Lisfranc's ligament is located between the medial cuneiform and the base of the second metatarsal. An avulsed fragment of bone between the first and second metatarsal bases may be seen if the ligament is injured.

The mechanism of injury to Lisfranc's joints in dancers has been described to include a fall off pointe position, missed jump landings, takeoff for a jump, and a foot catching a seam or irregularity in the floor. These injuries occur in ankle plantar flexion, with or without rotation, often with the metatarsal-phalangeal joints in maximal dorsiflexion (demi-pointe).[36,74–76] Most Lisfranc injuries require

surgical treatment, and only a simple dorsal ligament sprain with no instability should be treated nonsurgically. Any suspected Lisfranc injury should be referred to an orthopedic surgeon for evaluation. Recovery is prolonged, and immobilization with avoidance of weight-bearing activities for 6–12 weeks after surgery is required. Rehabilitation of the entire kinetic chain will be needed to return the dancer to full performance level.

### Cuboid Syndrome

Cuboid syndrome is an uncommon injury but may be seen in many forms of dance. Acute and chronic/overuse injuries have been described. Acute cuboid subluxation may occur with lateral ankle sprains or improper jump landings. The repetitive motions used when rising up to and down from relevé position are associated with this injury.

The dancer will complain of lateral midfoot pain and an inability to roll through the foot during the push-off phase of gait or to correctly achieve the demi-pointe or the full pointe position. Some dancers are unable to bear weight in acute injuries. Diagnosis is largely clinical, as radiographs, CT, and MRI scans rarely identify this subtle injury. Clinical tests including midtarsal adduction test, midtarsal supination test, and dorsal-plantar cuboid shear test have been described as reproducing the pain, but the specificity and sensitivity of these tests has not been determined.[77]

Tenderness may be dorsal or plantar in the lateral midfoot, over the surface of the cuboid and calcaneal cuboid joint. Mobility of the transverse tarsal joints may be diminished compared with the opposite foot. A step-off at the base of the fourth metatarsal may be palpable.

Treatment includes a manual reduction maneuver (cuboid whip) or passive mobilization of the rear and midfoot joints (cuboid squeeze); however, these maneuvers should not be performed repeatedly or with too much force. Taping may be used to stabilize the midfoot, often with a small felt pad under the cuboid to help maintain the reduction initially. Fibularis longus tightness should be addressed, as this is associated with the condition.[77–81] Pointe work and jumps should be restricted for 1–2 weeks or until the dancer can comfortably roll through the foot. Dancers may require orthotics in street shoes to control forefoot valgus if present.

### Fifth Metatarsal Fracture

Fractures of the fifth metatarsal are common in dance. The mechanism for injury is usually a missed jump landing or rolling over the outer border of the foot while on demi-pointe. The dancer will present with lateral foot pain, swelling, and ecchymosis. Physical examination findings include tenderness over the lateral metatarsal. Radiographs are needed for accurate diagnosis, as treatment is based on the location and type of fracture. A spiral shaft fracture, known as a "dancer's fracture," can be treated without surgery, regardless of displacement.[83] A removable cast boot, with weight-bearing as tolerated, is used until pain-free walking is possible, usually within 6 weeks. As soon as comfort allows, pool exercises and gentle active range of motion exercises are begun out of the boot. Return to dance is progressed slowly, first with barre work and pain-free exercises, and progression to center, turns, and jumps as symptoms resolve. Physical therapy focusing on proprioception, core, and foot intrinsic strength training is recommended. The clinician should evaluate the ankle for instability or ligament sprain, as both injuries may occur with this mechanism.

Avulsion fractures of the proximal fifth metatarsal are associated with the above mechanism of an ankle inversion injury. Typically extra-articular, the fracture line is through the tuberosity. Treatment with a stiff-soled shoe or removable cast boot to control symptoms is sufficient. Surgical treatment is reserved for the rare case of significant displacement or articular involvement. In skeletally immature dancers pain on the lateral border of the foot at the proximal end of the fifth metatarsal is more likely to be apophysitis (Iselin's disease), whether insidious or traumatic in onset.[36,62,64]

Jones fractures occur at the metaphyseal-diaphyseal junction of the fifth metatarsal in dancers and athletes. Because of poor blood supply in this area, these transverse fractures have a propensity for nonunion. Most common in modern and barefoot dancers, Jones fractures can be treated in a short leg cast for 6 to 8 weeks with non-weight-bearing. However, elite dancers and athletes typically are treated with bone stimulators and/or surgical treatment to avoid prolonged immobilization and reduce risk of nonunion.

Stress fractures of the proximal fifth metatarsal metaphyseal-diaphyseal area can be seen in dancers, who often report chronic lateral foot pain followed by an acute event. Radiographs demonstrate cortical thickening, periosteal reaction, and a wider fracture line than seen in the acute Jones fracture. These fractures require operative treatment, often with bone grafting and bone stimulator, due to poor healing potential similar to the acute Jones fracture.[47]

## Metatarsophalangeal Joints

Metatarsalgia is not exceptionally common in dancers, so in a dancer with forefoot pain Frieberg's infarction or MTPJ synovitis or instability should be suspected. Frieberg's infarction is an idiopathic osteonecrosis (most often of the second metatarsal head) more common in females and usually presents as metatarsalgia and MTPJ swelling and pain. Clinical symptoms often precede radiographic changes by 6 months, but a bone scan or MRI can provide an earlier diagnosis. Radiographs may reveal a flattening or fragmentation of the metatarsal head. Physical examination will demonstrate tenderness and often an effusion and decreased range of motion of the MTPJ. Conservative treatment including taping the toe, stiff-soled shoes out of class, and avoidance of painful activities should be employed.[84,85] Surgical debridement and cheilectomy are reserved for those who fail nonsurgical treatment.

**MTPJ instability** can be seen in dancers, as the demi-pointe position, with weight-bearing on the ball of the foot during demi-pointe position, transmits excess loads to the second and third metatarsal heads. Dancers will have plantar MTPJ tenderness on physical examination, yet report dorsal MTPJ pain with elevé. In addition, the painful MTPJ will have increased passive anterior/posterior translation (+MTPJ Lachman or Drawer test).[86] NSAIDS, padding, and taping the toe (to either the next toe "buddy taping" or to the plantar foot "hammertoe strapping") can be used to help alleviate symptoms. Strengthening of the foot intrinsic muscles with the doming exercise (Fig. 8.8) may help. Referral to an orthopedic foot and ankle specialist is recommended if symptoms persist.

## Sesamoid Injuries

The differential diagnosis for pain at the plantar aspect of the first metatarsophalangeal joint (1 MTPJ) in a dancer includes sesamoiditis, bursitis, osteonecrosis, stress or acute fracture of one or more sesamoid bone(s), or sprain of a bipartite sesamoid (of course infection, systemic inflammatory conditions, nerve entrapment, and tumor should be ruled out). Bipartite sesamoids are present in 10%–33% of feet.[47,64,84] The sesamoid bones are small bones imbedded within the flexor hallucis brevis (FHB) tendons and articulate with the plantar surface of the first metatarsal head. Their function is to stabilize the 1 MTPJ and to improve the power of the FHB tendons, much as the patella assists the quadriceps muscles. The sesamoids are subjected to high stress when the dancer rolls up

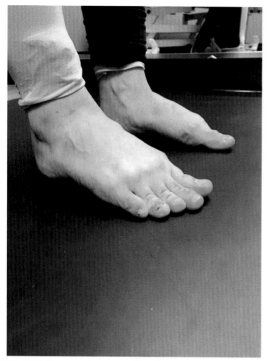

FIG. 8.8 Dancer demonstrating the "doming exercise" to strengthen foot intrinsic muscles.

onto demi-pointe or full pointe, or when taking off and landing a jump.

Presenting symptoms are pain under the first metatarsal head on the plantar forefoot, more so with relevé (rolling up onto the ball of the foot), running, and jumping. The dancer will be tender to palpation over the sesamoid bone, and a swollen and inflamed fluid-filled bursa may be palpable. The tibial sesamoid is most frequently involved. The sesamoids are embedded in the FHB tendons; therefore, the tenderness should move distally with dorsiflexion of the great toe on physical examination.

Injecting a small amount of local anesthetic will confirm the diagnosis. Bone scan and MRI may be needed to identify stress fractures or osteonecrosis. Plain radiographs (with sesamoid views) or CT scans can identity fractures. Ultrasound can demonstrate a fluid-filled bursa dynamically. Bipartite sesamoids will have rounded edges on a radiograph compared to the sharply defined edges of an acute sesamoid fracture. Technical errors such as rolling in, pronation, or forcing turnout can result in excessive loading of the sesamoids and must be corrected for successful resolution of symptoms. Improper jump landings without plié (slight bend in the knees) and the practice of walking with an out-toeing gait can contribute to sesamoid problems.[4]

Treatment includes a trial of padding to off-load the area. Felt dancer (sesamoid) pads with a cutout for the sesamoids may help, and use of a stiff-soled shoe such as a clog or hiking boot outside of class to limit hallux MTPJ motion may reduce symptoms. A removable cast boot can be used if symptoms are severe. Assessing and correcting alignment and technical problems is important for success. Corticosteroid injections in this area should be used rarely and only after technical errors are addressed. Sesamoid problems may take months to resolve fully, and surgical excision is not recommended in dancers as potential loss of plantar flexion strength could end a dance career.[47,84] Bone stimulators have been reported to improve healing in sesamoid fractures.[87]

### Hallux Rigidus

Hallux rigidus is an arthritic condition of the MTPJ. Dancers require 80–100 degrees of dorsiflexion when performing relevé onto demi-pointe; therefore, loss of motion in this joint can be disabling in a dancer. The stiffness in the joint causes the dancer to roll onto the lateral metatarsals in improper alignment (sickling) when rising to demi-pointe. Dancers with this condition report stiffness and pain of the 1 MTPJ and an inability to achieve full demi-pointe position. Dorsal fullness and a palpable osteophyte may be present. Radiographs reveal joint space narrowing, subchondral sclerosis, or dorsal osteophytes depending on the stage of the condition.

Early cases with stiffness, but few radiographic changes, should be treated with gentle traction and passive and active exercises that strengthen the intrinsic muscles of the foot. The "toe to toe" exercise can help achieve correct alignment. The dancer should avoid forcing the three-quarter pointe position, as this can exacerbate symptoms. Surgical cheilectomy with resection of the dorsal one-third of the joint, including the osteophytes, can improve symptoms, but as this is a degenerative condition of the joint, the dancer must be warned that surgery will not restore normal function. Recovery time may be as long as 3–6 months, and despite a technically successful surgery, some dancers will not achieve the required range of motion of the great toe.[47,84] There may be a role in the future for regenerative medicine techniques, but controlled studies are needed.

## Hallux Valgus/Bunions

Hallux valgus deformity occurs in dancers; however, there is conflicting data regarding whether the incidence of hallux valgus in dancers is greater than in the general population.[88–92] The cause of hallux valgus formation is multifactorial and likely results from a combination of genetic predisposition, foot shape, and shoe choice. Dancers with bunion-prone feet, those who force their turnout, and those with flexible pes planus may exacerbate an existing or developing bunion deformity. Young dancers with a bunion deformity likely have congenital metatarsus primus varus.[93]

Many dancers with bunions have little or no symptoms other than angular deformity of the hallux. Weight-bearing radiographs of the feet are used to diagnose hallux valgus and for surgical planning. Some dancers develop pain and swelling of the bursa over the medial 1 MTPJ. Acute inflammation (bursitis) of the 1 MTPJ should be treated with brief icing, NSAIDS, and taping to stabilize the hallux/1 MTPJ. Antibiotics may be required if an infection of the bursa develops. Dancers should be counseled to wear wide toe box and low-heeled or athletic type shoes outside of class if bunions are symptomatic. Use of toe spacers between the first and second toes, and in some instances a donut- or horseshoe-shaped pad over the medial prominence of the 1 MTPJ worn in the pointe shoes, can help to reduce symptoms while dancing. Some dancers find taping helpful. Intrinsic foot muscle strengthening exercises including the doming exercise, picking up marbles or pieces of makeup sponge with the toes, and hallux abduction exercises are important for all dancers, but especially so in dancers with hallux valgus prone feet. Attention to pointe shoe fit is critical for dancers with hallux valgus, as is emphasis on proper foot and leg alignment during technique class and avoidance of forced turnout. Dancers with bunions may find a pointe shoe style with a wider, square-shaped box and/or a higher than normal vamp or wings extending over the hallux MTPJ more supportive and comfortable. Avoiding over-turnout and pronation during training of young dancers can help to avoid exacerbation of bunion-prone feet.[4,30] It is recommended to avoid surgical intervention for bunions in professional dancers in the midst of their career. Any bunion surgery can lead to loss of dorsiflexion at the 1 MTPJ, and a minimum of 90 degrees of MTPJ dorsiflexion is required for the demi-pointe position.

## SUMMARY

To keep dancers healthy, the healthcare team and the dancer must work together. The physician must be an advocate for the dancer and work to provide an accurate diagnosis and an effective treatment strategy. The dancer's foot and ankle is subjected to high forces and unusual stresses in training and performance. The likelihood of a professional dancer having a foot or ankle injury is high.[18,21] Elite dancers often have a very high performance and rehearsal load, with little time for attention to aerobic fitness and general health. Unlike Little League Baseball, with defined pitch counts by age group, no similar recommended dance load limitations exist.[94] Monitoring performance and rehearsal load, fitness, and the general health of the dancer will help to maximize the dancer's healing potential. Adequate rest, fitness, recovery time, and nutrition are critical. Correction of muscle imbalances, attention to proper technique, sequential skill progression, and proper shoe fit may help limit acute injuries to the dancer. The physician must not limit his or her examination to the foot and ankle, but the entire kinetic chain of the dancer must be assessed. Injury or pain in the foot may predispose the dancer to problems further up the kinetic chain, and these must be addressed for successful return to performance.

The physician treating dancers must be sensitive to the fact that the dancer considers pain and injury a normal part of daily life. In their competitive world, dancers may fear treatments that could result in loss of audition, rehearsal, or performance. Creativity is needed to build trust with the dancer, and it is important whenever possible to modify treatment plans to accommodate the dancer's need to maintain strength, flexibility, and fitness during recovery.

## REFERENCES

1. Dozzi P, Winter D. Biomechanical analysis of the foot during rises to full pointe: implications for injuries to the metatarsal–phalangeal joints and shoe redesign. Kinesiology and Med for Dance.1993–1994;16(1):1–11. Available at: http://www.worldcat.org/title/biomechanical-analysis-of-the-foot-during-rises-tofull pointe-implications-for-injuries-to-the-metatarsal-phalangeal-joints-and shoeredesign/oclc/36937111.
2. Galea V, Norman R. Bone-on-bone forces at the ankle joint during a rapid dynamic movement. In: Winter DA, Norman RW, Wells RP, Hayes KC, Patla AE, eds. *Biomechanics IX-A*. Champaign, IL: Human Kinetics; 1985:71–76.

3. Russell J, McEwan I, Koutedakis Y, Wyon M. Clinical anatomy and biomechanics of the ankle in dance. *J Dance Med Sci*. 2008;12(3):75–82.

4. Kadel N. Foot and ankle injuries in the adolescent dancer. In: Solomon R, Solomon J, Micheli L, eds. *Prevention of Injuries in the Young Dancer*. Switzerland: Cham; 2017: 147–165. https://doi.org/10.1007/978-3-319-55047-3_9.

5. Bronner S, Ojofeitimi S, Rose D. Injuries in a modern dance company: effect of comprehensive management on injury incidence and time loss. *Am J Sports Med*. 2003; 31(3):365–373.

6. Bowling A. Injuries to dancers: prevalence, treatment, and perceptions of causes. *BMJ*. 1989;298:731–734.

7. Shah S, Weiss D, Burchette R. Injuries in professional modern dancers; incidence, risk factors, management. *J Dance Med Sci*. 2012;16(1):17–25.

8. Noon M, Hoch A, McNamara L, et al. Injury patterns in female Irish dancers. *PM R*. 2010;2(11):1030–1034.

9. Wanke E, Arendt M, Mill H, et al. Occupational accidents in professional dance with focus on gender differences. *J Occup Med Toxicol*. 2013;35:8. https://doi.org/10.1186/1745-6673-8-35.

10. Dobson R. Eight in ten dancers have an injury each year, survey shows. *BMJ*. 2005;331(7517):594.

11. Byhring S, Bø K. Musculoskeletal injuries in the Norwegian National Ballet: a prospective cohort study. *Scand J Med Sci Sports*. 2002;12:365–370.

12. Nilsson C, Leanderson J, Wykman J, et al. The injury panorama in a Swedish professional ballet company. *Knee Surg Sports Traumatol Arthrosc*. 2001;9(4):242–246.

13. Jacobs C, Cassidy JD, Côté P, et al. Musculoskeletal injury in professional dancers: prevalence and associated factors an international cross-sectional study. *Clin J Sport Med*. 2017;27(2):153–160.

14. Smith PJ, Gerrie BJ, Varner KE, McCullogh PC, Lintner DM, Harris JD. Incidence and prevalence of musculoskeletal injury in ballet. A systemic review. *Orthop J Sports Med*. 2015;3(7):2325967115592621. PMCID: PMC4622328.

15. Lloyd T, Triantafyllou SJ, Baker ER, et al. Women athletes with menstrual irregularity have increased musculoskeletal injuries. *Med Sci Sports Exerc*. 1986;18(4):374–379.

16. Warren MP, Brooks-Gunn J, Fox RP, et al. Persistent osteopenia in ballet dancers with amenorrhea and delayed menarche despite hormone therapy: a longitudinal study. *Fertil Steril*. 2003;80(2):398–404.

17. Steinberg N, Aujla I, Zeev A, Redding E. Injuries among talented young dancers: findings from the U.K. Centres for Advanced Training. *J Sports Med*. 2014;35(3):238–244. http://www.ncbi.nlm.nih.gov/pubmed/23900897.

18. Steinberg N, Siev-Ner I, Peleg S, et al. Injury patterns in young non-professional dancers. *J Sports Sci*. 2011;29(1):47–54. http://www.ncbi.nlm.nih.gov/?term=Siev-Ner%20I%5BAuthor%5D&cauthor=true&cauthor_uid=21086212.

19. Leanderson C, Leanderson J, Wykman A, Strender LE, Johansson SE, Sundquist K. Musculoskeletal injuries in young ballet dancers. *Knee Surg Sports Traumatol Arthrosc*. 2011;19:1531–1535.

20. Gamboa JM, Roberts LA, Maring J, Fergus A. Injury patterns in elite pre-professional ballet dancers and the utility of screening programs to identify risk characteristics. *J Orthop Sports Phys Ther*. 2008;38(3):126–136.

21. Ekegren CL, Quested R, Brodrick A. Injuries in pre-professional ballet dancers: Incidence, characteristics and consequences. *J Sci Med Sport*. 2014;17:271–275. From the U.K. Centres for Advanced Training. http://www.ncbi.nlm.nih.gov/pubmed/23900897. *J Sports Med*. 2014; 35(3):238–244.

22. Luke A, Kinney S, D'Hemecourt PA, Baum J, Owen M, Micheli LJ. Determinants of injuries in young dancers. *Med Probl Perform Art*. 2002;17:105–112.

23. Wiesler ER, Hunter DM, Martin DF, Curl WW, Hoen H. Ankle flexibility and injury patterns in dancers. *Am J Sports Med*. 1996;24:754–757.

24. Baxter-Jones A, Maffulli N, Helms P. Low injury rates in elite athletes. *Arch Dis Child*. 1993;68:130–132.

25. Hiller CE, Refshauge KM, Beard DJ. Sensorimotor control is impaired in dancers with functional ankle instability. *Am J Sports Med*. 2004;32(1):216–223.

26. Leanderson J, Eriksson E, Nilsson C, et al. Proprioception in classical ballet dancers. A study of the influence of an ankle sprain on proprioception in the ankle joint. *Am J Sports Med*. 1996;24(3):370–374.

27. Lin C, Lee I, Liao J, et al. Comparison of postural stability between injured and uninjured ballet dancers. *Am J Sports Med*. 2011;39(6):1324–1331.

28. Steib S, Zech A, Hentschke C, et al. Fatigue-induced alterations of static and dynamic postural control in athletes with a history of ankle sprain. *J Athl Train*. 2013;48(2): 203–208.

29. Schmitt H, Kuni B, Sabo D. Influence of professional dance training on peak torque and proprioception at the ankle. *Clin J Sport Med*. 2005;15(5):331–339.

30. Kadel N. Foot and ankle problems in dancers. *Phys Med Rehab Clin N Am*. 2014;25:829–844.

31. Elias I, Zoga A, Raikin S, et al. Bone stress injury of the ankle in professional ballet dancers seen on MRI. *BMC Musc Disord*. 2008;39:9. http://www.biomedcentral.com/1471-2474/9/39.

32. Peace K, Hillier JC, Hulme A, Healy J. MRI features of posterior ankle impingement syndrome in ballet dancers: a review of 25 cases. *Clin Radiol*. 2004;59(11):1025–1033.

33. McCormack M, Briggs J, Hakim A, Grahame R. A study of joint laxity and the impact of benign joint hypermobility syndrome in student and professional ballet dancers. *J Rheumatol*. 2001;31:173–178.

34. Briggs J, McCormack M, Hakim A, Grahame R. Injury and joint hypermobility syndrome in ballet dancers—a 5 year follow-up. *Rheumatology (Oxford)*. 2009;48(12): 1613–1614.

35. Moushine E, Crevoisier X, Leyvraz PF, Akiki A, Dutoit M, Garofalo R. Post-traumatic overload or acute syndrome of the os trigonum: a possible cause of posterior ankle impingement. *Knee Surg Sports Traumatol Arthrosc*. 2004; 12:250–253.

36. Malanga GA, Ramirez-Del Toro JA. Common injuries of the foot and ankle in the child and adolescent athlete. *Phy Med Rehabil Clin N Am.* 2008;19:347−371.

37. Hamilton W. Posterior ankle pain in dancers. *Clin Sports Med.* 2008;27:263−277.

38. Hamilton WG, Geppert MJ, Thompson FM. Pain in the posterior aspect of the ankle in dancers: differential diagnosis and operative treatment. *J Bone Joint Surg Am.* 1996;78:1491−1500.

39. Marotta J, Micheli LJ. Os trigonum impingement in dancers. *Am J Sports Med.* 1992;20:533−536.

40. Robinson P, White LM. Soft tissue and osseous impingement syndromes of the ankle: role of imaging in diagnosis and management. *Radiographics.* 2002;22:1457−1471.

41. Kadel N, Micheli L, Solomon R. Os trigonum impingement syndrome in dancers. *J Dance Med Sci.* 2000;4:99−102.

42. Russell J, Kruse D, Koutedakis Y, McEwan I, Wyon M. Pathoanatomy of posterior ankle impingement in ballet dancers. *Clin Anat.* 2010;23(6):613−621.

43. Albisetti W, Ometti M, Pascale V, DeBartolomeo O. Clinical evaluation and treatment of posterior impingement in dancers. *Am J Phys Med Rehabil.* 2009;88(5):349−354.

44. Giannini S, Buda R, Mosca M, Parma A, Di Caprio F. Posterior ankle impingement. *Foot Ank Int.* 2013;34(3):459−465.

45. Kolettis GJ, Micheli LJ, Klein JD. Release of the flexor hallucis longus tendon in ballet dancers. *J Bone Joint Surg Am.* 1996;78(9):1386−1390.

46. Michelson J, Dunn L. Tenosynovitis of the flexor hallucis longus: a clinical study of the spectrum of presentation and treatment. *Foot Ankle Int.* 2005;26(4):291−303.

47. Hamilton WG, Hamilton LH. Foot and ankle injuries in dancers. In: Mann R, Coughlin M, eds. *Surgery of the Foot and Ankle.* 7th ed. St. Louis (MO): Mosby Incorporated; 1999:1225−1256.

48. Abat F, Alfredson H, Cucchiarini M, et al. Current trends in tendinopathy: consensus of the ESSKA basic science committee. Part I: biology, biomechanics, anatomy and an exercise-based approach. *J Exp Orthop.* 2017;4:18. https://doi.org/10.1186/s40634-017-0092-6.

49. Rietveld A, Haitjema S. Posterior ankle impingement syndrome and m. flexor hallucis longus tendinopathy in dancers: results of open surgery. *J Dance Med Sci.* 2018; 22(1):3−10.

50. Rietveld A, Hagemans F. Operative treatment of posterior ankle impingement syndrome and flexor hallucis longus tendinopathy in dancers: open versus endoscopic approach. *J Dance Med Sci.* 2018;22(1):11−18.

51. Rietveld A, Hagemans F, Haitjema A, et al. Results of treatment of posterior ankle impingement syndrome and flexor hallucis longus tendinopathy in dancers: a systematic review. *J Dance Med Sci.* 2018;22(1):19−32.

52. O'Kane J, Kadel N. Anterior impingement syndrome in dancers. *Curr Rev Musculoskelet Med.* 2008;1:12−16.

53. van Dijk CN. Anterior and posterior ankle impingement. *Foot Ankle Clin.* 2006;11(3):663−683.

54. Kleiger B. Anterior tibiotalar impingement syndromes in dancers. *Foot Ankle.* 1982;3(2):69−73.

55. Stretanski MF, Weber GJ. Medical and rehabilitation issues in classical ballet: literature review. *Am J Phys Med Rehabil.* 2002;81:383−391.

56. Nihal A, Rose DJ, Trepman E. Arthroscopic treatment of anterior ankle impingement syndrome in dancers. *Foot Ankle Int.* 2005;26(11):908−912.

57. van Dijk C, Bergen C. Advancements in ankle arthroscopy. *J Am Acad Orthop Surg.* 2008;16(11):635−646.

58. van Dijk CN, van Sterkenburg MN, Wiegerinck JI, Karlsson J, Maffulli N. Terminology for Achilles tendon related disorders. *Knee Surg Sports Traumatol Arthrosc.* 2011;19(5):835−841. https://doi.org/10.1007/s00167-010-1374-z.

59. Comin J, Cook J, Malliaras P, et al. The prevalence and clinical significance of sonographic tendon abnormalities in asymptomatic ballet dancers: a 24 month longitudinal study. *Br J Sports Med.* 2013;47:89−92.

60. Mahieu N, Witvrouw E, Stevens V, et al. Intrinsic risk factors for the development of Achilles tendon overuse injury: a prospective study. *Am J Sports Med.* 2006;34(2):226−235.

61. Rehmani R, Endo Y, Bauman P, et al. Lower extremity injury patterns in elite ballet dancers: ultrasound/MRI imaging features and an institutional overview of therapeutic ultrasound guided percutaneous interventions. *HSSJ.* 2015;11:258−277. https://doi.org/10.1007/s11420-015-9442-z.

62. Frush TJ, Lindenfeld TN. Peri-epiphyseal and overuse injuries in adolescent athletes. *Sports Health.* 2009;1(3):201−211.

63. Walls R, Brennan S, Hodnett P, et al. Overuse ankle injuries in professional Irish dancers. *Foot Ankle Surg.* 2010;16(1):45−49.

64. Houghton KM. Review for the generalist: evaluation of pediatric foot and ankle pain. *Ped Rheum.* 2008;6:6. http://www.ped-rheum.com/content/6/1/6.

65. Schwartz E, Su J. Plantar fasciitis: a concise review. Perm J. *Winter.* 2014;18(1):e105−e107. https://doi.org/10.7812/TPP/13-113.

66. Yang W, Han Y, Cao X, et al. Platelet-rich plasma as a treatment for plantar fasciitis. A meta-analysis of randomized controlled trials. *Medicine.* 2017;96(44):e8475. https://doi.org/10.1097/MD.0000000000008475.

67. Kadel N, Teitz C, Kronmal R. Stress fractures in ballet dancers. *Am J Sports Med.* 1992;20(4):445−449.

68. O'Malley MJ, Hamilton WG, Munyak J. Stress fractures at the base of the second metatarsal in ballet dancers. *Foot Ankle Int.* 1996;17:89−94.

69. Micheli L, Sohn R, Solomon J. Stress fractures of the second metatarsal involving Lisfranc's joint in ballet dancers. *J Bone Joint Surg Am.* 1985;67:1372−1375.

70. Kadel N, Boenisch M, Teitz C, Trepman E. Stability of Lisfranc joints in ballet pointe position. *Foot Ankle Int.* 2005; 26(5):394−400.

71. Harrington T, Crichton K, Anderson I. Overuse ballet injury to the base of the second metatarsal a diagnostic problem. *Am J Sports Med.* 1993;21:591−598.

72. Nussbaum AR, Treves ST, Micheli L. Bone stress lesions in ballet dancers: scintigraphic assessment. *AJR Am J Roentgenol.* 1988;150(4):851−855.

73. Albisetti W, Perugia D, De Bartolomeo O, Tagliabue L, Camerucci E, Calori G. Stress fracture of the base of the metatarsal bones in young trainee ballet dancers. *Int Orthop.* 2010;34:51−55.

74. DellaValle C, Su E, Nihal A, Rosenberg Z, Trepman E. Acute disruption of the tarsometatarsal (Lisfranc's) joints in a ballet dancer. *J Dance Med Sci.* 2000;4(4):128−131.

75. Kadel N, Donaldson-Fletcher E. Lisfranc's fracture−dislocation in a male ballet dancer during take-off of a jump: a case report. *J Dance Med Sci.* 2004;8(2):56−58.

76. Gillespie P, Robertson A, George B, Nihal A. Acute Lisfranc joint disruption in a ballet dancer. *Foot Ankle Surg.* 2005; 11:105−108.

77. Durall C. Examination and treatment of cuboid syndrome: a literature review. *Sports Health.* 2011;3(6):514−519.

78. Adams E, Madden C. Cuboid subluxation: a case study and review. *Curr Sports Med Rep.* 2009;8(6):300−307.

79. Newell SG, Woodle A. Cuboid syndrome. *Phys Sportsmed.* 1981;9(4):71−76.

80. Marshall P. The rehabilitation of overuse foot injuries in athletes and dancers. *Clin Sports Med.* 1988;7(1):175−191.

81. Marshall P, Hamilton WG. Cuboid subluxation in ballet dancers. *Am J Sports Med.* 1982;20(2):169−175.

82. Patterson SM. Cuboid syndrome: a review of the literature. *J Sports Sci Med.* 2006;5:597−606.

83. O'Malley MJ, Hamilton WG, Munyak J. Fractures of the distal shaft of the fifth metatarsal."Dancer's fracture". *Am J Sports Med.* 1996;24(2):240−243.

84. Prisk V, O'Loughlin P, Kennedy J. Forefoot injuries in dancers. *Clin Sports Med.* 2008;27:305−320.

85. Air M, Rietveld A. Freiberg's disease as a rare cause of limited and painful relevé in dancers. *J Dance Med Sci.* 2010;14(1):32−36.

86. Thompson FM, Hamilton WG. Problems of the second metatarsophalangeal joint. *Orthopedics.* 1987;10(1): 83−89.

87. Bronner S, Novella T, Becica L. Management of a delayed-union sesamoid fracture in a dancer. *J Orth Sport Phys Ther.* 2007;37(9):529−537.

88. Davenport K, Simmel L, Kadel N. Hallux valgus in dancers: a closer look at dance technique and its impact on dancers' feet. *J Dance Med Sci.* 2014;18(2):86−92.

89. Desoille H, Bourguignon A, Chavy AL. Statistical study of the frequency of hallux valgus and of different forms of the foot in classical dancers. *Arch Mal Prof.* 1960;21: 343−349.

90. Einarsdóttir H, Troell S, Wykman A. Hallux valgus in ballet dancers: a myth? *Foot Ankle Int.* 1995 Feb;16(2):92−94.

91. van Dijk CN, Lim LS, Poortman A, et al. Degenerative joint disease in female ballet dancers. *Am J Sports Med.* 1995; 23(3):295−300.

92. Kennedy JG, Collumbier JA. Bunions in dancers. *Clin Sports Med.* 2008;27(2):321−328.

93. Coughlin MJ. Juvenile hallux valgus: etiology and treatment. *Foot Ankle Int.* 1995;16(11):682−697.

94. American Sports Medicine Institute. *Position statement for youth baseball pitchers updated;* 2013. http://www.asmi.org/research.php?page=research&section=positionStatement.

## CHAPTER 9

# The Professional Dancer's Hip

KATHLEEN L. DAVENPORT, MD, CAQSM

## INTRODUCTION

There is a high range of hip motion required for classical dance technique, which requires both mobility and stability of the hip joint to successfully complete these repetitive movements. Due to these high demands on the joint, the dancer's hip is at risk for injury with the incidence of hip pathology in professional dancers being reported at 15%−58%[1−4] with a higher incidence of overuse injuries,[2−4] and occurring in dance techniques requiring increased turnout.[3] There is an increased incidence of hip injuries in professional dancers compared to student dancers.[4]

Examination of the professional dancer's hip should be performed in standing, seated, supine, lateral, and prone positions.[5−7] All examinations should include inspection, palpation, range of motion, strength, and neurological testing. Special tests will be discussed below with their implications regarding specific pathology. Although this chapter discusses hip pathology, it must be remembered that surrounding structures, such as the sacroiliac joint, lumbosacral spine, nerve bundles, and pelvis, can refer pain to the hip and groin region, and these structures should be included in any differential diagnosis and hip examination.[8,9]

## OSTEOCHONDRAL PATHOLOGY
### Stress Fractures

Stress fractures of the femoral neck are uncommon, but are important to include in the differential diagnosis of hip pain in the dancer, as symptoms may be vague and an accurate and timely diagnosis often requires a high index of suspicion.[10] In dancers, fractures are considered to be caused by repetitive stress causing fatigue of normal bone.[11,12] New bone formation is unable to adequately respond to increased demands required by new or increased activity.[13] Dancers should be evaluated for relative energy deficiency in sport (RED-S), as athletes with RED-S are at increased risk of developing stress fractures.[14,15] Professional classical dancers have

traditionally maintained a low body weight and may be at risk for RED-S.[16−18] Additionally, the education in some dance communities regarding a "ramp up period" may be lacking and periods of increased activity, such as show rehearsals and summer camps, should increase the index of clinical suspicion of a stress fracture.[19]

Dancers with stress reactions and/or stress fractures of the hip may complain of anterior groin pain that worsens with activity, particularly while/after jumping and toward the end of class or rehearsal.[19] Pain is generally reported to improve with rest and decreasing high-impact activities. A stress fracture requires a high index of suspicion as symptoms are often vague and can be similar to other. Physical exam may demonstrate decreased hip range of motion,[13] antalgic gait, or inability to bear weight.[20] A hop test has increased sensitivity and should be considered in the physical examination to determine if the dancer has pain with a single jump on the affected side.[10] However, it is important to stress that caution is advised in including a hop test, as there is the risk of progression of a stress reaction or cause an outright fracture. Diagnostic work-up includes plain film X-rays, which are often negative in early presentation. MRI of the hip without contrast is definitive for diagnosis of a stress fracture or stress reaction. Work-up should also include nutritional evaluation with consideration of lab work, nutritional referral, potentially dual-energy x-ray absorptiometry (DEXA), and/or referral for full evaluation of metabolic bone health and RED-S.[15]

Treatment is contingent on the location of the fracture. Femoral neck fractures are classified as compression (inferior surface, less than 50% of the femoral neck) or tension (superior surface) types.[11,12,20,21] Compression-type stress fractures largely respond to conservative care, and the dancer should be placed nonweight bearing until asymptomatic, then weight bearing is slowly progressed, followed by gradually returning to full activity with high-impact movements, such as jumps, being added last.[13,14,20] Tension-sided

Performing Arts Medicine. https://doi.org/10.1016/B978-0-323-58182-0.00009-2

stress fractures require surgical fixation due to the high risk of poor outcomes, including avascular necrosis, malunion, and/or deformity.[14,20] Urgent surgical fixation should be considered for any displaced fracture.[13] In any stress reaction or stress fracture, it is essential to evaluate training factors, biomechanics, and nutritional balance.[14] Any diagnosis or concern of RED-S should be addressed with full work-up and appropriate referrals.[15] A gradual return to dance protocol may be allowed when the dancer has achieved pain free range of motion, asymptomatic full weight bearing, and treatment of any underlying risk factors.[21] Repeat MRI to monitor and assess healing.[21]

Pelvic stress fractures, most commonly the ischiopubic ramus, are rare but can occur in the highly athletic population. These stress fracture or stress reactions often present similarly to adductor tendinopathy, osteitis pubis, and/or athletic pubalgia. Similar to other stress fractures, there is an increased incidence in women with RED-S.[21] These fractures are often successfully treated with decreased weight bearing, activity modification, and treatment of underlying risk factors, followed by gradual activity progression.[21]

## INERT LAYER

### Capsular Injury

The hip capsule covers the majority of the femoral neck, extending from the intertrochanteric ridge to the acetabular rim, and is fortified by adjacent ligaments and muscles. Injury to the capsule can occur by traumatic hip dislocation, or in dance participation.[11] Classical ballet technique promotes axial loading with hip rotation, which can increase the risk for capsule stretch or rupture.[20,22] Capsular laxity, particularly if chronic in nature, can result in improper joint technique and increase the risk of secondary injuries, such as labral tears.[6] Additionally, laxity in the hip capsule from innate factors and/or prior injuries can result in surrounding structures, such as the iliopsoas muscle, compensating in an attempt to stabilize the joint. This compensation may result in the surrounding soft tissue structures becoming an independent source of anterior hip pain (see iliopsoas tendinopathy below).[6,20]

Groin pain, which worsens with passive external rotation and extension, is the primary presenting complaint of capsular injury.[20] This is a common position in classical ballet technique and can result in hip subluxation on imaging,[23] and therefore examination should include functional dance technique with observation of the hip biomechanics in these positions.

Treatment is conservative with movement modification for a short period of time, physical therapy, and antiinflammatory medications.[20] Arthroscopy for capsular plication is a treatment consideration if all conservative measures are unsuccessful and the dancer is unable to return to dance activity.[24] Capsular surgery should be considered as a last resort in the dancer athlete as tightening of the capsule may result in relative loss of range of motion and therefore inability to reach necessary dance positions.

### Labrum and Femoroacetabular Impingement

Femoroacetabular impingement (FAI) results from increased contact between the proximal femur and acetabulum, which is most evident in hip flexion and adduction.[25] In dancers, FAI may occur more often in the superior or posterior-superior where other athletes tend to impinge in the anterior-superior hip.[26,27] Regardless of activity, FAI is felt to be due to anatomical variants of the femoral head-neck junction (CAM), acetabular rim (pincer), or both.[7,28–31] CAM FAI can be considered as an inclusion injury with increased femoral head radius and decreased femoral head sphericity, causing acetabular and chondral injury.[28–30,32] Pincer impingement can be considered as an impaction-type injury and occurs in hips with acetabular overcoverage and/or retroversion, resulting in labral injury and acetabular rim bony deposition.[28–30,33] In many athletes, there is often a combination of both CAM- and pincer-type FAI.[31,32] Given the impaction mechanism, it has been shown that pincer-type FAI is more common in dancers compared to CAM-type FAI.[34–36] However, CAM-type FAI has been shown to be more common in males.[37] FAI can lead to injuries of the surrounding hip soft tissue structures from underlying abnormalities or direct mechanical stress.[25,28,31,38] The soft tissue pathology is dependent on the specific repetitive movements and can result in cartilage destruction, labral injury, and compensatory tendinopathies.

The clinical presentation of dancers with FAI tends to be gradual onset of decreased range of motion with anterior groin pain, which is worse with prolonged sitting.[25,30,31,39,40] FAI is more common in young, active athletes who participate in sports requiring repetitive hip flexion and rotation, such as dance.[29,39,41–43] When these positions are repeated frequently, the dancer may be at increased risk for early hip osteoarthritis or bone apposition at the acetabular rim, increasing the amount of impingement.[33,44] Therefore, a careful history regarding painful maneuvers, training techniques, cross-training activities, and hours of training is essential. Physical examination typically demonstrates decreased hip range of motion in flexion and internal rotation, and pain that is reproduced on physical exam with flexion-adduction-internal rotation (FADIR) maneuver.[29–31,43]

Initial treatment of FAI should be conservative with modifying activity to avoid exacerbated movements while optimizing stability of hip and core musculature.[29,30,43,45] In dancers, activity modification may include temporarily decreasing range of turnout, decreasing or eliminating *developé à la seconde* and other extension movements that are exacerbating the pain. It has been shown that compensated turnout has been predictive of lower extremity injury in dancers, including hip injury.[46] Antiinflammatory medications can be helpful to decrease pain and inflammation.[29] An intraarticular hip steroid injection may be considered for diagnostic and therapeutic pain relief,[29,47] although caution is advised given the risks of lidocaine chondrocytotoxicty[48–50] and rare risks of steroid to the hip joint,[51] which could be career ending in the professional dancer.

Surgical correction of FAI may be considered in high-level dancers who have failed extensive conservative care with the goal to provide increased clearance between the femoral head and the acetabulum.[30] With appropriate postoperative rehabilitation, there have been high rates of successful outcomes in athletes after FAI surgical correction.[20] Importantly, if surgery is considered for other concurrent soft tissue injuries, such as labral tears, it is essential that FAI correction is considered as part of the clinical discussion to address a potential underlying etiology.[7,32]

## Ischiofemoral Impingement
Ischiofemoral impingement refers to the compression of the quadratus femoris muscle between the ischium and the lesser trochanter in hip extension with external rotation and adduction.[52,53] The psoas insertion and hamstring origin may also be affected. A dancer may be susceptible to impingement due to congenital or acquired etiology, such as postfracture, degenerative arthritis, history of proximal femoral osteotomy, or history of total-hip arthroplasty.[52,54] Ischiofemoral impingement has been described in the setting of hamstring and gluteal injury in conjunction with snapping hip syndrome.[55]

Dancers may report buttock and medial thigh pain, particularly with external rotation and extension with adduction, such as *attitude en derrière* position. It has also been reported to mimic pain in the hamstring origin.[55] Physical examination should elicit reproduction of pain by placing the hip in extension, adduction, and external rotation.[52,53] Treatment is conservative including avoiding exacerbating movements with optimizing biomechanics, including specific attention to the quadratus femoris muscle stretching and strengthening.[55] Guided injection may be indicated for diagnostic and/or therapeutic pain relief. In some cases, partial tears have been demonstrated in the quadratus femoris muscle[52,54,55] and surgical resection of the lesser trochanter has been described to provide pain relief in a less active and older population.[56] Surgery in this higher risk area should be cautioned in young, active athletes.[53,55]

## Subspine Impingement
Subspine impingement may occur during hip flexion movements when the anterior inferior iliac spine (AIIS) is compressed inferiorly against the femoral neck.[57–59] This type of impingement has been described in patients with a prior history of AIIS avulsion fracture, at the origin of the rectus femoris muscle,[60] but has also been reported in the absence of prior AIIS injury.[57–59]

Dancers with subspine impingement may report pain with repetitive or prolonged hip flexion, which are common in many dance techniques and choreography. Physical examination typically reproduces pain with end range passive hip flexion, knee flexed, with or without loss of range of motion compared to the unaffected side. Examination includes AIIS palpation, which often reproduces pain. Lack of pain reproduction with resisted hip flexion can be useful to distinguish between passive painful structures (bony impingement) versus active structures (tendinitis, muscle injury, etc.). Conservative treatment includes activity modification, diagnostic intraarticular injection to rule out other pathology, and rehabilitation and may be sufficient and should be trialed prior to surgical consideration. Guided intraarticular hip injection can be considered if the diagnosis is unclear and/or the dancer has failed other treatments.[57–59] Ultimately, if the dancer has failed conservative treatment, arthroscopic decompression of the AIIS may be considered in rare cases to improve function and decrease pain.[57–59]

# ANTERIOR MUSCULAR PATHOLOGY
## Rectus Femoris and Sartorius
Injury to the rectus femoris and sartorius muscles is less common in the skeletally mature dancer, but any muscle crossing two joints may be at increased risk for injury to the myotendinous junction.[61] Apophyseal

avulsion injuries in skeletally immature patients can occur in both muscles.[61,62] Avulsion fracture of the rectus femoris can rarely occur in adults in the setting of strong eccentric contraction. This has been reported in National Football League (NFL) kickers.[63,64] These injuries can occur in the setting of a kick going from a hip extended/knee flexed starting point to hip flexed/knee extended endpoint.[64] Typically, avulsion fractures are managed conservatively, but surgical correction may be considered in rare cases.[64] One complication of avulsion fracture of the rectus femoris is a lengthened AIIS due to bony formation along the tract of injury, resulting in subspine impingement (see previous section).[58]

## Iliopsoas Tendinopathy

The iliopsoas muscle is one of the primary hip flexors.[65] The psoas and iliacus muscles have their origin on the lumbar spine and pelvis, respectively, and then combine prior to insertion onto the lesser trochanter.[65] Iliopsoas tendinopathy may be reported by dancers with repetitive hip flexion and/or hip hyperextension movements.[66,67] Iliopsoas tendinopathy may occur in the absence or presence of iliopsoas bursitis and/or internal snapping hip (internal coxa saltans).

The iliopsoas bursa is the largest bursa in the body and may become inflamed.[12,65] Ilopsoas bursitis can occur when the iliopsoas tendon tracts over the iliopectineal eminence, the anterior femoral head, and/or the anterior hip capsuloligamentous structures.[65,66] There may be audible or palpable snapping, and dancers may complain of a "snapping hip."[12,65] Snapping can occur from a variety of mechanisms, but is often due to the femur moving from flexion/external rotation into extension/internal rotation.[67,68]

Dancers will report anterior hip pain or groin pain that gets worse with activity, particularly hip rotation activity such as *grande ronde de jambe en l'air* or fan kicks.[65,66] An audible or palpable snap may be reported, which may or may not be painful. Positive physical exam findings may include tenderness to palpation over the iliopsoas myotendinous junction, pain with resisted hip flexion in slight external rotation, positive Thomas test, and/or pain with FADIR test.[65,66,69] In addition, if internal coxa saltans is present, the dancer may have a positive fan test where snapping and/or pain is reproduced when the limb is moved from flexion/external rotation into extension/internal rotation. If the pain and snapping is reproducible, it can often be palpated on physical examination.

Treatment is conservative and includes retraining muscle imbalances with targeted strengthening and stretching therapies.[46,65–67] If rehabilitation alone is insufficient, ultrasound-guided injections into the iliopsoas tendon bursa, or ultrasound guided saline peritenon hydrodissection may be considered.[65,66] Surgery should be avoided in the professional dancer at all costs, but hip arthroscopy can be discussed in rare cases when all conservative measures have failed.[65,66,69]

## LATERAL MUSCULAR PATHOLOGY
### Abductor Dysfunction

The greater trochanter is the attachment site for five muscles: the gluteus medius, gluteus minimus, piriformis, obturator externus, and obturator internus.[70] Overloading the "rotator cuff of the hip" can result in trochanteric bursitis, gluteus medius/minimus tendinopathy, and/or snapping iliotibial band (ITB) syndrome.[71] Hip abductor dysfunction has been shown to be more common in women compared to men, and it has been theorized that the wider female pelvis is a contributing factor.[70–73] This conglomeration of diagnoses with resultant lateral hip pain has been termed "greater trochanteric pain syndrome."[71,72]

Dancers will typically present with lateral hip pain, which they report is worse with direct pressure, walking, and repetitive hip movements such as stair climbing or fan kicks.[73,74] Lumbar spine pathology may be associated with hip abductor dysfunction, and treatment for both lumbar spine pain generators and greater trochanteric pain syndrome should be considered.[72,73] Physical examination should always include side lying positioning and often reproduces the dancer's presenting pain with direct palpation over the greater trochanter, flexion-abduction-external rotation (FABER) test, positive Ober test, and weakness with pain when tested resisted hip abduction.[70,73,74] It is imperative to make sure the dancer is using correct technique with resisted hip abduction to truly test the lateral musculature, as many patients will utilize tensor fascia latae and/or iliopsoas to compensate for weak hip abduction. A Trendelenburg sign or gait pattern may or may not be present and could be compensated.[74]

Conservative treatment with physical therapy and targeted exercises will resolve most patients' symptoms by correcting muscle imbalances, particularly gluteus medius/minimus weakness.[70,73,74] Antiinflammatory measures should be used with the functional goal of facilitating exercise participation and may include oral or topical antiinflammatory medications, or an ultrasound-guided peri-tenon or bursa steroid injection.[70,73,74] Recalcitrant cases are rare in the high-level athlete, but may include trochanteric bursectomy, with or without Iliotibial Band release.[70,73] Platelet-rich plasma (PRP) may be considered for treatment of gluteus minimus and medius tendinopathy and/or partial tears.[75] Rarely, surgery can be considered but should be reserved for patients with complete rupture of the tendon or chronic high-grade partial tendon tears that have failed to respond to nonoperative measures.[76]

## Iliotibial Band Dysfunction

ITB dysfunction can be a cause of lateral hip pain and lateral knee pain in dancers, although it is more common in runners and cyclists, who train preferentially in the sagittal plane.[77–79] The ITB originates from the outer aspect iliac crest and then inserts at Gerdy's tubercle, on the lateral tibial plateau.[79,80] It is a connective tissue sheath containing the tensor fascia lata (TFL) and gluteus maximus fascia. ITB pain may occur when the knee moves from flexion to extension, causing friction of the band when it moves over the lateral femoral condyle.[21,78,79] Contributing factors to ITB dysfunction include strength deficits, specifically hip abduction weakness, and increased ITB strain.[21,80,81]

ITB dysfunction can also be associated with external snapping hip.[82,83] External snapping hip most commonly occurs when the ITB snaps over the greater trochanter, but can also occur less commonly at the gluteus maximus tendon.[82,83] A snap in the lateral thigh may be felt and/or heard, and can be accentuated in the setting of posterior ITB or anterior gluteus maximus thickening.[83] The band is typically described as snapping from posterior to anterior over the greater trochanter as the hip moves from extension into flexion.[82] This may be able to be reproduced on dance specific physical examination with "fan kick" or *grande ronde de jambe en l'air* maneuvers.

Dancers typically localize their symptoms to the lateral hip and thigh, as well as the lateral knee.[21,80] Practitioners should inquire about training regimen, as often ITB symptoms are preceded by an increase in training, introduction of new movements, or a change in technique. Symptoms are typically exacerbated with activity, or shortly after exercise. On physical examination, there is often tenderness to palpation along the ITB, positive Ober's test, and weakness to resisted hip abduction.[77]

Treatment is conservative and focuses on restoration of hip abduction strength, fascial release, and addressing flexibility imbalances.[77] Decreasing inflammation can be considered to facilitate physical therapy participation with antiinflammatory medications, or a peri-fascial steroid injection. Surgical release has been documented in rare cases that have failed conservative treatments, but caution should be utilized in the dance population.[78] To successfully return the dancer to full activity, it is important to address biomechanics, muscle imbalances, and training factors, such as technique, cross training, and movement patterns.

## POSTERIOR MUSCULAR PATHOLOGY

### Hamstring Tendinopathy

Acute and chronic hamstring tendon pathology can significantly impair both professional and recreational dancers. The common hamstring tendon originates from the ischial tuberosity, with the exception of the short head of the biceps femoris, and comprises the semimembranosis, semitendinosis, and biceps femoris muscles.[84–86] The hamstring acts as a hip extensor and, to a lesser extent, as a knee flexor.[84,87–89] The mechanism of an acute hamstring injury is often a sudden eccentric hamstring muscle contraction or, more commonly in dancers, extreme hip flexion with knee extension, particularly in the setting of insufficient warm up.[84,85,87,90–92] Chronic hamstring tendinopathy develops in the setting of mild, low-grade microtrauma, which may occur in dancers, but is more common in long distance and mid-distance running.[86,92]

Injury, whether acute or chronic, typically occurs immediately adjacent to the myotendinous junction of the long head of the biceps femoris muscle.[12,85,86] Dancers commonly report loss of flexibility ("front split" of the affected leg), lower gluteal pain, "buttock pain," and/or posterior thigh pain that is exacerbated by activities such as hip flexion.[84,87] Physical exam findings include tenderness to palpation over the ischial tuberosity with bruising and/or palpable defect in the setting of acute complete or partial tear(s).[84,90,93] Risk factors for both acute and chronic hamstring tendinopathy include strength imbalances, insufficient warm up, and poor flexibility and treatments focus on restoration and correction of these elements.[85,87,89,92] Eccentric hamstring strengthening prevents both new and recurrent hamstring injuries and should be included in a home exercise and physical therapy program.[88] There is insufficient evidence to recommend steroid injections into this area, although any consideration of injection should be done under imaging guidance.[94] Injection of autologous blood products (whole blood, platelet rich plasma), followed by eccentric strengthening addressed in physical therapy can be considered.[95]

Complete rupture of the hamstring tendons can lead to significant disability with resultant pain, sciatic nerve irritation, and functional deficit. Surgical referral should occur in the setting of an acute two tendon rupture with 2-3 cm retraction or greater. A dancer should also be referred for surgical opinion in the setting of a three tendon complete rupture of any retraction distance.[96,97] Early referral is essential if possible, because a recommended repair should be completed acutely (within 3—4 weeks) to decrease scarring and adhesions, although allograft reconstruction of chronic tears has shown comparable functional outcomes in some cases.[98]

## MEDIAL MUSCULAR PATHOLOGY AND ATHLETIC PUBALGIA

### Adductor Tendinopathy

Six muscles make up the adductor group: the adductor longus, adductor brevis, adductor magnus, gracilis, pectineus, and obturator externus.[99] All adductor muscles have their origin at the pubis; the adductor magnus also has an origin on the ischium, and inserts along the medial femur. The most commonly injured muscle is the adductor longus and the mechanism of injury typically involves a sudden change in direction or momentum resulting in forceful eccentric contraction.[87,100,101] Risk factors for injury to the adductors should be assessed and treated, if present, and may include decreased strength, flexibility, and history of prior adductor injury.[99]

Dancers typically report acute or chronic groin pain, that is worse with passive hip abduction (stretching the adductor muscle group), resisted hip adduction, and worse with activity.[99,100] Dancers may also report subjective decreased performance because the adductor group is a hip stabilizer,[102] and may report focal weakness in the adductors.[100] Physical exam should include palpation and examination of any defect or ecchymosis that could indicate tear or rupture.[103] Examination should also include resisted adduction to assess for pain and weakness, which may be performed with the dancer supine and the extremity in the figure four position.[103]

Treatment is generally conservative and focuses on strengthening the adductor musculature with gradual progression back to performance.[99] Recurrent adductor injury is common,[104] and it is therefore essential to diligently restore function prior to full return to activity.[99]

### Osteitis Pubis

Osteitis pubis refers to an inflammatory pain syndrome of the pubic symphysis due to increased mobility at this typically immobile joint.[102,105] The exact etiology of this injury is unclear, but it typically occurs in the setting of repetitive, unequal stresses on the pubic symphysis with strain of the adductor attachment and irritation over the symphysis.[12,106,107] Pain can be reproduced by physical activity and is often seen in sports with cutting and twisting movements.[108] Decreased hip range of motion, with or without FAI, has been suggested as a risk factor for osteitis pubis.[105]

Dancers typically report pain at the anterior and medial groin.[105] It is important to keep a broad differential diagnosis, as there are frequently concomitant diagnoses of athletic pubalgia, adductor and/or iliopsoas strain, sacroiliac dysfunction, core musculature weakness, and/or FAI.105,108,59 To differentiate from other etiologies of groin pain, the pubic symphysis should be tender to direct palpation, although there may be concomitant tenderness over the adductor musculature, reproducible pain with hip adduction and lower abdominal musculature strength testing, and pubic symphysis pain with compression of the pelvis.[103,105,106] There may be loss of hip range motion, sacroiliac joint dysfunction, weakness in hip adductor or abductor musculature, and antalgic gait pattern.[105,109]

Treatment is conservative and typically requires an initial period of relative rest to decrease inflammation and irritation of the surrounding structures, although this can present a challenge in the professional dancer.[105,108] Physical therapy initially addresses range of motion and progresses to strengthening, focusing on core muscle reeducation and rehabilitation. Corticosteroid injection into the pubic symphysis can be considered if a dancer is unable to fully participate in physical therapy due to pain, and should be done under image guidance.[105,108,110] If a dancer has failed extensive conservative options, surgical stabilization of the pubic symphysis is rarely considered if pain continues to limit function.[109,111]

### Athletic Pubalgia ("Sports Hernia")

Athletic pubalgia, "sports hernia," or "core muscle dysfunction" refers to pathology involving the pubic joint, and is not a true inguinal hernia.[38,112] Diagnosis and etiology of athletic pubalgia are complicated due to historical challenges of definition and multiple sub-types being described.[112] This diagnosis has been described as injury to the conjoined tendon, rectus abdominus insertional, internal oblique musculature, and/or external oblique aponeurosis.[112—115] Although not fully understood, athletic pubalgia is considered to be an injury to the hip and lower abdominal flexion and adduction mechanism, resulting in lower abdominal and inguinal exertional pain.[38,112] Similar predisposing factors in adductor tendinopathy and osteitis pubis can also lead to athletic pubalgia.[115,116] Specifically, FAI is a strong risk factor for development and suboptimal outcomes of athletic pubalgia.[59]

Athletic pubalgia is more common in male athletes participating in sports that require cutting and turning motions.[112–116] Dancers will typically report insidious, gradual onset of anterior/medial groin and lower abdominal pain that is worse with activity and improves with rest.[38,113–115] Patients will predominantly complain of pain worsening with kicking, sneezing, abdominal core exercises (sit-ups), sprinting, and/or sudden movements.[38,113,114] Physical exam reveals tenderness to palpation over the pubic tubercle, conjoined tendon, and/or inguinal area.[113] There is no palpable inguinal hernia and thus the term "sports hernia" can be confusing.[117] Pain is reproduced with sit-up resisted on the ipsilateral side, resisted hip adduction, and with valsalva maneuver.[38,103,112,113]

Conservative treatment is typically initiated, similar to adductor strain and osteitis pubis, with relative rest followed by rehabilitation.[113,116] However, different from other causes of medial groin pain, athletic pubalgia is often recalcitrant to conservative treatments and surgery may be recommended.[38,112–116] If athletic pubalgia surgery is considered, any underlying predisposing intraarticular pathology, such as FAI, should also be considered for correction.[59] Postoperative recovery should include an adequate step-wise rehabilitation program to ensure full return to activities and to decrease the risk of recurrence.[111,112,116,118,119]

## CONCLUSIONS

Classical dance technique requires extreme range of motion of the hip joint, and injuries around the hip can vary in severity from mild muscle strains to fractures. Precise early treatment and diagnosis can be complicated by the overlapping hip anatomy and potential pathology. It is essential that the practitioner optimizes diagnosis and treatment by systematically analyzing each anatomical layer, including the osseous, intraarticular (capsule, labrum, and cartilage complex), muscular (core muscle dysfunction), and neural components.

## PHYSICAL EXAMINATION

The physical examination of the hip in the professional dancer is the same or similar to that of any athlete. The hip should be examined in supine, lateral, prone,

standing, and seated positions. In the supine position the dancer shoulder be examined with the hip flexed at 90 degrees to establish internal and external rotation. Professional ballet dancers often have retroverted hips to achieve the desired "turnout" or external rotation. It is imperative that the clinician maintains stability of the joint in range of motion to ensure accurate diagnosis. As many dancers have increased mobility or increased retroversion, maintenance of stability is imperative.

Palpation over the anterior superior iliac spine (ASIS), iliopsoas, adductor longus, public symphysis, and TFL is particularly important while the dancer is in the supine position. Special tests in the supine position include FADIR testing, which will evaluate some elements of FAI. Flexion can evaluate for subspine impingement. FABER testing can be done in figure four position or with the leg abducted somewhat laterally. This can assist in SI joint pathology diagnosis, compensatory muscular pathology. Resisted hip flexion, particularly with knee in extension, can be useful in examining the iliopsoas function and overactivation or weaknesses in the anterior hip complex. Resisted adduction can provide diagnostic information regarding adductor pathology. Additionally, a half sit-up or valsalva can give information regarding anterior abdominal musculature and fascial pathology.

In the lateral position, the examiner can assess the hip abductor musculature.

## IMAGING RECOMMENDATIONS
Treatment options
    Physical therapy
    Medications
    Injections
    Surgery

## REFERENCES

1. Smith PJ, Gerrie BJ, Varner KE, McCulloch PC, Lintner DM, Harris JD. Incidence and prevalence of musculoskeletal injury in ballet: a systematic review. *Orthop J Sports Med.* 2015;3(7):2325967115592621.
2. Smith TO, Davies L, de Medici A, Hakim A, Haddad F, Macgregor A. Prevalence and profile of musculoskeletal injuries in ballet dancers: a systematic review and meta-analysis. *Phys Ther Sport.* 2016;19:50–56.
3. Sobrino FJ, de la Cuadra C, Guillén P. Overuse injuries in professional ballet: injury-based differences among ballet disciplines. *Orthop J Sports Med.* 2015;3(6): 2325967115590114.

4. Trentacosta N, Sugimoto D, Micheli LJ. Hip and groin injuries in dancers: a systematic review. *Sports Health*. 2017; 9(9):422–427.

5. Martin HD, Kelly BT, Leunig M, et al. The pattern and technique in the clinical evaluation of the adult hip: the common physical examination tests of hip specialists. *Arthroscopy*. 2010;26(2):161–172.

6. Kelly BT, Williams 3rd RJ, Philippon MJ. Hip arthroscopy: current indications, treatment options, and management issues. *Am J Sports Med*. 2003;31(6): 1020–1037.

7. Leunig M, Beaule PE, Ganz R. The concept of femoroacetabular impingement: current status and future perspectives. *Clin Orthop Relat Res*. 2009;467(3): 616–622.

8. Byrd JW, Jones KS. Adhesive capsulitis of the hip. *Arthroscopy*. 2006;22(1):89–94.

9. Gwathmey FW, Byrd JWT. Hip pathology that can cause groin pain in athletes: diagnosis and management. In: Diduch DR, Brunt LM, eds. *Sports Hernia and Athletic Pubalgia: Diagnosis and Treatment*. Boston, MA: Springer US; 2014:31–54.

10. Clement DB, Ammann W, Taunton JE, et al. Exercise-induced stress injuries to the femur. *Int J Sports Med*. 1993;14(6):347–352.

11. Blankenbaker DG, De Smet AA. Hip injuries in athletes. *Radiol Clin North Am*. 2010;48(6):1155–1178.

12. Overdeck KH, Palmer WE. Imaging of hip and groin injuries in athletes. *Semin Musculoskelet Radiol*. 2004;8(1): 41–55.

13. Shin AY, Gillingham BL. Fatigue fractures of the femoral neck in athletes. *J Am Acad Orthop Surg*. 1997;5(6): 293–302.

14. Paluska SA. An overview of hip injuries in running. *Sports Med*. 2005;35(11):991–1014.

15. Mountjoy M, Sundgot-Borgen JK, Burke LM, et al. IOC consensus statement on relative energy deficiency in sport (RED-S): 2018 update. *Br J Sports Med*. 2018;52: 687–697.

16. Ravaldi C, Vannacci A, Zucchi T, et al. Eating disorders and body image disturbances among ballet dancers, gymnasium users and body builders. *Psychopathology*. 2003; 36(5):247–254.

17. Dotti A, Fioravanti M, Balotta M, Tozzi F, Cannella C, Lazzari R. Eating behavior of ballet dancers. *Eat Weight Disord*. 2002;7(1):60–67.

18. J1 A, Witcomb GL, Mitchell A. Prevalence of eating disorders amongst dancers: a systemic review and meta-analysis. *Eur Eat Disord Rev*. 2014;22(2):92–101.

19. Drew MK, Finch CF. The relationship between training load and injury, illness and soreness: a systematic and literature review. *Sports Med*. 2016;46(6):861–883.

20. Tibor LM, Sekiya JK. Differential diagnosis of pain around the hip joint. *Arthroscopy*. 2008;24(12): 1407–1421.

21. Fredericson M, Jennings F, Beaulieu C, Matheson GO. Stress fractures in athletes. *Top Magn Reson Imaging*. 2006;17(5):309–325.

22. Greenberg E, Wells L. Hip joint capsule disruption in a young female gymnast. *J Orthop Sports Phys Ther*. 2010; 40(11):761.

23. Mitchell RJ, Gerrie BJ, McCulloch PC, et al. Radiographic evidence of hip microinstability in elite ballet. *Arthroscopy*. 2016;32(6):1038–1044.

24. Philippon MJ. The role of arthroscopic thermal capsulorrhaphy in the hip. *Clin Sports Med*. 2001;20(4): 817–829.

25. Kuhlman GS, Domb BG. Hip impingement: identifying and treating a common cause of hip pain. *Am Fam Physician*. 2009;80(12):1429–1434.

26. Alradwan H, Philippon MJ, Farrokhyar F, et al. Return to preinjury activity levels after surgical management of femoroacetabular impingement in athletes. *Arthroscopy*. 2012;28(10):1567–1576.

27. Charbonnier C, Kolo FC, Duthon VB, et al. Assessment of congruence and impingement of the hip joint in professional ballet dancers: a motion capture study. *Am J Sports Med*. 2011;39(3):557–566.

28. Ganz R, Leunig M, Leunig-Ganz K, Harris WH. The etiology of osteoarthritis of the hip: an integrated mechanical concept. *Clin Orthop Relat Res*. 2008;466(2):264–272.

29. Lequesne M, Bellaiche L. Anterior femoroacetabular impingement: an update. *Joint Bone Spine*. 2012;79(3): 249–255.

30. Keogh MJ, Batt ME. A review of femoroacetabular impingement in athletes. *Sports Med*. 2008;38(10): 863–878.

31. Philippon MJ, Maxwell RB, Johnston TL, Schenker M, Briggs KK. Clinical presentation of femoroacetabular impingement. *Knee Surg Sports Traumatol Arthrosc*. 2007; 15(8):1041–1047.

32. Beck M, Kalhor M, Leunig M, Ganz R. Hip morphology influences the pattern of damage to the acetabular cartilage: femoroacetabular impingement as a cause of early osteoarthritis of the hip. *J Bone Joint Surg Br*. 2005; 87(7):1012–1018.

33. Corten K, Ganz R, Chosa E, Leunig M. Bone apposition of the acetabular rim in deep hips: a distinct finding of global pincer impingement. *J Bone Joint Surg Am*. 2011; 93(suppl 2):10–16.

34. Kolo FC, Charbonnier C, Pfirrmann CW, et al. Extreme hip motion in professional ballet dancers: dynamic and morphological evaluation based on magnetic resonance imaging. *Skelet Radiol*. 2013;42(5):689–698.

35. Duthon VB, Charbonnier C, Kolo FC, et al. Correlation of clinical and magnetic resonance imaging findings in hips of elite female ballet dancers. *Arthroscopy*. 2013;29(3): 411–419.

36. Harris JD, Gerrie BJ, Varner KE, Lintner DM, McCulloch PC. Radiographic prevalence of dysplasia, cam, and pincer deformities in elite ballet. *Am J Sports Med*. 2016;44(1):20–27.

37. Hetsroni I, Dela Torre K, Duke G, Lyman S, Kelly BT. Sex differences of hip morphology in young adults with hip pain and labral tears. *Arthroscopy*. 2013;29(1): 54–63.

38. Hammoud S, Bedi A, Magennis E, Meyers WC, Kelly BT. High incidence of athletic pubalgia symptoms in professional athletes with symptomatic femoroacetabular impingement. *Arthroscopy.* 2012;28(10):1388–1395.
39. Kassarjian A, Brisson M, Palmer WE. Femoroacetabular impingement. *Eur J Radiol.* 2007;63(1):29–35.
40. Laude F, Boyer T, Nogier A. Anterior femoroacetabular impingement. *Joint Bone Spine.* 2007;74(2):127–132.
41. Mason JB. Acetabular labral tears in the athlete. *Clin Sports Med.* 2001;20(4):779–790.
42. McCarthy JC, Noble PC, Schuck MR, Wright J, Lee J. The Otto E. Aufranc Award: the role of labral lesions to development of early degenerative hip disease. *Clin Orthop Relat Res.* 2001;(393):25–37.
43. Sink EL, Gralla J, Ryba A, Dayton M. Clinical presentation of femoroacetabular impingement in adolescents. *J Pediatr Orthop.* 2008;28(8):806–811.
44. Tannast M, Goricki D, Beck M, Murphy SB, Siebenrock KA. Hip damage occurs at the zone of femoroacetabular impingement. *Clin Orthop Relat Res.* 2008;466(2):273–280.
45. Jaberi FM, Parvizi J. Hip pain in young adults: femoroacetabular impingement. *J Arthroplasty.* 2007;22(7 suppl 3):37–42.
46. Bolia I, Utsunomiya H, Locks R, Briggs K, Philippon MJ. Twenty-year systematic review of the hip pathology, risk factors, treatment, and clinical outcomes in artistic athletes-dancers, figure skaters, and gymnasts. *Clin J Sport Med.* 2018;28(1):82–90.
47. Lee YK, Lee GY, Lee JW, Lee E, Kang HS. Intra-articular injections in patients with femoroacetabular impingement: a prospective, randomized, double-blind, cross-over study. *J Korean Med Sci.* 2016;31(11):1822–1827.
48. Dragoo JL, Braun HJ, Kim HJ, Phan HD, Golish SR. The in vitro chondrotoxicity of single-dose local anesthetics. *Am J Sports Med.* 2012;40(4):794–799.
49. Piper SL, Kramer JD, Kim HT, Feeley BT. Effects of local anesthetics on articular cartilage. *Am J Sports Med.* 2011;39(10):2245–2253.
50. Ravnihar K, Barlič A, Drobnič M. Effect of intra-articular local anesthesia on articular cartilage in the knee. *Arthroscopy.* 2014;30(5):607–612.
51. Wernecke C, Braun HJ, Dragoo JL. The effect of intra-articular corticosteroids on articular cartilage: a systematic review. *Orthop J Sports Med.* 2015;3(5):2325967115581163.
52. Patti JW, Ouellette H, Bredella MA, Torriani M. Impingement of lesser trochanter on ischium as a potential cause for hip pain. *Skeletal Radiol.* 2008;37(10):939–941.
53. Stafford GH, Villar RN. Ischiofemoral impingement. *J Bone Joint Surg Br.* 2011;93(10):1300–1302.
54. Torriani M, Souto SC, Thomas BJ, Ouellette H, Bredella MA. Ischiofemoral impingement syndrome: an entity with hip pain and abnormalities of the quadratus femoris muscle. *AJR Am J Roentgenol.* 2009;193(1):186–190.
55. O'Brien SD, Bui-Mansfield LT. MRI of quadratus femoris muscle tear: another cause of hip pain. *AJR Am J Roentgenol.* 2007;189(5):1185–1189.
56. Johnson KA. Impingement of the lesser trochanter on the ischial ramus after total hip arthroplasty. Report of three cases. *J Bone Joint Surg Am.* 1977;59(2):268–269.
57. Hetsroni I, Larson CM, Dela Torre K, Zbeda RM, Magennis E, Kelly BT. Anterior inferior iliac spine deformity as an extra-articular source for hip impingement: a series of 10 patients treated with arthroscopic decompression. *Arthroscopy.* 2012;28(11):1644–1653.
58. Larson CM, Kelly BT, Stone RM. Making a case for anterior inferior iliac spine/subspine hip impingement: three representative case reports and proposed concept. *Arthroscopy.* 2011;27(12):1732–1737.
59. Larson CM, Pierce BR, Giveans MR. Treatment of athletes with symptomatic intra-articular hip pathology and athletic pubalgia/sports hernia: a case series. *Arthroscopy.* 2011;27(6):768–775.
60. Pan H, Kawanabe K, Akiyama H, Goto K, Onishi E, Nakamura T. Operative treatment of hip impingement caused by hypertrophy of the anterior inferior iliac spine. *J Bone Joint Surg Br.* 2008;90(5):677–679.
61. Garrett Jr WE. Muscle strain injuries. *Am J Sports Med.* 1996;24(suppl 6):S2–S8.
62. Armfield DR, Kim DH, Towers JD, Bradley JP, Robertson DD. Sports-related muscle injury in the lower extremity. *Clin Sports Med.* 2006;25(4):803–842.
63. Hsu JC, Fischer DA, Wright RW. Proximal rectus femoris avulsions in national football league kickers: a report of 2 cases. *Am J Sports Med.* 2005;33(7):1085–1087.
64. Gamradt SC, Brophy RH, Barnes R, Warren RF, Thomas Byrd JW, Kelly BT. Nonoperative treatment for proximal avulsion of the rectus femoris in professional American football. *Am J Sports Med.* 2009;37(7):1370–1374.
65. Johnston CA, Wiley JP, Lindsay DM, Wiseman DA. Iliopsoas bursitis and tendinitis. A review. *Sports Med.* 1998;25(4):271–283.
66. Morelli V, Weaver V. Groin injuries and groin pain in athletes: part 1. *Prim Care.* 2005;32(1):163–183.
67. Wahl CJ, Warren RF, Adler RS, Hannafin JA, Hansen B. Internal coxa saltans (snapping hip) as a result of overtraining: a report of 3 cases in professional athletes with a review of causes and the role of ultrasound in early diagnosis and management. *Am J Sports Med.* 2004;32(5):1302–1309.
68. Deslandes M, Guillin R, Cardinal E, Hobden R, Bureau NJ. The snapping iliopsoas tendon: new mechanisms using dynamic sonography. *AJR Am J Roentgenol.* 2008;190(3):576–581.
69. Domb BG, Shindle MK, McArthur B, Voos JE, Magennis EM, Kelly BT. Iliopsoas impingement: a newly identified cause of labral pathology in the hip. *HSS J.* 2011;7(2):145–150.
70. Strauss EJ, Nho SJ, Kelly BT. Greater trochanteric pain syndrome. *Sports Med Arthrosc.* 2010;18(2):113–119.

71. Segal NA, Felson DT, Torner JC, et al. Greater trochanteric pain syndrome: epidemiology and associated factors. *Arch Phys Med Rehabil.* 2007;88(8):988–992.
72. Tortolani PJ, Carbone JJ, Quartararo LG. Greater trochanteric pain syndrome in patients referred to orthopedic spine specialists. *Spine J.* 2002;2(4):251–254.
73. Williams BS, Cohen SP. Greater trochanteric pain syndrome: a review of anatomy, diagnosis and treatment. *Anesth Analg.* 2009;108(5):1662–1670.
74. Bewyer DC, Bewyer KJ. Rationale for treatment of hip abductor pain syndrome. *Iowa Orthop J.* 2003;23:57–60.
75. Finnoff JT, Fowler SP, Lai JK, et al. Treatment of chronic tendinopathy with ultrasound-guided needle tenotomy and platelet-rich plasma injection. *PM R.* 2011;3(10):900–911.
76. Voos JE, Shindle MK, Pruett A, Asnis PD, Kelly BT. Endoscopic repair of gluteus medius tendon tears of the hip. *Am J Sports Med.* 2009;37(4):743–747.
77. Fredericson M, Weir A. Practical management of iliotibial band friction syndrome in runners. *Clin J Sport Med.* 2006;16(3):261–268.
78. Holmes JC, Pruitt AL, Whalen NJ. Iliotibial band syndrome in cyclists. *Am J Sports Med.* 1993;21(3):419–424.
79. Orchard JW, Fricker PA, Abud AT, Mason BR. Biomechanics of iliotibial band friction syndrome in runners. *Am J Sports Med.* 1996;24(3):375–379.
80. Hamill J, Miller R, Noehren B, Davis I. A prospective study of iliotibial band strain in runners. *Clin Biomech (Bristol, Avon).* 2008;23(8):1018–1025.
81. Noehren B, Davis I, Hamill J. ASB clinical biomechanics award winner 2006 prospective study of the biomechanical factors associated with iliotibial band syndrome. *Clin Biomech (Bristol, Avon).* 2007;22(9):951–956.
82. Allen WC, Cope R. Coxa saltans: the snapping hip revisited. *J Am Acad Orthop Surg.* 1995;3(5):303–308.
83. Lewis CL. Extra-articular snapping hip: a literature review. *Sports Health.* 2010;2(3):186–190.
84. Ali K, Leland JM. Hamstring strains and tears in the athlete. *Clin Sports Med.* 2012;31(2):263–272.
85. Clanton TO, Coupe KJ. Hamstring strains in athletes: diagnosis and treatment. *J Am Acad Orthop Surg.* 1998;6(4):237–248.
86. Linklater JM, Hamilton B, Carmichael J, Orchard J, Wood DG. Hamstring injuries: anatomy, imaging, and intervention. *Semin Musculoskelet Radiol.* 2010;14(2):131–161.
87. Heiderscheit BC, Sherry MA, Silder A, Chumanov ES, Thelen DG. Hamstring strain injuries: recommendations for diagnosis, rehabilitation, and injury prevention. *J Orthop Sports Phys Ther.* 2010;40(2):67–81.
88. Petersen J, Thorborg K, Nielsen MB, Budtz-Jorgensen E, Holmich P. Preventive effect of eccentric training on acute hamstring injuries in men's soccer: a cluster-randomized controlled trial. *Am J Sports Med.* 2011;39(11):2296–2303.
89. Reurink G, Goudswaard GJ, Tol JL, Verhaar JA, Weir A, Moen MH. Therapeutic interventions for acute hamstring injuries: a systematic review. *Br J Sports Med.* 2012;46(2):103–109.
90. Askling CM, Tengvar M, Saartok T, Thorstensson A. Acute first-time hamstring strains during high-speed running: a longitudinal study including clinical and magnetic resonance imaging findings. *Am J Sports Med.* 2007;35(2):197–206.
91. McSweeney SE, Naraghi A, Salonen D, Theodoropoulos J, White LM. Hip and groin pain in the professional athlete. *Can Assoc Radiol J.* 2012;63(2):87–99.
92. Opar DA, Williams MD, Shield AJ. Hamstring strain injuries: factors that lead to injury and re-injury. *Sports Med.* 2012;42(3):209–226.
93. Anderson K, Strickland SM, Warren R. Hip and groin injuries in athletes. *Am J Sports Med.* 2001;29(4):521–533.
94. Hoeber S, Aly AR, Ashworth N, Rajasekaran S. Ultrasound-guided hip joint injections are more accurate than landmark-guided injections: a systematic review and meta-analysis. *Br J Sports Med.* 2016;50(7):392–396.
95. Davenport KL, Campos JS, Nguyen J, Saboeiro G, Adler RS, Moley PJ. Ultrasound-guided intratendinous injections with platelet-rich plasma or autologous whole blood for treatment of proximal hamstring tendinopathy: a double-blind randomized controlled trial. *J Ultrasound Med.* 2015;34(8):1455–1463.
96. Cohen S, Bradley J. Acute proximal hamstring rupture. *J Am Acad Orthop Surg.* 2007;15(6):350–355.
97. Cohen SB, Rangavajjula A, Vyas D, Bradley JP. Functional results and outcomes after repair of proximal hamstring avulsions. *Am J Sports Med.* 2012;40(9):2092–2098.
98. Folsom GJ, Larson CM. Surgical treatment of acute versus chronic complete proximal hamstring ruptures: results of a new allograft technique for chronic reconstructions. *Am J Sports Med.* 2008;36(1):104–109.
99. Nicholas SJ, Tyler TF. Adductor muscle strains in sport. *Sports Med.* 2002;32(5):339–344.
100. Grote K, Lincoln TL, Gamble JG. Hip adductor injury in competitive swimmers. *Am J Sports Med.* 2004;32(1):104–108.
101. Morelli V, Smith V. Groin injuries in athletes. *Am Fam Physician.* 2001;64(8):1405–1414.
102. Prather H, Cheng A. Diagnosis and treatment of hip girdle pain in the athlete. *PM R.* 2016;8(suppl 3):S45–S60.
103. Trofa DP, Mayeux SE, Parisien RL, Ahmad CS, Lynch TS. Mastering the physical examination of the athlete's hip. *Am J Orthop.* 2017;46(1):10–16.
104. Ekstrand J, Hägglund M, Waldén M. Epidemiology of muscle injuries in professional football (soccer). *Am J Sports Med.* 2011;39(6):1226–1232.
105. Hiti CJ, Stevens KJ, Jamati MK, Garza D, Matheson GO. Athletic osteitis pubis. *Sports Med.* 2011;41(5):361–376.

106. Choi H, McCartney M, Best TM. Treatment of osteitis pubis and osteomyelitis of the pubic symphysis in athletes: a systematic review. *Br J Sports Med.* 2011;45(1):57–64.
107. Angoules AG. Osteitis pubis in elite athletes: diagnostic and therapeutic approach. *World J Orthop.* 2015;6(9):672–679.
108. Beatty T. Osteitis pubis in athletes. *Curr Sports Med Rep.* 2012;11(2):96–98.
109. Mehin R, Meek R, O'Brien P, Blachut P. Surgery for osteitis pubis. *Can J Surg.* 2006;49(3):170–176.
110. Byrne CA, Bowden DJ, Alkhayat A, Kavanagh EC, Eustace SJ. Sports-related groin pain secondary to symphysis pubis disorders: correlation between MRI findings and outcome after fluoroscopy-guided injection of steroid and local anesthetic. *Am J Roentgenol.* 2017;209(2):380–388.
111. Kajetanek C, Benoît O, Granger B, et al. Athletic pubalgia: return to play after targeted surgery. *Orthop Traumatol Surg Res.* 2018;104(4):469–472.
112. Meyers WC, McKechnie A, Philippon MJ, Horner MA, Zoga AC, Devon ON. Experience with "sports hernia" spanning two decades. *Ann Surg.* 2008;248(4):656–665.
113. Farber AJ, Wilckens JH. Sports hernia: diagnosis and therapeutic approach. *J Am Acad Orthop Surg.* 2007;15(8):507–514.
114. Litwin DE, Sneider EB, McEnaney PM, Busconi BD. Athletic pubalgia (sports hernia). *Clin Sports Med.* 2011;30(2):417–434.
115. Swan Jr KG, Wolcott M. The athletic hernia: a systematic review. *Clin Orthop Relat Res.* 2007;455:78–87.
116. Caudill P, Nyland J, Smith C, Yerasimides J, Lach J. Sports hernias: a systematic literature review. *Br J Sports Med.* 2008;42(12):954–964.
117. Zoga AC, Kavanagh EC, Omar IM, et al. Athletic pubalgia and the "sports hernia": MR imaging findings. *Radiology.* 2008;247(3):797–807.
118. Knapik DM, Gebhart JJ, Nho SJ, Tanenbaum JE, Voos JE, Salata MJ. Prevalence of surgical repair for athletic pubalgia and impact on performance in football athletes participating in the national football league combine. *Arthroscopy.* 2017;33(5):1044–1049.
119. Jack RA, Evans DC, Echo A, et al. Performance and return to sport after sports hernia surgery in NFL players. *Orthop J Sports Med.* 2017;5(4):2325967117699590.

## CHAPTER 10

# Management of the Dancer's Spine

MATTHEW GRIERSON, MD

## INTRODUCTION

The aesthetics of dance culture, obvious in performance and reinforced throughout popular media, emphasizes perfection as the dancer moves her body through space. The legs must be high, the hips maximally turned out, and the spine must bend in every direction. There is a palpable influence on the young dancer struggling to emulate the seasoned professional. Clinicians must learn to pick up on subtle clues that provide insight into how this culture affects a dancer's identity. Something as fundamental as a dancer's relationship to "turn out" can have significant biomechanical consequences for other areas of the body, including the spine.

Lumbar injuries are common, both in dancers and the general population, and these injuries often resolve before a definitive diagnosis is achieved or interventional options are necessary. Understanding that the natural history of most causes of low back pain is benign, the real clinical value from an evaluation for this issue may come more directly from work helping the dancer to develop lifelong strategies for healthy movement. Simple gestures, such as installing a ballet barre in a clinic room or taking an interest in the dancer's choreography, can go a long way in helping to build trust within the dancer–clinician relationship (see Fig. 10.1). Dancers seek both an accurate diagnosis and realistic treatment plan,[1] but if the assessment space feels less clinical, they may feel more comfortable sharing subtle details that could influence clinical decision-making and help reduce the risk for future injury.

## EPIDEMIOLOGY FOR LOW BACK PAIN

The spine ranks second among the most prominent areas of dance injury and is implicated in about 30% of injuries.[2–4] Dancers perform repetitive extensions, high velocity twisting, and bending movements, all of which require sophisticated levels of motor control at the end ranges of motion.[5] It is therefore not surprising when studies have found that more than 70% of professional dancers and 63% of preprofessional dancers report experiencing low back pain within the preceding 12 months.[5,6]

There is rarely one single factor that predisposes a dancer to injury. However, clinicians commonly find evidence of repeated overload, impaired biomechanics, or improper technique.[5,7–13] One theory is that dancers develop impaired lumbopelvic motor control in the setting of multiple injuries, degenerative changes, or repetitive end-range motions, leading to compensation patterns that predispose to further tissue stress.[14] Dancer hypermobility has also been implicated, although more recent studies suggest that the quality of movement, rather than the quantity of hypermobility, may be the more important issue.[5] Impairments in core strength have also been implicated, but there is not yet a simple or straightforward way to screen for this in dancers in a way that predicts injury.[15]

## HISTORY AND EXAMINATION

The history and physical examination not only assists in narrowing the differential when diagnosing spinal injuries, but more importantly gives the clinician an opportunity to identify risk factors for injury or other issues that may impact a dancer's career. Experienced clinicians instinctively reference common patterns of injury, such as whether a particular concern is exacerbated by flexion- or extension-based movements or whether the injury is present in an adolescent dancer or dancer toward the end of her career.

The standard orthopedic examination consists of inspection, palpation, range of motion assessment, and special testing, but dancer-specific functional testing is also important to identify subtle muscular imbalances and help establish trust between dancer and clinician.

### Inspection/Posture

Postural deviations are often implicated when a dancer presents with pain, with concern that changes in alignment could lead to increased injury risk.[16–18] Evaluation

Performing Arts Medicine. https://doi.org/10.1016/B978-0-323-58182-0.00010-9

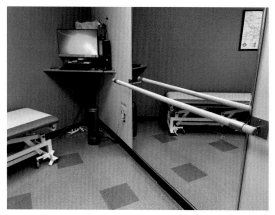

FIG. 10.1 Example of a dancer-centered clinic room, with ballet barre and mirror.

of the dancer in multiple planes is important, but one of the most common analyses involves assessing for lumbar lordosis, as anterior pelvic tilt and lumbar hyperlordosis are very common in dancers. To obtain extreme external rotation of the hip, some dancers will compensate by rolling in at the foot (pronating), which sends forces up the leg that can lead to exaggerated forward tilting of the pelvis. Hyperlordosis may also be a sign of weak abdominals. Head position, shoulder height, scapular symmetry, scoliotic curves, muscular bulk, and pelvic obliquity should all be assessed, preferably with the dancer dressed in attire where the clinician can easily visualize the scapula and spine.

## Palpation

This part of the examination usually begins with the patient standing as the examiner palpates the top of the iliac crest for symmetry. Palpation of the spinous processes can identify a step-off, which may indicate a spondylolisthesis. Attention is turned to any tender areas, including a survey of the paraspinal muscles, to determine if there are any tender or trigger points and whether muscle spasms are present. Depending on the patient's symptoms, it can also be helpful to palpate the Posterior Superior Iliac Spine (PSIS), ischial tuberosity, piriformis and gluteal musculature, and greater trochanter to identify areas of tenderness that may help narrow the differential.

## ROM

During range of motion assessments of the lumbar spine, identifying a "direction preference" can be helpful if there is pain. As the dancer bends forward and returns to neutral, an asymmetric spine may indicate a mild scoliosis that was more elusive during postural

assessment. There is no "gold standard" for assessing lumbar range of motion in the general population,[19] much less in dancers, and thus is an opportunity for the clinician to qualitatively assess the motion and identify asymmetry or compensation patterns that may be relevant to the presenting injury.

## Special Testing

Special testing for individual diagnoses are discussed later in this chapter. Generalized joint hypermobility can be assessed using the Beighton criteria.[20] There are nine points possible, with one point given for each side if the dancer can passively bend her thumb forward to touch the volar forearm, extend her short finger greater than 90°, hyperextend her elbow beyond 10°, or hyperextend her knee beyond 10°. One final point is given if the dancer is able to place the palm of her hand flat on the floor with the legs straight, something most trained dancers can easily perform without difficulty.

Dancers can be considered as being "tight" (0−3), "hypermobile" (4−6), or "extremely hypermobile" (7−9).[21] It is beyond the scope of this chapter to discuss hypermobility in detail, but about 20%−60% of professional dancers are considered hypermobile,[22,23] which is not a modifiable condition, but may have implications for rehabilitation or risk of injury. There is concern that this could lead to instability at the end range of motion and subsequent cumulative microtrauma could lead to impaired proprioception and motor control.[5] Studies of dancers with joint hyperlaxity have demonstrated lower muscle strength, lower submaximal energy capacity, and decreased functional walking distance.[24] Fortunately, they have also shown that enhancing physical fitness and strength can be beneficial in regards to enhancing dancers' functional ability and motor competence.

## Functional

There are several functional measures of core strength that are easy to perform in clinic, including the knee lift abdominal test (KLAT) and the bent knee fall out (BKFO). The KLAT is performed from a resting position supine with both knees bent and feet flat on the table. The dancer is asked to lift one foot off the table to 90° and is evaluated by their ability to maintain a stable spine and neutral pelvis. The BKFO is also performed with the dancer lying supine on a table, but this time one leg is resting flat on the table and the other resting with the knee bent and foot flat on the table. The dancer is observed as their leg is lowered laterally to approximately 45° of abduction/external rotation and then returned to the starting position. The dancer is again observed to see how well they maintain good trunk stabilization. This can be performed subjectively by placing a hand under the small of a dancer's back or more objectively (typically in studies) using a pressure biofeedback unit inflated behind the dancer's spine.

Depending on the dancer's preferred movement style, it can also be helpful to evaluate basic dance motions, paying careful attention to alignment of the spine. If the dancer is able to reproduce the type of movement that aggravates her typical pain (or show a video), this can also be helpful. For ballet and modern dancers, it is useful to observe demi plié in both parallel and first position, observing how successful the dancer is at maintaining optimal alignment with a neutral pelvis and without significant genu valgus or foot pronation. For more advanced dancers, the "airplane test" is also a very good test of lumbopelvic alignment and stability.[25] In this test, the dancer is instructed to stand in parallel position and extend one leg back, keeping the other leg straight. The trunk is pitched forward, keeping the pelvis square to the ground. The dancer performs five controlled plies while bringing the arms forward to touch the ground five times.

## CLINICAL DIAGNOSES AND SYNDROMES
### Muscle Strain/Spasm

Treatment of muscular low back pain in dancers is similar to other athletes and has not changed drastically over the last several decades.[12,26] A paper documenting injuries among the 1976 Canadian Olympic team described a "five-point attack" for treating muscular low back pain, which included achieving pain relief, stretching tight muscles (when appropriate), strengthening areas of relative imbalance, optimizing training habits, and offering education on how to prevent recurrence.[27]

Although muscle strains and muscle spasms are considered a benign category of injury, representing little permanent tissue damage, the pain can be significant, symptoms can last 4–6 weeks, and can recur throughout a dancer's career.[4] This may lead to anxiety, fear of movement, and subsequent dysfunctional movement compensation patterns. Muscle strains in the low back are a diagnosis of exclusion in adolescent dancers, where there is a higher concern for stress injury to the spine.

On examination, the clinician will find taut, rope-like bands of tissue localized to the lumbar paraspinals and quadratus lumborum. Depending on the extent of the injury, the cervical, thoracic, gluteal, and periscapular musculature may be involved as well. Palpation of the "myofascial trigger points" can refer pain in predictable patterns. The pain may respond acutely to oral analgesia (limited use of Non-steroidal anti-inflammatory drugs (NSAIDs) or "muscle relaxants"), stretching, and manual therapies. For refractory cases, trigger point injections (with local anesthetic or normal saline) or "dry needling" can also be considered, but dance medicine clinicians typically exercise caution when providing interventional treatment within days of an important rehearsal or performance. Longer-term benefit is often achieved through physiotherapy and dance technique assessments to correct biomechanical factors that predisposed to the initial muscular stress.

### Scoliosis

Scoliosis is a spinal deformity, most commonly idiopathic, resulting in a lateral and rotatory curve to the spine. Curves, especially those less than 20°, produce few symptoms or complaints, and fewer than 0.25% of cases in the general population require specific treatment.[28] Thus, dancers do not typically present to the clinic naming "scoliosis" as their primary concern. It is more often detected during examination for a musculoskeletal complaint or as an incidental finding during a preseason assessment. Adolescents with mild scoliosis can be monitored for progression until skeletal maturity, bracing (or even less common surgery) is reserved for higher risk curves. In general, physical therapy and other rehabilitative approaches are emphasized to address any underlying musculoskeletal stresses.

### Spondylolysis

Spondylolysis is a fatigue or stress injury to the pars interarticularis in the posterior spine, an area of relative weakness during spinal maturity. It should be considered high on the differential diagnosis any time an adolescent dancer presents with low back pain. The mechanism of injury involves repeated extension and rotational stresses on the spine, found in many common dance positions such as a cambré or an arabesque derrière. Examination findings have low specificity, including lumbar hyperlordosis, paraspinal muscle spasms, pain during extension, and tenderness to palpation throughout the lumbar spine.[29,30] The single leg hyperextension test, where the dancer leans backward while standing on one leg, is often used in clinical evaluations, but little association has been found between this test and the presence of a confirmed stress fracture on imaging.[31]

A definitive diagnosis can only be made with appropriate imaging. To limit radiation exposure, initial radiographs can be limited to AP and lateral views.

Oblique or "coned down" views at the lumbosacral junction do not appear to confer any additional diagnostic benefit.[32] Due to concerns about radiation exposure with the more sensitive bone scan with Single Photon Emission Computed Tomography (SPECT), many clinicians rely on magnetic resonance imaging (MRI) to achieve the diagnosis. However, not all bony defects are visible on MRI, and one must exercise caution when interpreting the results of a normal MRI in a dancer at high risk of spondylolysis. The sensitivity of standard 1.5T MRI sequences has been estimated at 80%,[31] and greatly depends on image slice thickness, spacing, and orientation (see Fig. 10.2). Stronger 3T MRIs may one day prove to be as sensitive as SPECT with CT, but they have not been studied thoroughly and are not yet standard in all practice settings. If using an MRI, specific protocols to evaluate for this diagnosis should be used.

The primary focus of treatment for spondylolysis involves rest and rehabilitation, with the clinician tailoring treatment to the goals of the dancer. Athletes who rest from their sport for at least 12 weeks have

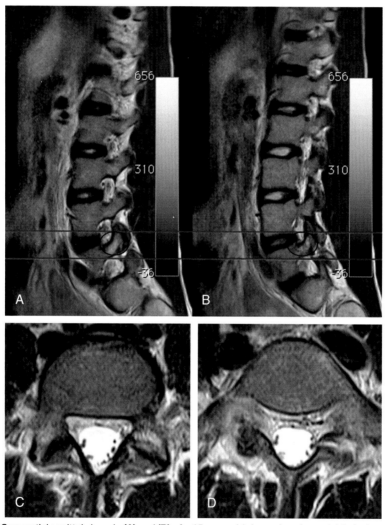

FIG. 10.2 Sequential sagittal views in **(A)** and **(B)** of a 15-year-old dancer's spine notable for increased signal in the pars interarticularis (black circle). Red lines correspond the levels taken for cross-sectional views (axial) on MRI. Axial views in **(C)** and **(D)** were normal due to the type of sequence used for MRI (which did not take a detailed look at the pars in this view).

been shown to be 16.4 times more likely to have a favorable clinical outcome compared to those who return early.[33] However, a dancer with a terminal (or complete) fracture through the pars would not be expected to ever achieve bony union, regardless of time spent resting, and may not require as much time away from dance. Fortunately, they tend to do well clinically even with nonunion. The decision on whether or not to prescribe a brace is based to some extent on where a physician has trained and other regional preferences. In communities where bracing is not common, the treating physician must weigh the social stigma of wearing the brace with the benefits of treatment. So far, no study has definitively demonstrated a greater benefit of bracing over simple activity restriction. Studies investigating different bracing protocols have shown similar long-term outcomes even when athletes admit to not consistently using their brace.[33–37]

### Facetogenic Pain

The lumbar zygapophysial joints (or "facet" joints) are paired synovial joints that are formed between the superior and inferior articular processes of each vertebra.[38] The facets are not a common pain generator in young dancers, but dancers may experience pain at these joints as they advance in their career. It can occur either in the setting of normal "wear and tear" of the joints, or possibly from a traumatic event, such as a fall.

Typically, the pain is more prominent during extension-based activities, but physical examination alone is often insufficient at establishing a definitive diagnosis. In the nondancer population, the gold-standard for diagnosing facet pain involves numbing the affected joint with local anesthetic on two separate occasions (using an anesthetic with two different lengths of action). The patient completes a pain diary, and if greater than 80% of the pain is relived while the numbing medication is in effect, then more lasting therapeutic options are considered.

One treatment to consider is an intraarticular injection with a steroid, but this has not necessarily been shown to provide better symptom control than placebo.[39] Radiofrequency ablation, or cauterization of the nerves to the painful joint, is well tolerated for facet-mediated pain in the nondancer population, but the nerves to the multifidi are denervated in the process. The resulting weakness, which would be more subtle in a nondancer, in conjunction with loss of proprioception from the denervated joint may have implications for the dancer's performance. Even subtle changes in sensory feedback from the joint or associated strength deficits in the deep muscles of the spine may have a big effect on performance. Regenerative medicine

techniques including prolotherapy or injection of platelet rich plasma (PRP) to stimulate the body's natural ability to heal are currently on the cutting edge of clinical research, and we may have more information about their clinical utility in the years ahead.

### Discogenic Pain

As dancers age, they would be expected to experience conditions also common in the general population. The outer ring of the spinal discs are highly innervated, and occasionally a dancer may develop a fissure between the circumferential layers of the annulus fibrosis. Typically, this is treated similarly to other causes of lumbar pain, and does not generally require or respond well to interventional treatment strategies.[40] For severe discogenic pain, lumbar epidural steroid injections are sometimes considered, but they are typically more effective when there is a pinched nerve from a herniated disc and leg pain is present.

### Sacroiliac Joint

The sacroiliac joint helps distribute forces from the trunk to the pelvis and lower extremities. Biomechanical stresses can be transmitted from the lumbar spine, and pain can be the result of either excessive or reduced motion at the joint. Pain is often localized to the low back and gluteal region, and a dancer may point within 1 cm inferomedial to the PSIS (a "positive" Fortin finger test).[41,42] Sacroiliac joint mediated pain is typically assessed using a cluster of examination maneuvers, as no one test has sufficient sensitivity/specificity for Sacroiliac (SI) joint dysfunction. These examination maneuvers include the Fortin finger test, posterior pelvic pain provocation test (P4), Patrick or Flexion, Abduction, External Rotation (FABER) test, Gaenslen Test, compression test, and distraction test (or gapping).[43]

In addition to the standard rehabilitative considerations of optimizing technique and biomechanics through the spine and pelvis, many physical therapists utilize manual techniques, and can teach dancers how to perform these techniques at home to reduce pain. Some sacroiliac joint belts can also provide support during a difficult pain episode and, depending on the choreography, may provide a low enough profile to be tolerated during rehearsal or performance. For refractory cases, cortisone injections can be considered to reduce tissue sensitivity while working on more long-term plans from a rehabilitation perspective. Prolotherapy, where an irritating dextrose solution is injected to reduce ligament laxity, has been recommended by some reports, but the quality of evidence so far is poor and further study is needed.[44]

## Piriformis Syndrome

Piriformis syndrome is often considered a diagnosis of exclusion, as the presentation is similar to the more common syndrome that occurs when there is a pinched nerve from a herniated disc, with pain that starts in the gluteal area and radiates down the leg.[45] The sciatic-like pain is explained considering that the proximal sciatic nerve can be compressed by anatomic variations of the piriformis or muscle hypertonicity exaggerated by hip and leg maneuvers.[46] For patients with refractory symptoms despite work with a physical therapist and an unremarkable lumbar MRI, an ultrasound-guided diagnostic injection into the piriformis can help confirm the diagnosis. The injection may also provide some therapeutic benefit by reducing tone in the muscle and thus facilitating participation in therapy. In some cases, botulinum toxin injections can be considered, although again one must exercise caution when performing this type of treatment, as dancers may be more sensitive to the effects of muscle denervation than other patients.[47]

## CONCLUSION

Although in this chapter we have only highlighted the most common causes of low back problems in dancers, as with any person, it is important to keep a broad differential diagnosis, especially if someone is not improving at the rate expected. Helping the dancer cultivate a strong rehabilitation team is important, particularly to facilitate long-term strategies to reduce risk of future injury. Dancers do recognize the time and effort it takes to carefully evaluate an injury and develop a plan for recovery. They appreciate knowing more about their anatomy and generally take a very active role in rehabilitative treatment. Getting to understand them as artists and helping them return to performance can be very rewarding, especially after prolonged periods away from dance.

## REFERENCES

1. Air ME, Grierson MJ, Davenport KL, Krabak BJ. Dissecting the doctor-dancer relationship: health care decision making among American collegiate dancers. PM R. 2014; 6(3):241–249.
2. Bowling A. Injuries to dancers: prevalence, treatment, and perceptions of causes. BMJ. 1989;298(6675):731–734.
3. Garrick JG, Requa RK. Ballet injuries. An analysis of epidemiology and financial outcome. Am J Sports Med. 1993; 21(4):586–590.
4. Gottschlich LM, Young CC. Spine injuries in dancers. Curr Sports Med Rep. 2011;10(1):40–44.
5. Roussel NA, Nijs J, Mottram S, Van Moorsel A, Truijen S, Stassijns G. Altered lumbopelvic movement control but not generalized joint hypermobility is associated with increased injury in dancers. A prospective study. Man Ther. 2009;14(6):630–635.
6. Ramel E, Moritz U. Self-reported musculoskeletal pain and discomfort in professional ballet dancers in Sweden. Scand J Rehabil Med. 1994;26(1):11–16.
7. Bachrach RM. Team physician #3. The relationship of low back/pelvic somatic dysfunctions to dance injuries. Orthop Rev. 1988;17(10):1037–1043.
8. (a) Bryan N, Smith B. The ballet dancer. Occup Med. 1992; 7(1):67–75.
   (b) Coplan J. Ballet dancer's turnout and its relationship to self-reported injury. J Orthop Sports Phys Ther. 200232(11): 579–584.
9. Gamboa JM, Roberts LA, Maring J, Fergus A. Injury patterns in elite pre-professional ballet dancers and the utility of screening programs to identify risk characteristics. J Orthop Sports Phys Ther. 2008;38(3):126–136.
10. Hincapié CA, Morton EJ, Cassidy JD. Musculoskeletal injuries and pain in dancers: a systematic review. Arch Phys Med Rehabil. 2008;89:1819–1829.
11. Kelman B. Occupational hazards in female ballet dancers, advocate for a forgotten population. AAOHN J. 2000; 48(9):430–434.
12. Khan K, Brown J, Way S, et al. Overuse injuries in classical ballet. Sports Med. 1995;19(5):341–357.
13. Shah S. Caring for the dancer: special considerations for the performer and troupe. Curr Sports Med Rep. 2008; 7(3):128–132.
14. Roussel N, De Kooning M, Schutt A, et al. Motor control and low back pain in dancers. Int J Sports Med. 2013; 34(2):138–143.
15. Davenport KL, Air M, Grierson MJ, Krabak BJ. Examination of Static and Dynamic core strength and rates of reported dance related injury in collegiate dancers: a cross-Sectional study. J Dance Med Sci. 2016;20(4):151–161.
16. O'Sullivan PB, Mitchell T, Bulich P, et al. The relationship between posture and back muscle endurance in industrial workers with flexion-related low back pain. Man Ther. 2006;11(4):264–271.
17. Riegger-Krugh C, Keysor JJ. Skeletal malalignments of the lower quarter: correlated and compensatory motions and postures. J Orthop Sports Phys Ther. 1996;23(2):164–170.
18. Cowan DN, Jones BH, Frykman PN, et al. Lower limb morphology and risk of overuse injury among male infantry trainees. Med Sci Sports Exerc. 1996;28(8):945–952.
19. Solomon J, Nadler SF, Press J. Physical examination of the lumbar spine. In: Malanga GA, Nadler SF, eds. Musculoskeletal Physical Examination: An Evidence-based Approach. 1st ed. Philadelphia, PA: Elsevier Mosby; 2006.
20. Beighton P, Grahame R, Bird H. Hypermobility of Joints. London: Springer Verlag; 1999.
21. Stewart DR, Burden SB. Does generalised ligamentous laxity increase seasonal incidence of injuries in male first division club rugby players? Br J Sports Med. 2004;38(4): 457–460.

22. Moser BR. Hip pain in dancers. *Curr Sports Med Rep.* 2014; 13(6):383−389.

23. Hamilton WG, Hamilton LH, Marshall P, Molnar M. A profile of the musculoskeletal characteristics of elite professional ballet dancers. *Am J Sports Med.* 1992;20(3): 267−273.

24. McCormack M, Briggs J, Hakim A, Grahame R. Joint laxity and the benign joint hypermobility syndrome in student and professional ballet dancers. *J Rheumatol.* 2004;31(1): 173−178.

25. Richardson M, Liederbach M, Sandow E. Functional criteria for assessing pointe-readiness. *J Dance Med Sci.* 2010;14(3):82−88.

26. Baker RJ, Patel D. Lower back pain in the athlete: common conditions and treatment. *Prim Care.* 2005;32(1): 201−229.

27. Smith CF. Physical management of muscular low back pain in the athlete. *Can Med Assoc J.* 1977;117(6): 632−635.

28. Asher MA, Burton DC. Adolescent idiopathic scoliosis: natural history and long term treatment effects. *Scoliosis.* 2006; 1(1):2.

29. McCleary MD, Congeni JA. Current concepts in the diagnosis and treatment of spondylolysis in young athletes. *Curr Sports Med Rep.* 2007;6(1):62−66.

30. Anderson S. Assessment and management of the pediatric and adolescent patient with low back pain. *Phys Med Rehabil Clin North Am.* 1991;2:157−185.

31. Masci L, Pike J, Malara F, Phillips B, Bennell K, Brukner P. Use of the one-legged hyperextension test and magnetic resonance imaging in the diagnosis of active spondylolysis. *Br J Sports Med.* 2006;40(11):940−946.

32. Beck NA, Miller R, Baldwin K, et al. Do oblique views add value in the diagnosis of spondylolysis in adolescents? *J Bone Joint Surg Am.* 2013;95(10):e65.

33. El Rassi G, Takemitsu M, Glutting J, Shah SA. Effect of sports modification on clinical outcome in children and adolescent athletes with symptomatic lumbar spondylolysis. *Am J Phys Med Rehabil.* 2013;92(12): 1070−1074.

34. Fujii K, Katoh S, Sairyo K, Ikata T, Yasui N. Union of defects in the pars interarticularis of the lumbar spine in children and adolescents: the radiological outcome after conservative treatment. *J Bone Joint Surg Br.* 2004;86(2): 225−231.

35. Steiner M, Micheli LJ. Treatment of symptomatic spondylolysis and spondylolisthesis with the modified Boston brace. *Spine (Phila Pa 1976).* 1985;10(10):937−943.

36. Standaert C, Herring S. Expert opinion and controversies in sports and musculoskeletal medicine: the diagnosis and treatment of spondylolysis in adolescent athletes. *Arch Phys Med Rehabil.* 2007;88(4):537−540.

37. Ruiz-Cotorro A, Balius-Matas R, Estruch-Massana A, Vilaró Angulo J. Spondylolysis in young tennis 1042 players. *Br J Sports Med.* 2006;40(5):441−446.

38. Bogduk N. A narrative review of intra-articular corticosteroid injections for low back pain. *Pain Med.* 2005;6(4): 287−296.

39. Bogduk N. Evidence-informed management of chronic back pain with facet injections and radiofrequency neurotomy. *Spine J.* 2008;8(1):56−64.

40. Simon J, McAuliffe M, Shamim F, et al. Discogenic low back pain. *Phys Med Rehabil Clin N Am.* 2014;25(2): 305−317.

41. DeMann LE. Sacroiliac dysfunction in dancers with low back pain. *Man Ther.* 1997;2(1):2−10.

42. Fortin JD, Falco FJ. The Fortin Finger Test: an indicator of sacroiliac pain. *Am J Orthop (Belle Mead NJ).* 1997;24(7): 477−480.

43. Robinson HS, Brox JI, Robinson R, Bjelland E, Solem S, Telje T. The reliability of selected motion- and pain provocation tests for the sacroiliac joint. *Man Ther.* 2007;12: 72−79.

44. Dagenais S, Haldeman S, Wooley JR. Intraligamentous injection of sclerosing solutions (prolotherapy) for spinal pain: a critical review of the literature. *Spine J.* 2005;5(3): 310−328.

45. Kirschner J, Foye P, Cole J. Piriformis syndrome, diagnosis and treatment. *Muscle Nerve.* 2009;40(1):10−18.

46. Foster MR. Piriformis syndrome. *Orthopedics.* 2002;25(8): 821−825.

47. Santamato A, Micello MF, Valeno G, et al. Ultrasound-guided injection of botulinum toxin type a for piriformis muscle syndrome: a case report and review of the literature. *Toxins (Basel).* 2015;7(8):3045−3056.

## CHAPTER 11

# Unique Considerations in the Child and Adolescent Dancer

MARINA GEARHART, BA • AMY X. YIN, MD • ANDREA STRACCIOLINI, MD, FAAP, FACSM

## INTRODUCTION

The adolescent years are met with the *perfect storm* for injury to young dancers. It is a time when the demands of dance become more challenging physically and technically, coincident with periods of rapid physical and biomechanical changes to the body as growth progress and puberty ensues. All too often the result is injury, time loss from dance, and adverse health outcomes. Moreover, caring for the child and adolescent dancer presents many unique challenges to dance teachers, parents, and healthcare practitioners. Specifically, during the adolescent years, young dancers are required to navigate through different psychosocial aspects of growth, development, and puberty. Maintaining a healthy balance is important, and includes managing sleep requirements and adequate nutrition patterns as well as participating in multimodal exercise and cross training. Minimizing unhealthy habits during these formative years for the young dancer requires attention to sedentary behaviors and screen time, and use of dietary supplements and tobacco use.

This chapter highlights some of the special considerations for healthcare professionals, teachers, and parents caring for, and training, youth dancers. Specifically, injury risk factors including growth and development, overuse and technical issues, and early specialization are discussed. Unique issues pertaining to adolescent dancer health are highlighted including nutrition and energy balance, sleep and sedentary behaviors, smoking, and concussion.

### Epidemiology

Millions of children and adolescents participate in dance. A survey conducted between 2003 and 2006 by O'Neill et al. noted that dance participation had a 20% prevalence in US adolescents, specifically 34.8% of girls and 8.4% of boys.[1] Unfortunately, dance injuries seem to disproportionally affect young and adolescent dancers compared with adult dancers. Preprofessional dancers 9−18 years old report higher rates of injury (0.77−4.71/1000 dance hours)[2−5] than both adult professional ballet and modern dancers (0.51−4.4/1000 dance hours).[6−9] 42.1%−77% of preprofessional ballet students aged 9−20 years report an injury at least once during their training.[3−5] In addition, recreational adolescent dancers are also affected by high rates of injury. A 2012 study of 1336 nonprofessional female dancers 8−16 years old reported a dance injury rate of 42.6%.[10]

Injury epidemiology research in youth dancers is scarce. The majority of injuries in the young dancer are in the lower extremity, 53% being of the foot/ankle, 21.6% being in the hip, 16.1% being in the knee, and 9.4% being in the back.[4] Yin et al., in a retrospective review of dance injuries presenting to a pediatric sports/dance medicine clinic, found that the most common injuries to the young dancers aged 5−17 years were tendonitis/tendinopathy, patellofemoral pain syndrome, apophysitis, ankle impingement syndrome, and hip labral tear; the majority of the injuries occurred in the lower extremities, with knee and ankle injuries being the most common.[11] With such prevalence of dance participation and significant rates of injury in the young dancer, understanding population specific risk factors and health issues is critical.

### Risk Factors for Adolescent Dancers

Injuries are common in the dance world, and some clear intrinsic and extrinsic risk factors have been previously reported in the literature. Risk factors that may be involved in a given injury include training errors, musculotendinous imbalance, anatomic malalignment of the lower extremity, shoe wear, and floor surface.[12] Steinberg et al., in a study of 1336 nonprofessional female dancers, found that 43% of the study cohort were injured and, precursors to injury included range of motion, anatomical anomalies, technique, and dance discipline.[10] For the pediatric and young dancer specifically, growth,[13,14] overuse,[15,16] technique errors,[15,16] and early specialization[17] may all play a large role in injury risk. Furthermore, among the dancer population, it is quite common for dancers to delay seeking medical attention for injuries until they completely lose function,[16] placing them at further risk of adverse consequences.

### Growth

The child and adolescent dancer is in a vital growth period. Although peak growth occurs generally around 12 years of age for girls and 14 years for boys, biological maturity differs greatly for children of the same age. During the period of rapid growth, injuries can endure and be irreversible through adulthood.[18] Risk factor for injury includes strength and flexibility imbalances that develop during this time. Furthermore, coincident and even preceding this time of growth and development, many dancers start intense training at the age of 6–8 or even younger.[19] Stracciolini et al., in a study investigating injury patterns in young dancers throughout growth, showed that the proportion of injuries to the foot-ankle/lower leg/knee in prepubescent dancers was significantly greater than injuries to the thigh/hip-pelvis/spine/upper extremity; in comparison, the proportion of injuries to the thigh/hip-pelvis/spine/upper extremity was greater in the pubescent dancers.[20] The findings of this study support the notion that during the period of rapid growth and skeletal immaturity in the dancer, gains in height are not met with significant gains in peri-pelvic and core strength resulting in poor neuromuscular control about the hip and pelvis, resulting in increased injury risk to the hips and spine.

### Technique and overuse injury

Literature suggests that injury mechanism and prevention needs will vary between dance styles and techniques. In ballet, knee injuries are most common due to the "turned out" position. Those who do not naturally have "turn out" from the hips will often "force" their hips, knees, and ankles into a 180-degree turn out.[16] Biomechanical issues in the dancer can also increase the risk of injury; for example, range of motion, hypermobility, anatomical anomalies, and body structure.[10] Proper technique and training may help reduce injury as well as strengthening of the intrinsic foot and ankle muscles.[4]

In modern dance, there are many subset techniques within the overarching style with different injury risks.

To illustrate, the Horton technique and Graham technique vary greatly in their movement quality.[15,21] According to Solomon and Micheli (1986), the Horton technique tends to be more precarious on the lower back than the Graham technique.[15] Rapid growth combined with dance uniquely sets up the young dancer for stress injury to the spine.[22] In young athletes/dancers, patterns of injury to the spine differ as compared to the adult. Posterior column stress injuries are more common in young dancers/athletes, and back injuries are more common in male dancers than female dancers.[12] In comparison, adult athletes tend to succumb to discogenic and degenerative spine processes.[23] In professional level dancers, stress injuries to the spine are reported to occur in 7% of 54 professional ballet dancers.[22] The incidence of spine stress fractures in young dancers is unknown and is presumed to be under diagnosed.

Overuse injuries are the most common injuries in dancers; this was found to be true in three styles: ballet, modern, and aerobic dance.[16] Overuse injuries occur due to repetitive submaximal loading of the musculoskeletal system when rest is not adequate to allow for structural adaptation to take place and can occur to the muscle-tendon unit, bone, articular cartilage, physis, bursa, and/or neurovascular structures.[24] Repetition is needed to obtain particular skills in dance, and may serve to strengthen compensatory muscles and stimulate balance and reduce the risk of injury[15]; however, all too often, repetition results in muscle exhaustion[16] with resultant sacrifice in technique. Repetitiveness, even in the correct form, of any muscle group may result in overuse injury.[15] It is particularly important during times of high demand when dancers are fatigued and stressed in preparation for a show, that overuse and repetition are monitored. This is especially true for the dancer in training, as the young dancer has not yet developed the skill set required to monitor fatigue, and may not advocate for rest as needed for fear of reprimand and discrimination by peers and teachers. To this point, Liederbach et al. investigated fatigue related injury in dancers versus team sport athletes. The researchers found that dancers took more time than team sport athletes to reach fatigue as demonstrated with landing biomechanical data, and all groups landed with worse alignment after being fatigued after more hours of training, placing them at increased risk for injury.[25]

### Early specialization

Early sports specialization is defined as high-intensity training focused on a single sport from a young age with the hopes of mastering particular skills needed to succeed in the future.[26] Participating in many sports allows for well-rounded motor skills, training of opposing muscle groups, and improvement in flexibility patterns all serving to increase athletic success and decrease the risk of injury.[27] No studies have looked at early specialization in dancers, but there are studies that have examined sport specialization.[17,28]

Overuse injuries such as spondyloysis, osteochondritis dessecans, and stress fractures are all very common in athletes who specialize early.[27] Females playing single sport had four times greater risk of injury than those females who play multiple sports.[17] In addition, a study in Russia found that out of those that went to a high-level training institution only 0.14% became elite athletes.[27] The limited success of athletes participating in early specialization was echoed in a German study, where researchers found that early athletic success may come of early specialization, but to see longer senior-level success, multi-sport participation is warranted.[27] It is only logical to infer that these patterns may also apply to dancers, with early intense training and specializing increasing their risk of overuse injury. More research must be conducted to look at whether participating in many styles of dance is sufficient, or if the dancer should be participating in an additional cross-training or organized sport other than dance to avoid the injuries associated with specialization.

## CONCUSSION IN DANCE

Among possible unique injuries of the adolescent dancer, concussions are low in likelihood and understudied within the dance medicine field. Generally, dancers are aware of concussion symptomology.[29] The difficulty is that the ethos of dance is to "tough it out" when dealing with pain and injury. It is important that physicians and teachers of dance maintain an increased awareness of dance-related concussions, as the symptoms of concussion are often subtle, difficult to detect, and can be easily overlooked.[30]

To date, no studies have investigated the most beneficial way to treat concussions in dancers. The number of dancers present with concussions is extremely low. In one study, an on-site athletic trainer who saw a cohort of 137 university dance conservatory students over the course of the year saw only seven dance-related concussions.[29] In a retrospective chart review of a large teaching hospital over a 5.5-year period, only 11 dancers presented with dance-related concussions.[31]

In a case series by Stein et al. (2014), the mechanisms behind each concussion were not consistent. Each of these mechanisms occurred across a span of dance genres, including ballet, modern, hip-hop, musical theater, and acrobatics.[31] Concussions can vary by the individual,[30] the style of dance, and the movement being performed.[29]

The duration of the symptoms is not consistent either. Duration of concussion symptoms in dancers can range anywhere from 3 weeks to 2 years.[31] Although loss of consciousness at the time of the concussion does not occur in most cases, immediate symptoms tend to be headaches, migraine- or tension-type, and paresthesias.[30] Dizziness, poor balance, nausea, fatigue, confusion, sleep disturbance, emotional changes, difficulty with concentration and memory, and sensitivity to light and noise are all further symptoms that can arise. It is important to note that each dancer or athlete will present with different symptomology. In addition, it is important to consider other previous or present diagnoses, injuries, or medications that the dancer or athlete is taking at the time.[30]

As per established in return to play protocols for athletes, dancers that have been diagnosed or questioned to have a concussion should be removed from their activity.[32] It is most critical for the individual to rest, both physically and cognitively. Rest time varies person to person. Walking, stationary bicycling, or other light activity is suggested when returning to activity slowly. It is important that screen time, including computer use and texting, be limited during recovery time.[30,33] Full recovery usually happens within a month period.[30] Recently, it has been noted that there are psychosocial consequences that come along with extended periods of rest post-concussion. For example, feelings of worthlessness, social adjustment, and maintenance of independence.[34] Although the steps pertain to sport, they may be applicable to dance as well.

## SEDENTARY BEHAVIORS AND SLEEP

Sedentary behaviors and the impact on health in athletes have received more attention in the literature. Although dancers are generally considered to be immune to the ill effects of sedentary behaviors, this may not be the case. Sedentary behaviors in adolescents has been shown to be associated with elevated body mass index (BMI), blood pressure, and total cholesterol, in addition to lowered self-esteem, physical fitness, and lack of academic achievement.[35–37]

One measure of sedentary behavior is screen time. The American Academy of Pediatrics currently recommends that parents limit their children's total media time to 1–2 h/day.[38] In a recent study published in the *Journal of Dance Medicine and Science*, the authors investigated associations between sedentary behaviors, sleep hours, and BMI among young dancers participating in a summer intensive dance training program. The mean total screen time for the dancers in the study was reported to be 3.4 ± 2.1 h/day, ranging from 0 to 11 h/day. The total screen time was independently positively associated with BMI.[39] Furthermore, this same study revealed that almost two-thirds of the dancers got less than or equal to 8 h of sleep per night, and that the older dancers tended to sleep less than the younger dancers.[39] The Center for Disease and Prevention (CDC) currently recommends 9–10 h of sleep per night for all teenagers.[40] The National Sleep Foundation's Sleep in America Poll found that by the 12th grade 75% of students self-reported sleep durations of less than 8 h/night compared with 16% of sixth graders. Although 30%–41% of sixth through eighth graders were getting nine or more hours of sleep, only 3% of 12th graders reported doing so.[41] Finally, given the extreme physical demands of dance, coupled with high academic and social pressures, sleep requirements for young dancers may very well be even greater than the sleep requirements for others.

Although no studies to date exist that link sleep deprivation and injury in dancers, an association between amount of sleep and injury has been reported by Milewski et al., who found that sleep duration in athletes was an independent factor associated with injury, and the athletes who slept on average less than 8 h/night were 1.7 times more likely to have had an injury when compared with those who slept more than 8 h.[42]

## NUTRITION AND ENERGY BALANCE

The topic of nutrition and energy balance in adolescent dancers requires some focused discussion. Nutritional imbalance and low energy availability, especially in the growing and adolescent dancer, can lead to significant long-term health consequences. The idea of female athletic triad has been well known traditionally as the triad of energy deficiency with or without disordered eating, menstrual disturbance/amenorrhea, and bone loss/osteoporosis.[43] More recently, the terminology of "Relative Energy Deficiency in Sport" (RED-S) has taken hold. This new description of the syndrome of RED-S is to encompass the complexity of energy imbalance on healthy, performance, and function of both female and male athletes. As defined by the International Olympic Committee (IOC) consensus statement, the syndrome of RED-S refers to "impaired physiological

function including, but not limited to, metabolic rate, menstrual function, bone health, immunity, protein synthesis, cardiovascular health caused by relative energy deficiency."[44] Low dietary intake is abundantly prevalent among dancers, and the health consequences of this must not be underestimated.

The dance aesthetic, specifically ballet, places a high value on specific body shapes and sizes, and it is a widespread concern that dancers may have insufficient energy intake and be predisposed to disordered eating to maintain those aesthetics. In a meta-analysis by Arcelus et al. of 33 studies published between 1966 and 2013 on this topic, the overall prevalence of disordered eating in dancers was noted to be 12.0% (16.4% for ballet dancers), with anorexia affecting 2.0% (4% for ballet dancers), bulimia affecting 4.4% (2% for ballet dancers), and eating disorders not otherwise specified (EDNOS) affecting 9.5% (14.9% for ballet dancers).[45] This study found that dancers had a three times higher risk of suffering from eating disorders.[45] Furthermore, the risk to ballet dancers specifically is also highlighted in a survey study by Ringham of 29 female ballet dancers, which reported that 83% of all the dancers met criteria for anorexia nervosa (9.6%), bulimia nervosa (10.3%), anorexia and bulimia nervosa (10.3%), or EDNOS (55.0%).[46] In fact, dancers had assessments more similar to eating-disordered individuals than to controls in this study.[46]

The risk of low energy availability and disordered eating is very much a problem in the adolescent dancer, as nutrition is a key factor in healthy growth. Adolescent is a period of accelerated development. By age 18, approximately 90% of total peak bone mass has been gained. The last 10% occurs in the next 10 years, varying by gender and genetics, as bones mature to a fully ossified skeleton.[47] A balanced and sufficient diet is absolutely critical in achieving good growth and health[48,49] as well as decreasing fatigue and risk of injury.[50] Low energy intake or availability may cause a gamut of issues including delayed puberty, menstrual irregularity, decreased muscle mass, and higher risk of fatigue and injury.[51] Dancers and dance teachers often perceive the physical logical pubertal changes in weight and shape as a "make-or-break" in their potential professional ballet career[52] creating a nidus for poor self-image and disordered eating. The pervasiveness of this was demonstrated in a study by Burckhardt et al., who examined 127 female dancers with an average age of 16.7 at an internationally renowned ballet competition for preprofessional dancers. Food intake by the dancers was found to be below the recommendations for a normally active population in all food groups except animal proteins.[53] In addition, BMI for age was normal in only 43% of the dancers, with 16% of dancers having severe degree of thinness (12.6% Grade 2% and 3.1% Grade 3 thinness via Tanner scores).[53] Among those 127 female dancers, 117 had late average age for menarche at 13.9 years of age, with 10 dancers found to have primary amenorrhea, and one secondary amenorrhea. The relationship between BMI and menstrual patterns in dancers was echoed in Stracciolini et al.'s study of 105 female dancers, average age of 14.8 years. Not only was there a significant negative correlation between BMI and age of first menses, but also 44% of these dancers surveyed reported menstrual irregularities.[54] Even worse, this pattern of disordered eating and menstrual irregularity can follow these young dancers to adulthood, as noted by Peric et al. who reported patterns of disordered eating and amenorrhea in professional ballet dancers.[55]

The interplay between dancing and nutrition and bone health is slightly more complex. In Burckhardt's study, bone mineral content (BMC) as evaluated by bone densitometry (DEXA scan) was found to be low in preprofessional dancers and associated with nutritional factors, with dairy products having a positive influence.[53] However, low BMC is not universally found in adolescent dancers. One study by Yang et al. compared BMC in 60 dancers and 77 controls between the ages of 15—17 found that, after adjusting for age and BMI, dancers showed higher total body bone mineral content and leg length/height.[56] This was also noted in a study by Matthews et al., who monitored the effects of ballet dancing on BMC in female nonelite dancers and normally active controls for 3 years across puberty. Comparing 82 ballet dancers and 61 controls starting at age 8—11 years at baseline found that, after adjusting for growth and maturation, dancers had significantly greater BMC of the total body, lower limbs, femoral neck, and lumbar spine than controls by DEXA.[57] It is possible that, although dance as a weight-bearing exercise can promote bone growth, this effect is mitigated by low energy bioavailability and disordered eating commonly found in dancers.

Ultimately, what is clear is that energy availability and nutrition have a critical role in the development of adolescent dancer. Dancers, parents, teachers, and healthcare providers all must be vigilante in monitoring for signs of relative energy deficiency, and more research is essential to further understand how best to mitigate risk of negative consequences as well as optimize growth, health, and performance of adolescent dancers.

## TOBACCO AND SUBSTANCE USE

Social pressures, stress relief, and the drive to maintain weight may lead to the abuse of substances by the young dancer. Studies in adult retired ballet dancers found a greater prevalence of smoking among ballet dancers versus control.[58] Lewis et al. in England found that 46% of retired ballet dancers studied had smoked during the time that they worked as professional dancers. Furthermore, patterns of smoking may differ among the dance disciplines and training level.[59] Bronner et al. studied 211 professional dancers in the United States and found that only 2.5% of modern dancers smoked compared with 18% of ballet dancers. Stein et al. investigated cigarette use among dancers at varying levels of training (high school, college, professional), 8.7% of dancers were current smokers and 9.4% were former smokers. Moreover, 51.8% of the dancers believed that at least half of all dancers smoked. Furthermore, 79.9% indicated that they had had a dance teacher or choreographer who smoked.[60] Finally, Peric et al. reported in a sample of 21 professional ballet dancers in Croatia that 40% of dancers smoked (25% smoke on a daily basis), 36% often used analgesics, and 25% engaged in binge drinking at least once a month.[55] Continued awareness and education, especially in the vulnerable child and adolescent dancer, is critical to offset the increased potential of substance use in this population.

## INJURY PREVENTION AND MANAGEMENT
### Screening

There a several reasons to screen dancers, that being to determine if dancer possesses characteristics needed for dance, to disclose pathology, quantify risk, to establish the characteristics for given levels, and to establish a baseline in data with the goal of setting educational and training or rehabilitative strategies.[61] To prevent injury, it is crucial to screen dancers for existing or future injury.[4] Steinberg et al. suggest that screening should be mandatory to identify current injury or identify risk factors for future injury.[10] History forms should be examined prior to physical screening to identify previous injury or illness. Screening often has a measure of flexibility, general posture, body type per dance style, evaluation of the feet, ankles, hips, knees, and back.[4] Flexibility measures are often made for the general public, which can inaccurately describe the dancer, because of the greater flexibility in dancers than the general public. Posture can be examined by having the dancer stand feet together, evaluating the level of the shoulders, and bend forward to scan for scoliosis. Following this test, it is important and straightforward to evaluate the knees. Hyperextension, bowlegs, knock-knees, and femoral anteversion are easily identifiable. Misalignment such as these, can lead to lateral tendinitis. Next is to evaluate the ankles, which should not supinate or pronate. From the ankles, the feet should be examined next. Screening of the feet should be performed in turned out relevé to look for supination, and flat foot turn out to look for pronation. Weight and height should also be taken down, but in the evaluation, should not be seen by the dancer, as this is a taxing process.[16] It is important to use screening measures that are specific to dancers, and not to overall athletes, because average results may vary from the general population.[61]

Preparticipation screening can be time consuming and labor intensive. Screening, although tedious, can surface issues of malalignment before they become problematic.[16] Although no difference in injury rate was found between a group of dancers who were screened and those who were not, future studies should look at the preventative measures taken after the time of being screened and compare this with dancers who did not take preventative measures post-screening.[21]

### Resistance Training and Rehabilitation

Resistance training (also referred to as strength training) is a progressive use of varying loads, movements, and velocities to improve muscle strength power, and endurance.[62] To prevent injury in the young dancer, it can be beneficial to incorporate strength and integrative resistance training, as well as flexibility work.[13] There is a new shift from post injury rehabilitation to injury prevention using resistance training. However, many dancers are hesitant to participate in resistance training with the fear that it will increase muscle bulk, while taking away from ballet aesthetic. Integrating resistance training into dance training will help improve core stability and lower extremity strength, without dramatic increase in muscle bulk or change in aesthetics.[62]

It is important to understand that resistance training in children is safe and will not negatively impact growth or be injurious to immature skeletons, as long as conducted with a qualified instructor who monitors technique and progression. Finally, most young dancers should participate in resistance training as an integral part of their routine dance training. Although dancers have been found to have strong lower extremities, supplemental resistance training can improve both muscular and anaerobic power, as well as serve to prevent future injury. There is a need in the dance community to dispel the myths surrounding resistance training

and to continue to be informed of the significant benefits, effectiveness, and safety of strength and resistance training.

### CONCLUSION

Dance training in the youth has many physical and psychosocial benefits including the health benefits of strength and sustained physical activity, confidence building, and the beauty of the dance itself. Awareness of the unique health issues facing the child and adolescent dancer including risk factors for injury, nutrition and bone health, sedentary behaviors, and substance use is critical to health maintenance. Incorporating resistance training and early education surrounding risks for injury, such as nutrition education, into routine youth dance training is recommended to improve youth dancer's overall health and well-being.

### REFERENCES

1. O'Neill JR, Pate RR, Liese AD. Descriptive epidemiology of dance participation in adolescents. *Res Q Exerc Sport.* 2011; 82(3):373−380. https://doi.org/10.1080/02701367.2011. 10599769.
2. Luke AC, Kinney SA, D'Hemecourt PA, et al. Determinants of injuries in young dancers. *Med Problems Perform Artists*; September 1, 2002. http://link.galegroup.com/apps/doc/ A173187315/AONE?sid=googlescholar.
3. Leanderson C, Leanderson J, Wykman A, Strender L-E, Johansson S-E, Sundquist K. Musculoskeletal injuries in young ballet dancers. *Knee Surg Sports Traumatol Arthrosc.* 2011;19(9):1531−1535. https://doi.org/10.1007/s00167-011-1445-9.
4. Injury patterns in elite Preprofessional ballet dancers and the Utility of screening Programs to identify risk characteristics. *J Orthop Sports Phys Ther.* 2008;38(3): 126−136. https://doi.org/10.2519/jospt.2008.2390.
5. Ekegren CL, Quested R, Brodrick A. Injuries in preprofessional ballet dancers: incidence, characteristics and consequences. *J Sci Med Sport.* 2014;17(3):271−275. https://doi.org/10.1016/j.jsams.2013.07.013.
6. Shah S, Weiss DS, Burchette RJ. Injuries in professional modern dancers: incidence, risk factors, and Management. *J Dance Med Sci.* 2012;16(1):17−25.
7. Nilsson C, Leanderson J, Wykman A, Strender L-E. The injury panorama in a Swedish professional ballet company. *Knee Surg Sports Traumatol Arthrosc.* 2001;9(4): 242−246. https://doi.org/10.1007/s001670100195.
8. Bronner S, Worthen L. The demographics of dance in the United States. *J Dance Med Sci.* 1999;3(4):151−153.
9. Ballet injuries: injury incidence and severity over 1 year. *J Orthop Sports Phys Ther.* 2012;42(9):781−790. https:// doi.org/10.2519/jospt.2012.3893.
10. Steinberg N, Siev-ner I, Peleg S, et al. Extrinsic and intrinsic risk factors associated with injuries in young dancers aged

8−16 years. *J Sports Sci.* 2012;30(5):485−495. https://doi.org/10.1080/02640414.2011.647705.

11. Yin AX, Sugimoto D, Martin DJ, Stracciolini A. Pediatric dance injuries: a cross-sectional epidemiological study. *PM&R.* 2016;8(4):348−355. https://doi.org/10.1016/j.pmrj.2015.08.012.

12. Micheli LJ. Back injuries in dancers. *Clin Sports Med.* 1983;2(3):473−484.

13. Gerbino PG, Stracciolini A, Gearhart MG. Knee problems in the young dancer. In: *Prevention of Injuries in the Young Dancer.* Contemporary Pediatric and Adolescent Sports Medicine. Cham: Springer; 2017:129−145. https://doi.org/10.1007/978-3-319-55047-3_8.

14. Micheli LJ. Overuse injuries in children's sports: the growth factor. *Orthop Clin North Am.* 1983;14(2):337−360.

15. Solomon RL, Micheli LJ. Technique as a consideration in modern dance injuries. *Phys Sportsmed.* 1986;14(8):83−90. https://doi.org/10.1080/00913847.1986.11709150.

16. Solomon R, American Alliance for Health, Physical Education, Recreation, Dance, National Dance Association. *Preventing Dance Injuries: An Interdisciplinary Perspective.* Reston, VA: AAHPERD Publication Sales Office; 1990.

17. Jayanthi NA, LaBella CR, Fischer D, Pasulka J, Dugas LR. Sports-specialized intensive training and the risk of injury in young athletes: a clinical case-control study. *Am J Sports Med.* 2015;43(4):794−801. https://doi.org/10.1177/0363546514567298.

18. Phillips C. Strength training of dancers during the adolescent growth Spurt. *J Dance Med Sci.* 1999;3(2):66−72.

19. Kadel NJ, Teitz CC, Kronmal RA. Stress fractures in ballet dancers. *The Am J Sports Med*; 1992. http://journals.sagepub.com/doi/abs/10.1177/036354659202000414.

20. Stracciolini A, Yin AX, Sugimoto D. Etiology and body area of injuries in young female dancers presenting to sports medicine clinic: a comparison by age group. *Phys Sportsmed.* 2015;43(4):342−347. https://doi.org/10.1080/00913847.2015.1076326.

21. Weigert BJ, Erikson M. Incidence of injuries in female university-level modern dancers and the effectiveness of a screening Program in Altering injury patterns. *ProQuest.* 2007;22. https://search.proquest.com/openview/3182e4d586503238/1?pq-origsite=gscholar&cbl=12230.

22. Micheli LJ, Curtis C. Stress fractures in the spine and Sacrum. *Clin Sports Med.* 2006;25(1):75−88. https://doi.org/10.1016/j.csm.2005.08.001.

23. Micheli LJ, Wood R. Back pain in young athletes: significant differences from adults in causes and patterns. *Arch Pediatr Adolesc Med.* 1995;149(1):15−18. https://doi.org/10.1001/archpedi.1995.02170130017004.

24. DiFiori JP, Benjamin HJ, Brenner JS, et al. Overuse injuries and burnout in youth sports: a position statement from the American Medical Society for Sports Medicine. *Br J Sports Med.* 2014;48(4):287−288. https://doi.org/10.1136/bjsports-2013-093299.

25. Liederbach M, Kremenic IJ, Orishimo KF, Pappas E, Hagins M. Comparison of landing Biomechanics between male and female dancers and athletes, part 2: influence of fatigue and implications for anterior cruciate ligament injury. *Am J Sports Med.* 2014;42(5):1089−1095. https://doi.org/10.1177/0363546514524525.

26. LaPrade RF, Agel J, Baker J, et al. AOSSM early sport specialization consensus statement. *Orthop J Sports Med.* 2016;4(4):2325967116644241. https://doi.org/10.1177/2325967116644241.

27. Sugimoto D, Stracciolini A, Dawkins CI, Meehan WPI, Micheli LJ. Implications for training in youth: is specialization benefiting Kids? *Strength Cond J.* 2017;39(2):77. https://doi.org/10.1519/SSC.0000000000000289.

28. Pasulka J, Jayanthi N, McCann A, Dugas LR, LaBella C. Specialization patterns across various youth sports and relationship to injury risk. *Phys Sportsmed.* 2017;45(3):344−352. https://doi.org/10.1080/00913847.2017.1313077.

29. McIntyre L, Liederbach M. Concussion knowledge and behaviors in a sample of the dance community. *J Dance Med Sci.* 2016;20(2):79−88. https://doi.org/10.12678/1089-313X.20.2.79.

30. Stein CJ, Meehan WP. Concussion and the female athlete. In: *The Young Female Athlete.* Contemporary Pediatric and Adolescent Sports Medicine. Cham: Springer; 2016:135−145. https://doi.org/10.1007/978-3-319-21632-4_10.

31. Stein CJ, Kinney SA, McCrystal T, et al. Dance-related concussion: a case series. *J Dance Med Sci.* 2014;18(2):53−61. https://doi.org/10.12678/1089-313X.18.2.53.

32. Bazarian JJ, Veenema T, Brayer AF, Lee E. Knowledge of concussion guidelines among practitioners caring for children. *Clin Pediatr (Phila).* 2001;40(4):207−212. https://doi.org/10.1177/000992280104000405.

33. Kerrigan JM, Giza CC. When in doubt, sit it out! Pediatric concussion—an update. *Childs Nerv Syst.* 2017;33(10):1669−1675. https://doi.org/10.1007/s00381-017-3537-4.

34. Pelczar M, Polityńska B. [Pathogenesis and psychosocial consequences of post-concussion syndrome]. *Neurol Neurochir Pol.* 1997;31(5):989−998.

35. de Rezende LF, Lopes MR, Rey-López JP, Matsudo VKR, Luiz Odo C. Sedentary behavior and health outcomes: an overview of systematic reviews. *PLoS One.* 2014;9(8):e105620. https://doi.org/10.1371/journal.pone.0105620.

36. Trinh L, Wong B, Faulkner GE. The independent and Interactive associations of screen time and physical activity on mental health, school connectedness and academic achievement among a population-based sample of youth. *J Can Acad Child Adolesc Psychiatry.* 2015;24(1):17−24.

37. van Ekris E, Altenburg TM, Singh AS, Proper KI, Heymans MW, Chinapaw MJM. An evidence-update on the prospective relationship between childhood sedentary behaviour and biomedical health indicators: a systematic review and meta-analysis. *Obes Rev.* 2016;17(9):833−849. https://doi.org/10.1111/obr.12426.

38. Bar-On ME, Broughton DD, Buttross S, et al. Children, adolescents, and television. *Pediatrics.* 2001;107(2):423−426. https://doi.org/10.1542/peds.107.2.423.

39. Stracciolini A, Stein CJ, Kinney S, McCrystal T, Pepin MJ, Meehan III WP. Associations between sedentary behaviors, sleep patterns, and BMI in young dancers Attending a

summer intensive dance training Program. *J Dance Med Sci.* 2017;21(3):102−108. https://doi.org/10.12678/1089-313X.21.3.102.

40. CDC—How Much Sleep Do I Need?—Sleep and Sleep Disorders; 2015. https://www.cdc.gov/sleep/about_sleep/how_much_sleep.html. Accessed January 5, 2018.

41. 2006 Teens and Sleep; 2006. https://sleepfoundation.org/sleep-polls-data/sleep-in-america-poll/2006-teens-and-sleep. Accessed January 4, 2018.

42. Milewski MD, Skaggs DL, Bishop GA, et al. Chronic lack of sleep is associated with increased sports injuries in adolescent athletes. *J Pediatr Orthop.* 2014;34(2):129. https://doi.org/10.1097/BPO.0000000000000151.

43. What is the Triad?. *Female Athlete Triad Coalit;* June 2017. http://www.femaleathletetriad.org/athletes/what-is-the-triad/.

44. Mountjoy M, Sundgot-Borgen J, Burke L, et al. The IOC consensus statement: beyond the female athlete triad—relative energy deficiency in sport (RED-S). *Br J Sports Med.* 2014;48(7):491−497. https://doi.org/10.1136/bjsports-2014-093502.

45. Arcelus J, Witcomb GL, Mitchell A. Prevalence of eating disorders amongst dancers: a systemic review and meta-analysis. *Eur Eat Disord Rev.* 2014;22(2):92−101. https://doi.org/10.1002/erv.2271.

46. Ringham R, Klump K, Kaye W, et al. Eating disorder symptomatology among ballet dancers. *Int J Eat Disord.* 2006;39(6):503−508. https://doi.org/10.1002/eat.20299.

47. Parfitt AM, Travers R, Rauch F, Glorieux FH. Structural and cellular changes during bone growth in healthy children. *Bone.* 2000;27(4):487−494. https://doi.org/10.1016/S8756-3282(00)00353-7.

48. Bianchi S. Ultrasound of the peripheral nerves. *Joint Bone Spine.* 2008;75(6):643−649. https://doi.org/10.1016/j.jbspin.2008.07.002.

49. Cromer B, Harel Z. Adolescents: at increased risk for osteoporosis? *Clin Pediatr (Phila).* 2000;39(10):565−574. https://doi.org/10.1177/000992280003901001.

50. Brown DD, Challis J. *Optimal nutrition for dancers.* 2017; 111. http://repository.ubn.ru.nl/handle/2066/168349.

51. Rogol AD, Clark PA, Roemmich JN. Growth and pubertal development in children and adolescents: effects of diet and physical activity. *Am J Clin Nutr.* 2000;72(2):521s−528s.

52. Mitchell SB, Haase AM, Malina RM, Cumming SP. The role of puberty in the making and breaking of young ballet dancers: perspectives of dance teachers. *J Adolesc.* 2016;

47(suppl C):81−89. https://doi.org/10.1016/j.adolescence.2015.12.007.

53. Burckhardt P, Wynn E, Krieg M-A, Bagutti C, Faouzi M. The effects of nutrition, puberty and dancing on bone density in adolescent ballet dancers. *J Dance Med Sci.* 2011;15(2):51−60.

54. Stracciolini A, Quinn BJ, Geminiani E, et al. Body mass index and menstrual patterns in dancers. *Clin Pediatr (Phila).* 2017;56(1):49−54. https://doi.org/10.1177/0009922816642202.

55. Peric M, Zenic N, Sekulic D, Kondric M, Zaletel P. Disordered eating, amenorrhea, and substance use and misuse among professional ballet dancers: preliminary analysis. *Med Pr.* 2016;67(1):21−27. https://doi.org/10.13075/mp.5893.00294.

56. Yang LC, Hu J, Lan Y, Yang YH, Zhang Q, Piao JH. The differences in bone mineral content between female dancers and controls aged 15-17 years old and its relationship with physical activity level. *Zhonghua Yu Fang Yi Xue Za Zhi.* 2009;43(12):1077−1080.

57. Matthews BL, Bennell KL, McKay HA, et al. Dancing for bone health: a 3-year longitudinal study of bone mineral accrual across puberty in female non-elite dancers and controls. *Osteoporos Int.* 2006;17(7):1043−1054. https://doi.org/10.1007/s00198-006-0093-2.

58. Khan KM, Green RM, Saul A, et al. Retired elite female ballet dancers and nonathletic controls have similar bone mineral density at weightbearing sites. *J Bone Miner Res.* 1996;11(10):1566−1574. https://doi.org/10.1002/jbmr.5650111025.

59. Lewis RL, Dickerson JWT, Davies GJ. Lifestyle and injuries of professional ballet dancers: reflections in retirement. *J R Soc Health.* 1997;117(1):23−31. https://doi.org/10.1177/146642409711700107.

60. Stein CJ, Gleason CN, Pepin MJ, et al. Cigarette smoking among dancers of different ages and levels of training. *J Dance Med Sci.* 2016;20(4):174−180. https://doi.org/10.12678/1089-313X.20.4.174.

61. Liederbach M. Screening for functional capacity in dancers designing standardized, dance-specific injury prevention screening tools. *J Dance Med Sci.* 1997;1(3):93−106.

62. Stracciolini A, Myer GD, Faigenbaum AD. Resistance training for pediatric female dancers. In: *Prevention of Injuries in the Young Dancer.* Contemporary Pediatric and Adolescent Sports Medicine. Cham: Springer; 2017:79−93. https://doi.org/10.1007/978-3-319-55047-3_5.

## CHAPTER 12

# Considerations for Screening Professional Dancers

HEATHER SOUTHWICK, PT, MSPT

## INTRODUCTION

Dancing at the professional level requires intensity of training and performing that is generally more than 45 exposure hours per week.[1] Inevitably, this intensity is accompanied by a rising rate of injury mandating the need for specialized healthcare.[2] Participation in professional dance training and performing is physically and psychologically demanding and injuries are an expected outcome.[3,4] Professional dance differs from students at the preprofessional and college level in many ways, but most significantly the professional dancer is being paid to do a job that requires keeping his or her body healthy. All dancers tend to push their physical limits, often considered a hallmark of professional dance. However, illness and injury can be expensive, so it is in the financial interest of a company to have healthy dancers.

As a preliminary step toward injury prevention, preparticipation screenings for athletes have been utilized since the 1980s in an effort to determine readiness for play and to reduce injury.[5] Given that participation in sports programs from the amateur to professional level often requires a preparticipation physical examination by a physician, it is a matter of concern that professional dancers, who may be training at higher levels of intensity and exposure, generally have no such requirement. In the dance medicine literature, there is agreement that while screenings are not intended to substitute for a dancer's healthcare, they can be used to identify intrinsic risk factors for illness or injury.[3] There is also agreement among healthcare professionals who care for dancers that the initial phase of injury prevention is to have a formal process to uncover intrinsic risk factors that contribute to injury and illness and to counsel each dancer, recommending interventions based on the information gathered.

Statistically, 67%—95% of dancers in professional companies have been reported to be injured annually.[2,6,7] Multiple intrinsic and extrinsic factors contribute to these statistics in complicated ways. Intrinsic risk factors include age, sex, personality type, previous injury, posture and alignment, hypermobility, cardiovascular fitness level, muscular flexibility, strength, and functional movement patterns. A screening assessment allows for review of past and current intrinsic attributes that can impact future health and injury. It can also help healthcare practitioners establish baselines for a dancer in a variety of physical areas. Instituting a mechanism and format for identifying issues that may cause a dancer to be unable to work certainly has the potential to save dance companies' money. The benefits of screening professional dancers are numerous, even though the identification of risk factors has not always shown to be a predictor of injury.[2] Until a robust and comprehensive injury surveillance system is standardized and utilized, it is difficult to confidently link risk factors from a screening to injury. Recent studies are making an effort to implement valid and reliable screening tools that do determine dancer readiness for participation in various settings and can identify risk for injury. However, these studies often have small sample sizes, varying injury definitions, and self-report of injury versus diagnosis by a healthcare practitioner.[8]

## OBJECTIVES OF SCREENING

There are many goals of screening in professional dance; however, the priority is to improve safe participation. A screening tool in the professional health setting should be designed to detect potentially life-threatening or disabling medical or musculoskeletal conditions that may limit a dancer's safe participation, while also aiming to detect medical or musculoskeletal conditions that may predispose dancers to injury or illness during their season. Specifically, the screening tool should help

Performing Arts Medicine. https://doi.org/10.1016/B978-0-323-58182-0.00012-2

medical practitioners gain an understanding of the baseline profile of an individual dancer's medical, psychologic, nutritional, and physical status. Determining a dancer's general health is very important, yet this remains uncommon for most professional dance companies. Assessing an individual's fitness level and identifying prior health issues or chronic issues such as asthma, diabetes, or thyroid problems allows healthcare providers to make recommendations for interventions and referrals as appropriate. Without a screen, there may be no opportunity to review underlying pathology in a professional company setting. The screening process also allows education of the dancer on his/her individual strengths and weaknesses while promoting self-awareness of the areas that can be addressed with exercise to improve function and training. Ultimately, the most important objective of screening is to prevent potential injury, not predict injury, by identifying risks and underlying pathologies that would not have otherwise been exposed.[2,3]

## BENEFITS OF SCREENING

There are many benefits to implementing a screening program in a professional company. Allowing a dancer to meet and establish a relationship with a healthcare team of physicians, physical therapists, and athletic trainers who are knowledgeable in dance can create trust and allow earlier problem recognition and injury reporting. Removing the well-known stigma of seeking healthcare among professional dancers can help them feel more comfortable accessing services for prevention, as opposed to waiting until they sustain an injury.[9] A screen can also provide the opportunity for counseling and timely referral to specialties in fields like nutrition and sports psychology and to educate dancers on the importance of these areas to their overall health and performance. The education that accompanies the screen can motivate dancers to improve their overall fitness and performance on certain tests and measures. Most importantly, while the screen may be broad-based, it should always conclude with individual recommendations, exercises to improve areas of weakness, and referrals for further evaluation as indicated.

## FACTORS SIGNIFICANT TO SUCCESS

In order for a screening program to be successful at the professional level, many factors need to be addressed and communicated to the dancers. The most essential is privacy and confidentiality. In some cases, the artistic and company management may need to be educated on the laws around personal health information. In a professional company setting, while the management may be paying for the dancer and practitioner time, thus bearing the cost of the screening program, they do not have access to the dancer's private medical information. Companies need to compensate both the dancers and the healthcare practitioners. In practice, the dancer cost is absorbed into salaries like a costume fitting, while the noticeable cost is the day or two of time for the medical teams.

Assessing the whole dancer is critical. Health risks in professional dance are not limited to physical injury, and it is helpful for practitioners responsible for a company to have prior knowledge of past medical histories, allergies, and medications in the event of a medical emergency. Psychologic and psychosocial factors likely have significant influence on the occurrence, recovery, and outcome of work-related injuries.[10] In medicine, psychosocial factors have been shown to be at least as important as physical factors in determining health.[11] A comprehensive screen should include physical, emotional, nutritional, and general heath assessments. Success also depends on broad company participation and support from the leadership in the company. Having full company participation is important, and preseason, posthire screenings should be treated as a routine part of company life.

For a screening program to have the greatest impact, it should take place early in the company season, ideally during the first week of rehearsals, so there is time for deficits in strength and flexibility to be identified and corrective training initiated before the dancer is fully engrossed in rehearsals and performances. In addition, helping to facilitate appointments with primary care physicians and dentists for annual well visits can also help prevent health issues at more intense times in the dance season. It is not appropriate to utilize screens as a test of acceptability into a company or for casting.[12,13] It should be a posthire assessment to assure all parties that the screening has no relation to employment status, but rather is intended to help each dancer achieve a safer, healthier, and more productive season.

## LOCATION OF SCREENING ASSESSMENTS

Screening locations vary depending on the needs and goals of the dancers. Sometimes screens are performed in a physician's office or physical therapy clinic, which allows for consistency, privacy, and a setting outside of the work environment. This may help dancers feel more comfortable about revealing themselves. However, to promote convenience and compliance, more often screening assessments are conducted in the company studios. Larger numbers of dancers are screened in stations set up by a healthcare team that may be comprised of physicians, physical therapists, athletic trainers, sports psychologists, nutritionists, and healthcare providers with backgrounds in dance technique and movement analysis. In the professional setting, it is not advised that artistic staff have any direct involvement with the screening process.

## STANDARDIZING THE SCREENING TOOL

The professional dance population has similarities in age range, health risks, physical presentation, and general goals so a standardized protocol based on the premise that there are basic principles of functional movement common to all types of dancers has many benefits. In addition, basic aspects of general health, nutrition, substance use and abuse, and emotional status need to be reviewed. Issues in any one of these areas can increase risk of injury and illness for a dancer. Utilizing a standardized protocol with specific guidelines for use allows consistency and reliability in the information collected and the opportunity to evaluate larger trends and health patterns among professional dancers. The process should be efficient and effective, addressing the most significant issues for overall health and musculoskeletal issues commonly seen in dancers at the professional level. When the goals of the screening process are clear, the tests and measures to be selected become more obvious. At the professional level, screening tool assessments should include a comprehensive medical history and a combination of physical tests that efficiently examine a dancer's posture and alignment, flexibility, strength, cardiovascular parameters, and issues with motor patterns and muscle recruitment functionally.

## HEALTH HISTORY

In a professional company, one of the most significant areas of the screen is the health history. If a dance company has no time or budget for a full screening process that includes physical assessments, obtaining a health history that addresses multiple areas of past and present health issues is highly recommended. General health questions and medical history should be comprehensive and inquire if there is an ongoing or chronic illness, such as asthma, allergies, diabetes, and history of concussion which can help identify the need for further information or referral. In professional dancers, cardiac questions should be included, as over 95% of all sudden deaths in athletes under 30 years of age are due to structural cardiac problems.[14] Questioning of this

kind is consistent with the Preparticipation Physical Evaluation published by the American College of Sports Medicine and used for athletes in high schools and colleges throughout the United States.[15,16]

In the dance population, there is a higher than normal incidence of menstrual dysfunction, musculoskeletal injury, and lower bone density that is all interrelated. (Referred to as the female athlete triad or Relative Energy Deficiency.) Including questions regarding the onset of menses and frequency of menstruation can help the healthcare practitioner uncover areas that not only can lead to injuries but also can have potentially serious and detrimental health consequences. Dancers who demonstrate amenorrhea for more than 6 months have been shown to be more likely to sustain a stress injury than dancers with normal menstruation.[17] A thorough history of past injuries is also important, as these are risk factors for recurrent injury. Ankle sprains, which are often dismissed as insignificant by dancers, offer a perfect example of this requirement, as research provides ample evidence of future injury with history of prior ankle sprain.[18] Previous injury is the most frequently cited risk for future injury in the literature and can include reinjury of the same issue or a new injury that may arise from inadequate rehabilitation and prevention from an original injury.[8]

The health history questionnaire also provides an excellent opportunity for addressing mental health questions regarding depression, anxiety, and requests for counseling. Psychologic risk factors for injury are often overlooked and should be a priority when screening. These risk factors have been show in the literature to influence both the occurrence and outcomes of injury.[19–22] Stress, psychologic distress, disordered eating patterns, and poor coping skills are all associated with both risk and outcomes of dance injuries.[23] Other issues including sleep, personality, and social support have been associated with increased risk of injury. More emphasis is being placed on the inclusion of patient perspectives in the assessment of outcomes and treatment effects in medicine. In order to gather this information effectively, the use of psychometric patient-reported outcome instruments should be utilized more often. Validated instruments such as the EAT-26, Profile of Mood States and disability scales such as the DFOS-36 (adapted for dance) are gaining more reliability and validity as potential predictors of injury.[1–3]

Nutrition questions should address concerns around weight and eating for optimal performance. All dancers can benefit from individual nutritional counseling to optimize performance, and asking dancers if that type of counseling would be helpful can help facilitate services available for a myriad of nutritional issues. Athletes aged 16–35 (the range of professional dancers) years generally do not feel they need to see a primary care physician or a dentist on an annual basis. A screening program gives healthcare practitioners the opportunity to inquire about recent healthcare visits and to provide resources for services under healthcare systems and insurance that may be new for a dancer starting in a company or a country with a system that differs from what they have previously known.

## PHYSICAL ASSESSMENT

What should be included in the physical assessment will depend on the goals of the screen. Time constraints and resources at the professional level are always significant factors. Unless there is the opportunity to spend 2–3 hours screening each dancer, every test and measurement discussed in this chapter may not be included in one screening assessment. For the Dance/USA Task Force on Dancer Health, a standardized screen was created with the goal that the physical assessment and the appropriate recommendations following the screen could be completed within 30 minutes. Generally, in a professional setting, if the time of the dancers and the practitioners is paid time, then this time limit needs to be a priority. In addition, the areas that are thought to present the most risk for injury should be analyzed and prioritized. As has already been stated, risk factors are still under review in the literature and in clinical practice, so physical assessment tests are likely to change as evidence-based practices evolve.

### Height, Weight, and Body Mass Index

Obtaining anthropometric measurements such as height and weight provide a baseline for the individual dancer and the information required to calculate body mass index (BMI). It is important that clinicians and dancers understand that the purpose of obtaining these measurements is to help identify dancers who are at risk of injury because their BMI is too low. The approach to these measurements should be handled with sensitivity in this population because in ballet, where thinness is the generally valued esthetic, dancers are often preoccupied with weight and body image. A proper screening not only helps identify dancers at risk due to a low BMI but also assesses any issues with menstrual cycles, as this combination can lead to dangerous health issues and multiple injuries, such as stress fractures.[24] In addition, it has been established in the literature that dancers at the professional level often lose body fat during intense performance times such as during *Nutcracker*

season.[25] Having baseline information on individual dancers can be imperative to identifying an issue later in the performance year. In cases where inadequate energy intake is a concern, or where a dancer appears too thin, referral to multiple practitioners to insure safety and to address any underlying issues with health, diet, and psychologic issues is indicated.

### Alignment and Posture

Integral to all dance styles and esthetic values is a dancer's technique and alignment. Faulty technique and compromised alignment lead to injury.[26] Knowledge of a dancer's baseline posture and structure can be imperative to help understand these issues as they pertain to injury prevention. A quick observational review or the use of more comprehensive parameters to assess how a dancer is built can help highlight areas of weakness, unbalanced strength, or joint hyper/hypomobility. The goal is to identify areas that may benefit from exercises or other interventions or to facilitate referral for further evaluation.

Any structural issue identified with a postural screen is likely to be more apparent when dance technique or functional movement is added. As the observation of posture is often subjective and relates more to evaluation than screening, it is often limited to looking for asymmetry in the spine with the Adams Forward Bend Test, a decreased or absent thoracic kyphosis and/or an increased lumbar lordosis (as observed with an anterior pelvic tilt). Generally, for efficiency, postural issues may be observed as part of functional testing, rather than a separate area on the screen.

### Cardiovascular Fitness

Screening tests for cardiovascular fitness vary according to the parameters assessed and how the information is applied. Research in this area has provided a better understanding of the physiologic demands of dancing. In general, dance is categorized as a high-intensity, intermittent form of exercise.[27] Cardiovascular testing in performance has shown that both the aerobic and anaerobic energy systems may be utilized, while dance classes seem to stimulate only the anaerobic system, producing energy bursts for 10–12 s.[28] If class has lower cardiovascular demands than performance, a dancer's aerobic fitness may not be adequate for the demands of repetitive rehearsals or performances, potentially leading to fatigue and injury.[29,30] Screening tests that assess cardiovascular health, fitness, and recovery can be very helpful in establishing a baseline and motivating dancers to perform supplemental cardiovascular cross-training.

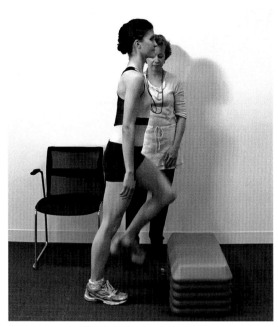

FIG. 12.1  3-Minute step test.

The accelerated 3-minute step test is used by many professional companies as a measure of cardiovascular fitness, as it is simple and quick to implement (Fig. 12.1, *step test*). In addition to other parameters, physical fitness is measured by the postexercise heart rate, considered to be an indicator of cardiorespiratory fitness. Bronner and Rakov have compared an accelerated 3-minute step test (112 beats/min) to the well-studied YMCA step test (96 beats/min) and a benchmark standard, the incremental treadmill test, using heart rate (HR) and oxygen consumption (VO2) as variables.[31] They have repeatedly found the accelerated 3-minute step test to be an efficient, acceptable tool for testing cardiac recovery in dance populations when compared to other validated testing.

There are many other screening tests that examine cardiovascular fitness, such as the dance-specific aerobic fitness test, that can be implemented when appropriate for the screening goals and if time and resources allow.[32,33]

### Range of Motion/Flexibility

Dancers generally work at the extremes of joint motion; many studies demonstrate greater range of motion than what is observed in the general population.[34,35] Most dancers will have greater than "normal" motion at most joints, therefore, when assessing range of motion, it is generally more helpful to screen for passive range of motion as it relates to flexibility. In the younger student population, screening for passive range of motion is imperative and can help establish if the dancer possesses enough flexibility to achieve proper technique, especially in a growing body. Some screens will actually measure range with a goniometer to track changes, but full measurements constitute an evaluation, not a screening. A screening that includes flexibility should only have yes or no answers when establishing if enough flexibility is present. Generally, when range of motion tests are performed to establish flexibility, they are done passively and stopped at the "first end feel," defined as the first onset of resistance or compensatory adjacent joint movement. In the professional dancer, assessing muscle tightness through passive range of motion is generally more helpful in an evaluation for a specific issue, rather than a screening. In general, deficits in range can often be noted through functional screening tests as well.

Owing to the extreme range of motion needed around the hips coupled with the need for lumbo-pelvic stability, flexibility in the hamstrings, iliopsoas, quadriceps, and Iliotibial band (ITB) are all significant to maintaining proper alignment and control. Screening for tightness of the iliopsoas with a Thomas test will reveal that most dancers are tight in the deep hip flexors, which can make it difficult to correct an anterior pelvic tilt, increase lumbar lordosis, place the lower abdominals in an inefficient position, and restrict the height of arabesque. The Ely test for quadriceps and the Ober test for the ITB also demonstrate tightness in this population. For efficiency, a modified Thomas test is generally used and the iliopsoas is considered tight if the hip cannot achieve 0° extension, the rectus femoris tight if the knee is not at 90° passively, and the ITB tight if the hip remains abducted. Restrictions in hamstring and quadriceps flexibility have been identified as risk factors for injury in other athletic populations.[8] Hamstring length is often assessed with a passive straight leg raise. A dancer should possess >90° of passive hip flexion before the pelvis moves and generally it is expected that professional females have at least 120° of passive hip flexion with the straight leg test. Clinically, tightness in the hamstrings can contribute to anterior hip pain and pathology by effecting alignment and increased use of hip flexors overworking to increase the leg height against hamstring tightness.

Another area that is useful is screening passive range of motion for hip external and internal rotation, with the hip in extension, to establish baseline motion. Screening for motion in this area can indicate if a dancer is using all available motion. Internal rotation is often limited, as many professional-level dancers present with 10° or less of internal rotation. This also provides an opportunity to educate the dancer on the importance of incorporating internal rotation stretches and strengthening exercises to balance rotation around the hip joint. Lack of internal rotation can lead to various injuries in the lower back, SI joint, and hips. Also, screening for significant asymmetries in hip rotation is important, as many dancers will present with differences in range between their hips. Dancers will often force the less mobile side to meet the side with more range when turning out. It is actually safer to work to the lesser side instead.

Screening for tightness in the lower leg at the ankle and foot is also extremely important to assess for imbalance or lack of sufficient motion for proper technique. The most common injuries in dance are at the ankle, due to limitations in dorsiflexion or plantar flexion. Studies have shown that dorsiflexion range decreases with increasing dance experience and ability, while plantar flexion is observed to increase with enhanced dance proficiency.[35] Adequate ankle dorsiflexion is important to achieve proper demi-plié (hip and knee flexion with ankle dorsiflexion), allowing for proper shock absorption in both preparation and recovery for jumps and turns.[36] To more accurately reflect the available range of motion necessary during functional activities, weight bearing measures such as the knee to wall test are recommended. This test has also been shown to be more reliable than measurements in non–weight bearing positions.[37,38]

### Hypermobility

It has been demonstrated in the literature that hypermobile dancers are at risk for increased injury,[39] and assessment for hypermobility is a key component in the screening of all dancers. Many practitioners who care for dancers have noted anecdotally that extreme hypermobility is more common at the professional level that it was 20 years ago. Joint hypermobility is a simple term that can include a number of etiologies for excessive joint movement. It may be related to bone structure, such as in shallow joint sockets, the result of changes in collagen of joint capsules and ligaments, or neuropathic differences resulting in muscle weakness or reduced joint proprioception.[40] Excessive joint mobility may be due to a general benign tendency toward increased laxity of the ligaments or can indicate more serious conditions such as Ehlers-Danlos or Marfan syndromes.[40] It is estimated that 44% of dancers present with some type of joint hypermobility, depending on the screening tool that is used.[38] Most

commonly, the 9-point Beighton Assessment of Hypermobility is used as it is a quick screen. A dancer is considered hypermobile if the Beighton score is 5/9 or greater. Higher scores should be referred for physical therapy and further medical evaluation as indicated.[39] Some studies are also finding that dancers with low Beighton scores, in the 0–2 range, are also more susceptible to injury. Bronner and Bauer found that dancers with low (0–2) and high (5–9) Beighton scores were 1.5 times more likely to sustain time loss injuries as those with medium scores (3,4).[8] This is definitely an area for further study to better understand the impact that joint stiffness and laxity can both have on injury.

Hypermobile dancers must be educated on the need to increase strength and stability to reduce shearing forces at their joints. The hypermobile dancer will frequently complain of feeling tightness. Their muscles may be quite tight as they are working harder just to maintain postural stability and control at looser joints which lack adequate passive restraint of the ligaments. Screening for hypermobility offers the opportunity to facilitate referral to a physical therapist who will teach her or him how to safely release stiffness in the muscles, and how to avoid pushing into extreme ranges of motion where they are more likely to be overstretching already loose and compromised joint ligaments and capsules. Attention to promoting stability around the joints is paramount to help the hypermobile dancer avoid injury.

### Strength

Methods for evaluating strength objectively in a quick screen are often debated. In dancers, it is most important to examine dynamic strength through the full range of motion, as they generally need the most power at the end range when the muscle is in its most contracted state. For example, the external rotators of the hip need to be very strong at their shortest end range, which is not typical for the strength-tension relationship of muscle. The current standard for muscle strength assessment is the manual muscle testing method, using a 5-point grading scale.[41] The reliability and accuracy of manual muscle testing is often called into question in the literature, even though it has been a clinically useful tool for many years. In most research today, isometric handheld dynamometers are often utilized and have been shown to have good reliability across varied patient populations.[42,43] However, they are expensive and can only assess strength at one joint angle administered as a break test, rather than through the entire range of motion. Break testing may miss areas of weakness through the range of motion in a dancer at the professional level. In addition, the strength and angle of the tester are parameters that can affect reliability and validity. The gold standard of muscle testing includes isokinetic dynamometers such as a Cybex or BioEx and is not practical or affordable for a screen. Until newer devices such as the IRL handheld dynamometer,[44] which measures dynamic strength, are more affordable and accessible, manual muscle testing may need to suffice for a standardized screening in the professional dance population. With screening, a grade lower than 5/5 should be considered a positive result, and manual muscle testing needs to be performed through the full and available range of motion. Asymmetry and side-to-side differences in strength should be noted. Deficits between sides that are greater than 10% have been shown to be a risk factor for injury. Asymmetry in strength between sides may be found to be a more important indicator of risk for injury than general weakness, and for reliability and accuracy the handheld dynamometer may be needed.

Poor core stability and inadequate neuromuscular control have been identified as risk factors for both upper and lower extremity injury in athletes. Assessing core strength and pelvic stability through both muscle and functional testing is arguably the most important aspect of any screening process. Proximal control of the hip and trunk are important indicators of lower extremity stability, as a dancer needs to be able to control his or her center of gravity over a small base of support. Testing should focus on strength and recruitment of the transversus abdominis and lower abdominal area, as some professional dancers are surprisingly weak in these muscles. The gold standard for testing lower abdominal strength is the Kendall and Kendall double leg lowering test, but its reliability has been called into question.[45] It is imperative that this test be done correctly and that dancers know it is a test and not an exercise. Holding a plank or side planks for more than 2 min can also be used as a strength and endurance test for the core muscles.

Screening for strength at the hip can be instrumental in identifying areas of potential risk factors for injury. Athletes with weak hip abductors and hip external rotator muscles have been shown to be more likely to sustain an ankle injury during a sports season.[46] Side-to-side difference in strength has also been shown to be a risk factor for injury. Female athletes with self-reported low back pain had greater side-to-side differences in proximal hip muscular strength than healthy females.[47,48] Weakness in the hip abductors and adductors can be screened with functional testing such as the step down test or Trendelenburg test. Testing hip

external rotation strength provides the opportunity to compare active to passive turnout range. In addition, many lower extremity injuries have been shown to be related to a lack of external rotator strength, in particular patellofemoral pain syndromes.[49,50]

## Balance
The ability to control balance during activity is critical to prevent lower extremity injury. Screening for postural control and balance can be an efficient way to discover areas of weakness, lack of range of motion, and decreased proprioception. Impaired balance is a risk factor for traumatic ankle sprains and non−contact ACL injuries.[51,52] The ability to control balance during activity has been shown to be critical in prevention of lower extremity injury.[52,53] Testing can also help the practitioner detect residual deficits that remain following a previous injury. Balance consists of the visual system, the vestibular system, and the somatosensory system, which includes touch, nociception, and proprioception. Screening to evaluate balance can involve decreasing the input of one system, such as vision in the single leg stance with eyes closed. In the professional dancer a, single leg balance test with eyes closed for 60 s is the gold standard.[52] Screening with a movement-based test, such as the Star Excursion Test, is often used to test dynamic balance.

## Functional Testing
The use of functional tests can be an efficient way to evaluate flexibility, strength, balance, and technique. Functional testing can help establish a baseline, as a measure to allow for return to dance, or an indicator that progression during rehabilitation is appropriate to more vigorous dancing such as jumping. Many functional tests evaluate whole body mechanics and motor control using regionally interdependent musculoskeletal relationships and observation models. The premise of this approach is that dysfunctional movement patterns and poor alignment in nearby joints can lead to musculoskeletal disorders and injury. The regional interdependence theory suggests the need to address not only the injured area but also proximal and distal deficits that may increase risk for subsequent injury.[10] Generally, functional testing for dancers is performed in parallel positions, as the goal is to identify deviations from functional movement patterns that are common in an anatomic neutral position. In addition, ballet dancers at least are more accustomed to standing in a turned out position so compensation patterns can be more obvious in a parallel position as it is less familiar.

The majority of injuries arises from cumulative microtrauma and is therefore multifactorial due to chronic joint position faults and muscle imbalances that result from training. Motor control screening tests such as shifting weight from two legs to one, limb dissociation from the trunk in a single leg stance, and developmental sequences that start in quadruped or kneeling and progress to high kneeling, to half kneeling, to single leg balance have been shown to be useful in identifying areas of poor core control and adaptations to suboptimal strength or flexibility.[10] Each stage in this progression is dependent upon successful sensory-motor integration, appropriate weight shifts, and limb dissociation from a stable trunk. Zazulak (2007) has correlated an inability to sustain neutral trunk position to athletic injury, as a neutral pelvis is important for optimizing lumbosacral and hip joint motions during dance activities to reduce compression and force on spinal and joint tissues. Skilled acquisition of motor control is essential for safe participation as the demands of choreography generally require shifting bases of support and center of mass levels in varying ways and speeds while interacting with other dancers, lights, costumes, and shoe wear.[10]

The single leg step-down test, performed in parallel off an 8″ step to the depth of the dancer's deepest plié, can be an efficient way to screen for neuromuscular control (Fig. 12.2A). Observing five repetitions of this test with attention to pelvic alignment, excessive hip adduction or internal rotation, knee valgus, and foot pronation can identify risks for injury that need to be addressed with physical therapy intervention and conditioning to avoid future issues.[54] (Fig. 12.2A–C).

The airplane test is another functional measure that is often included to screen for neuromuscular control.[54] (Fig. 12.3). The triplanar nature and combined dynamic movement of this test allows for quick assessment of cervical stability, lumbopelvic control, ability to maintain lower limb alignment, and compensations at the ankle and foot. Horizontal positioning of the trunk and visual field demands significant control of multiple planes of motion during a plié with the long lever arm of the trunk and leg in the sagittal plane therefore testing fundamental, dance specific technique demands.

### Technique

Assessing technique as part of a screening is also a form of functional testing. While it is generally the most subjective aspect of the screen, it can yield important information regarding areas that need to be addressed to prevent injury. However, at the professional level, technique analysis may be more appropriate for evaluation

and analysis of regional interdependent factors than in a quick screen. Risk of injury is certainly increased when any step is performed with suboptimal recruitment of muscles or poor alignment. Often compensations seen in professional dancers are well-established motor control patterns that are very subjective and can be difficult to discern. Studies in younger dancers have examined pelvic and knee alignment in specific dance steps such as single leg plié and single leg jumps and found a correlation between poor alignment and increased risk for overuse injury.

One test often used in professional dancers and students is the Single-leg Sauté Test. It consists of 16 consecutive single-leg jumps with the legs externally rotated in a turned out position. Successful execution requires maintaining a neutral pelvis with an upright, stable trunk and neutral lower extremity alignment, along with toe-heel landing each repetition with a fully extended knee and pointed foot when in the air. The pass criterion is defined as demonstrating proper execution of at least 8 of the 16 jumps. This test is challenging and can demonstrate a number of compensations to be further evaluated with physical therapy.

As previously mentioned, the tests and measurements selected for any tool screen will depend on the type, level, and setting for professional dancers, but working with a standardized screen across the professional dance population is preferable. Many of the screening tests discussed are included in the Dance/USA Task Force on Dancer Health screen, which was specifically developed for professional level dancers with a company setting and constraints in mind. The Task Force on Dancer Health is consistently working to change the screen based on current evidence-based practice and literature, along with the experience of the companies using the screen.

## RECOMMENDATIONS

Providing timely feedback for dancers on the results of the screen significantly affects the success of the program. Elite athletes need to have a good understanding of their own strengths and weaknesses. Discussion of results should be handled carefully and delivered positively, sensitively, and without judgment. The focus of recommendations should be on enhancing ability, rather than an obstacle to performance or a greater risk of injury. Also, feedback should emphasize that the goal of any exercises recommended is to improve their dance technique and overall health.

It should be recognized that recommendations from a screen are designed to raise "red flags," so referral to

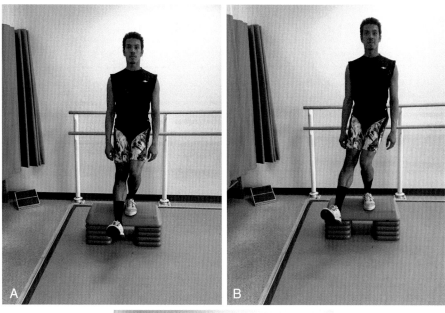

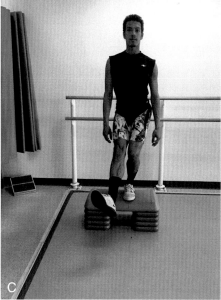

FIG. 12.2 Proper alignment and movement dysfunctions with step down test. **(A)** Proper alignment. **(B)** Left knee valgus collapse. **(C)** Positive Trendelenburg (hip drop).

appropriate practitioners can be made as indicated. As part of the planning process, it is important to identify a group of practitioners in the community that can be helpful in dealing with areas of risk noted with the screening. From the health history section, there may be issues identified that should be further addressed by the primary care physician or a sports medicine specialist (preferably with experience in dance). Depending on the response, referral to a sports psychologist or nutritionist may be warranted. Frequently, the physical assessment may identify areas to be addressed with an additional comprehensive physical therapy evaluation and treatment. Providing exercises and concrete suggestions for improvement is important to begin

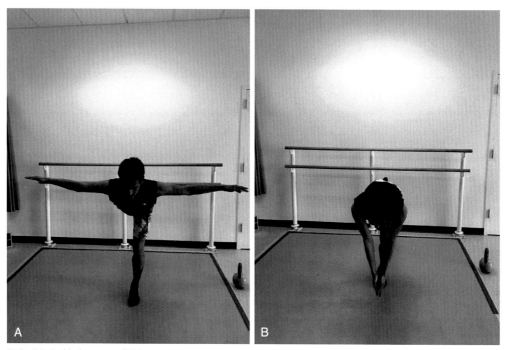

FIG. 12.3  Airplane test. **(A)** Proper alignment of leg extended and arms in second. **(B)** Proper alignment into plié with arms coming down and together.

addressing any physical issues regarding flexibility, strength, or balance immediately.

## SCREENING POTENTIAL FOR RESEARCH

Ideally, a standardized screen will enable the dance medicine community to identify and understand the various attributes necessary for optimal function and safety of professional dancers. To truly establish the value of identifying characteristics in dancers thought to be risk factors for injury, a comprehensive and standardized injury tracking system also needs to be established. Screening tools need to be adaptable and change as research evolves. As more evidence-based work is produced in dance and sports medicine, changes are proposed for validated tests and measures that are shown to explore a musculoskeletal issue more accurately. Research promotes adaptations in sports screening tests to make them more specific to dancers. Currently the literature does not identify any data to support one specific screen or to establish the best practices for risk factor identification.[5] Many potential benefits have been discussed, and if one injury is prevented or a single life-threatening situation such as an eating disorder is discovered, all the efforts are validated.

## CONCLUSION

Either a comprehensive screen or a simple health history questionnaire can be effective as an initial step in understanding a dancer's strengths and weaknesses to provide education and recommendations to both reduce injury and maximize a dancer's capabilities. It has been well established that screening programs are most effective when coupled with ongoing educational programs and interventions.[13] It is evident that screening will continue to be a significant area for study and research, especially if the intrinsic factors that include health history, psychologic influences, and physical attributes identified can be linked to the prevention of future injuries.

## REFERENCES

1. Junck E, Richardson M, Dilgen F, Liederbach MJ. A retrospective assessment of return to function in dance after physical therapy for common dance injuries. *J Dance Med Sci.* 2017;21(4):156–167.
2. Gamboa J, Roberts L, Fergus M. Injury patterns in elite pre-professional ballet dancers and the utility of screening programs to identify risk characteristics. *J Orthop Sports Phys Ther.* 2008;38:126–136.

3. Liederbach MJ. Screening for functional capacity in dancers: designing standardized, dance-specific injury prevention screening tools. *J Dance Med Sci.* 1997;1(3):93–106.

4. Hamilton L, Hamitlon W, Meltzer J, et al. Personality, stress and injuries in professional dancers. *Am J Sports Med.* 1989;17(2):263–267.

5. Sanders B, Blackburn T, Boucher B. Clinical commentary: pre-participation screening the sports physical therapy perspective. *Int J Sports Phys Ther.* 2013;8(2):180–193.

6. Bronner S, Ojofeitimi S, Rose D. Injuries in a modern dance company: effect of comprehensive management on injury incidence and time loss. *Am J Sports Med.* 2003; 31:365–373.

7. Solomon R, Solomon J, Micheli LJ, McGray E. The cost of injuries in a professional ballet company: a five-year study. *Med Probl Perform Art.* 1999;14:164–169.

8. Bronner S, Bauer N. Risk factors for muscluloskeletal injury in elite pre-professional modern dancers: a prospective cohort prognostic study. *Phys Ther Sport.* 2018;31:42–51.

9. Lai R, Krasnow D, Thomas M. Communication between medical practitioners and dancers. *J Dance Med Sci.* 2008; 12(2):47–53.

10. Liederbach MJ. Perspectives on dance science rehabilitation, understanding whole body mechanics and four key principles of motor control as a basis for healthy movement. *J Dance Med Sci.* 2010;14(3):114–124.

11. Wadell G, Newton M, Henderson I, et al. A fear avoidance beliefs questionnaire (FABQ) and the role of fear—avoidance beliefs in chronic low back pain and disability. *Pain.* 1993;52:157–168.

12. Potter K, Galbraith G, Baas J. Screening for improved dance function. *IADMS Bull Teach.* 2011;3(1):14–17.

13. Clark T, Gupta A, Chester H. Developing a dancer wellness program employing developmental evaluation. *Front Psychol.* 2014;5:731.

14. Van Camp S. Sudden death in athletes. In: Grana WA, Lombardo JA, eds. *Advances in Sports Medicine and Fitness.* Chicago: Year Book Medical Publishers; 1988:121–142.

15. Riebe D, Franklin B, Thompson P, et al. Updating ACSM's recommendations for exercise pre-participation health screening. *Med Sci Sports Exerc.* 2015;47(11):2473–2479.

16. Pre-Participation Screening. https://www.aap.org/en-us/professionalresources/practice-support/Documents/Preparticipation-Physical-Exam-Form.pdf.

17. Benson CA, Kessler HA. Update: Epstein-Barr virus-related disease. *Compri Ther.* 1988;14:58–64.

18. Brinkman R, Evans T. History of ankle sprain as a risk factor of future lateral ankle sprain in athletes. *J Sport Rehabil.* 2011;20(3):384–388.

19. Liederbach MJ, Compagno JM. Psychological aspects of fatigue related injuries in dancers. *J Dance Med Sci.* 2001; 5(4):116–120.

20. Mainwaring L, Krasnow D, Kerr G. And the dance goes on: psychological impact of injury. *J Dance Med Sci.* 2001;5(4): 105–115.

21. Hamilton LH, Solomon R, Solomon J. A proposal for standardized psychological screening of dancers. *J Dance Med Sci.* 2006;10:40–45.

22. Adam MU, Brassington GS, Matheson GO, Steiner H. Psychological factors associated with performance-limiting injuries in professional ballet dancers. *J Dance Med Sci.* 2004;8(2):43–46.

23. Mainwaring L, Finney C. Psychological risk factors and outcomes of dance injury: a systematic review. *J Dance Med Sci.* 2017;21(3):87–96.

24. Stokic E, Srdic B, Barak O. Body mass index, body fat mass and the occurrence of amenorrhea in ballet dancers. *Gynecol Endocrinol.* 2005;20(4):195–199.

25. Micheli L, Cassella M, Faigenbaum A, Southwick H, Ho V. Pre-season to post-season changes in body composition of professional ballet dancers. *J Dance Med Sci.* 2005;9(2): 56–59.

26. Howse J, McCormack M. *Dance Technique and Injury Prevention.* 3rd ed. London: A & C Black Publishers; 2000.

27. Wyon M, Redding E. Physiological monitoring of cardiorespiratory adaptations during rehearsal and performance of contemporary dance. *J Strength Cond Res.* 2005;19(3): 611–614.

28. Wyon M, Redding E, Head A, Sharp C, Craig S. Oxygen uptake during modern dance class, rehearsal, and performance. *J Strength Cond Res.* 2004;18(4):646–649.

29. Liederbach M, Schanfein L, Kremenic I. What is known about the effect of fatigue on injury occurrence among dancers? *J Dance Med Sci.* 2013;17(3):101–108.

30. Wyon MA, Koutedakis Y. Muscular fatigue: considerations for dance. *J Dance Med Sci.* 2013;17(2):63–69.

31. Bronner SJ, Rakov S. An accelerated step test to assess dancer pre-season aerobic fitness. *J Dance Med Sci.* 2014; 18(1):12–21.

32. Wyon M, Redding E, Head A, Craig S. Development, reliability, and validity of a multistage dance specific aerobic fitness test (DAFT). *J Dance Med Sci.* 2003;7(3):80–84.

33. Redding E, Weler P, Ehrenberg D, et al. The development of a high intensity dance performance test. *J Dance Med Sci.* 2009;13(1):3–9.

34. Gannon LM, Bird HA. The quantification of joint laxity in dancers and gymnasts. *J Sports Sci.* 1999;17(9):743–750.

35. Russell JA, Kruse DW, Nevill AM, Koutedakis Y, Wyon MA. Measurement of the extreme ankle range of motion required by female ballet dancers. *Foot Ankle Spec.* 2010;3(6):324–330.

36. Dickson D, Hollman-Gage K, Ojofeitimi S, Bornner S. Comparison of functional ankle motion measures in modern dancers. *J Dance Med Sci.* 2012;16(3):116–125.

37. Konor M, Morton S, Eckerson J, Grindstaff T. Reliability of three measures of ankle dorsiflexion range of motion. *Int J Sports Phys Ther.* 2012;7(3):279–287.

38. Baurnbach S, Braunstein M, Seelinger F, Borgmann L, Polzer H. Ankle dorsiflexion: what is normal? Development of a decision pathway for diagnosing impaired ankle dorsiflexion and medical gastrocnemius tightness. *Arch Orthop Traum Su.* 2016;136(3):1203–1211.

39. Day H, Koutedakis Y, Wyon M. Hypermobility and dance: a review. *Int J Sports Med.* 2011;32(7):485–489.

40. Knight IA. *A Guide to Living with Hypermobility Syndrome; Bending without Breaking.* London: Kingsley Publishers; 2011:22–23.

41. Clarkson HM. *Musculoskeletal Assessment: Joint Range of Motion and Manual Muscle Strength*. Lippincott, Williams & Wilkins; 2000.
42. Andrews A. Hand-held dynamometry for measuring muscle strength. *J Hum Muscle Perf*. 1991;1:35–50.
43. Stark T, Walker B, Philips J, Fejer R, Beck R. Hand-held dynamometry correlation with the gold standard isokinetic dynometry: a systemic review. *Phys Med Rehab*. 2011;3(5):472–479.
44. Le-Ngoc L, Janssen J. Validity and reliability of a hand-held dynamometer for dynamic muscle strength assessment. In: *Rehabilitation Medicine*. Christchurch, New Zealand: In Tech; 2012:53–66.
45. Zannotti CM, Bohannon RW, Tiberio D, Dewberry MJ, Murray R. Kinematics of the double-leg-lowering test for abdominal muscle strength. *J Orthop Sports Phys Ther*. 2002;32(9):432–436.
46. Leetun DT, Ireland ML, Willson JD, Ballantyne BT, McClay I. Core stability measures as risk factors for lower extremity injury in athletes. *Med Sci Sports Exerc*. 2004; 36(6):926–934.
47. Bowerman E, Whatman C, Harris N, Bradshaw E. A review of the risk factors for lower extremity overuse injuries in young elite female ballet dancers. *J Dance Med Sci*. 2015; 19(2):51–56.
48. Jacobs C, Ulh T, Mattacola C, Shapiro R, Rayens W. Hip abductor function and lower extremity landing kinematics: sex differences. *J Athl Train*. 2007;42(1):76–83.
49. Dolak K, Silkman C, Medina McKeon J, Hosey R, Lattermann C. Hip strengthening prior to functional exercises reduces pain sooner than quadriceps strengthening in females with patellofemoral pain syndrome: a randomized clinical trial. *J Orthop Sports Phys Ther*. 2011;41(8): 560–570.
50. Khayambashi K, Mohammadkhani Z, Ghaznavi K, Lyle MA, Powers CM. The effects of isolated hip abductor and external rotator muscle strengthening on pain, health status, and hip strength in females with patellofemoral pain. *J Orthop Sports Phys Ther*. 2012;42(1):22–29.
51. Hertel J, Buckley WE, Denegar CR. Serial testing of postural control after acute lateral ankle sprain. *J Athl Train*. 2001; 36(4):363–368.
52. Richardson M, Leiderbach MJ, Sandow E. Functional criteria for assessing pointe readiness. *J Dance Med Sci*. 2010;14(3):6–7.
53. Hewett TE, Meyer GD, Ford KR, et al. Biomechanical measures of neuromuscular control and valgus loading of the knee predict anterior cruciate ligament injury risk in female athletes: a prospective study. *Am J Sports Med*. 2005; 33:492–501.
54. Park K, Cynn H, Choung S. Musculoskeletal predictors of movement quality for the forward step-down test in asymptomatic women. *J Orthop Sports Phys Ther*. 2013; 43(7):504–510.

## CHAPTER 13

# Bone Health of the Dancer

MEGHAN L. KEATING, MPAS, PA-C • ALLYSON L. PARZIALE, BS • KATHRYN E. ACKERMAN, MD, MPH

## INTRODUCTION

Many determinants of osteoporosis begin in childhood and adolescence, emphasizing the importance of optimizing bone health from a young age. Osteoporosis, a condition of fragile and weak bones, is predicted to cost over $25.3 billion annually by 2025.[1] Roughly, one in four men and one in two women over the age of 50 are at risk of breaking a bone due to the disease.[1,2] Participating in weight-bearing activities, such as dance, can aid in building strong and healthy bones.[3] Paradoxically, dancers are at risk for developing poor bone health. Many dancers undertake rigorous training routines beginning at a young age and are pressured to meet certain body ideals, heightening their risk for developing eating disorders (ED) or disordered eating (DE).[4] This combination of physical and mental stressors, coupled with low energy availability (EA), can lead to hormonal changes, resulting in low bone mineral density (BMD) and increased injury risk.[5] Thus, it is important to understand the relationships among physical activity, diet, the endocrine system, and bone health to improve clinical care for dancers. This chapter provides an overview of the epidemiology, clinical presentation, and current management of bone health in dancers.

## KEY DEFINITIONS

*Dual Energy X-ray Absorptiometry (DXA):* a standard research and clinical technology used to measure bone mineral content (BMC, in grams) and bone mineral density (BMD, in g/m$^2$) using two X-ray beams.[6]

*DXA Z-Score:* A measure of BMD that indicates the standard deviation compared to a gender- and age-matched control group. Z-scores are used for children, premenopausal women, and men <50 years of age.[7]

*DXA T-Score:* A measure of BMD that indicates the standard deviation compared to the mean for a young, healthy adult. T-scores are used for postmenopausal women and men ≥50 years of age.[7]

*Osteoporosis:* A condition of decreased BMD that is correlated to increased risk of fracture. In children and adolescents, it is defined as a Z-score ≤ −2.0 with a significant fracture history.[7] In postmenopausal women and men ≥50 years old, it is defined as a T-score ≤ −2.5.[7]

*Low Bone Density:* A Z-score between −1.0 and −2.0 in a young weight-bearing athlete or a T-score between −1.0 and −2.5 in a postmenopausal woman or man ≥50 years of age. The term "osteopenia" is used only for T-scores between −1 and −2.5 and not for young patients with low Z-scores.[7,8]

*Peak Bone Mass:* The amount of bone accrued by the time a stable skeletal state occurs during young adulthood. *Peak bone mass* is important for the concept of *peak bone strength*, which is characterized by bone mass, density, microarchitecture, microrepair mechanisms, and geometric properties that provide structural strength.[9]

*Energy Availability (EA):* The amount of energy consumed through diet that is left over for all other physiological functions after daily exercise.[10]

*Amenorrhea:* Absence of menstruation by the age of 15 years in those with normal secondary sexual characteristics (primary amenorrhea) or absence of menses ≥3 months in previously menstruating females (secondary amenorrhea).[11]

*Oligomenorrhea:* Fewer than nine menstrual cycles per year or cycle length greater than 35 days.[12]

*Female Athlete Triad:* A condition describing the interrelationship of EA, menstrual function, and BMD.[13]

*Relative Energy Deficiency in Sport (RED-S):* A syndrome describing the consequences of energy deficiency on exercise performance and physiological functioning in females and males, including (but not limited to) impairments to bone health, menstruation in women, and other aspects of the endocrine system.[14,15]

Performing Arts Medicine. https://doi.org/10.1016/B978-0-323-58182-0.00013-4

## BONE DEVELOPMENT AND RISK FACTORS FOR LOW BONE MINERAL DENSITY

Bone is a dynamic tissue composed of noncollagenous proteins, hydroxyapatite salts, and a matrix of collagen.[16] From birth to adulthood, bone mineral content (BMC) increases significantly and peak BMD is typically reached by the second or early 3rd decade of life, with minimal subsequent growth.[17] Nearly 40%−60% of adult BMD is attained during adolescence, with substantial gains occurring just after peak height velocity (PHV).[18,19] PHV, when the maximum rate of growth occurs, happens around age $11.5 \pm 1.8$ and $13.5 \pm 1.8$ years in American girls and boys, respectively.[20] During the lag time between PHV and peak bone mass accrual, there may be an increased vulnerability for bone fragility, possibly explaining the increased rate of forearm fractures seen in girls 8−12 years of age and boys around the age of 11 years.[21−23] By the age of 18, roughly 90% of peak bone mass has been accrued.[24]

Throughout life, the skeleton continues to undergo remodeling. The process of remodeling involves both bone formation and resorption, and the relative rates of these mechanisms change depending on factors such as nutrition, health status, and age.[25] During childhood and adolescence, bone formation must exceed resorption to build bone mass. Peak BMD and bone strength are achieved around age 30.[17] In females, bone mass is mostly maintained until menopause. During menopause, rapid bone loss occurs, and this loss gradually slows in the postmenopausal years.[26] In males, bone loss occurs gradually and later in life.[27] This decline in bone mass in both males and females contributes to increased risk of fracture in the elderly compared to younger populations.[28]

Over 9 million Americans are affected by osteoporosis with an additional 43.1 million having low bone density.[29] There is an inverse relationship between fracture risk and BMD at multiple measured sites, emphasizing the importance of building strong bones early in life.[30,31] Reaching adequate peak bone mass should be prioritized to optimize bone health, which can be achieved by addressing modifiable components of bone acquisition, including participation in weight-bearing exercise, eating well, and avoiding smoking. However, genetic determinants account for approximately 70% of the variation in bone mass; the various genes responsible for low BMD are poorly characterized.[32] For example, females whose mothers have a history of osteoporotic fractures are more likely to have lower BMD.[33,34] Sex influences bone growth potential, with males typically having greater BMD than

**TABLE 13.1**
**Factors Affecting Bone Mass[16]**

| |
|---|
| **Nonmodifiable** |
| Genetics |
| Gender |
| Ethnicity |
| **Modifiable** |
| Nutrition |
|   Calcium |
|    Vitamin D |
|    Sodium |
|    Protein |
| Soda |
| Exercise and lifestyle |
| Body weight and composition |
| Hormonal status |

females.[35] Ethnicity is a nonmodifiable risk factor; some differences include white- and Asian-Americans having lower BMD than black Americans.[36] Although much of a dancer's bone health is determined by his/her parents, it is important to address the modifiable factors. Table 13.1 lists various modifiable and nonmodifiable risk factors for low BMD.

## BUILDING AND MAINTAINING HEALTHY BONES THROUGH WEIGHT-BEARING EXERCISE

Participation in weight-bearing physical activity throughout childhood is a key component to building healthy bones.[3] Osteogenic effects are achieved when the activity provides significant impact loading to the skeleton, thus increasing bone formation and improving BMC.[37,38] Girls who begin strenuous exercise during prepubescence typically gain twice as much BMC compared to those who begin similar types of exercise after puberty.[39] Similar effects have also been observed in male populations: males (mean age: 18.9 years) who began participating in sports before the age of 13 had higher areal BMD, cortical bone size, and trabecular volumetric BMD.[40]

Weight-bearing athletes typically have 5%−30% higher BMD compared to nonathletes, and this improved BMD can translate to reduced fracture risk later in life.[41,42] Female and male adolescents who participate in high- or odd-impact loading activities, such as soccer, basketball, and volleyball, have significantly greater BMD compared to those who participate in nonimpact sports or who are sedentary.[43]

Residual skeletal benefits of competitive athletics, such as increased BMC and BMD, have been observed 20 years after retirement from competition.[44,45] Continued involvement in physical activity throughout the lifespan is recommended to maintain BMD/BMC, as the effects of historical weight-bearing physical activity diminish. Fracture risk over the age of 35 years has been shown to be lower in retired male athletes versus nonathletes (8.5% vs. 12.9%).[46]

Dance is considered a loaded physical activity that should provide adequate mechanical strain to achieve osteogenic benefit during development.[47] In a 3-year longitudinal study of female ballet dancers and controls ages 8–11 years at baseline, after controlling for maturation and growth, the dancers demonstrated higher BMC at the total body, lumbar spine, femoral neck, and lower limbs compared to normally active, nondancers.[48] Except for the femoral neck, these differences were first noted 1 year after PHV, the peri-pubertal years. At the femoral neck, the mean BMC difference between groups was more robust and noted earlier (4% and prepuberty). This difference was maintained through the study and attributed to beginning dance training prior to puberty.[48] The nondancers, however, had 4.5% greater BMC in the upper extremities compared to the dancers, supporting the concept that bone accrual is enhanced with site-specific loading and dancers may need to focus on more strength training with their arms.[48]

In a study of female preprofessional ballet dancers ages 15–18 years, mean bone mineral apparent density (BMAD, BMD adjusted for height) was 37% below the fifth percentile of reference data at the lumbar spine.[49] The dancers had significantly greater BMAD of the femoral neck compared to the mean of the reference population, again suggesting the long-term benefits of early training on the weight-bearing femoral neck and the need for cross-training and adequate nutrition to benefit the entire skeleton.[49]

Poor nutritional and other habits may mitigate osteogenic benefits of long-term dance. Site-specific BMD has been observed to be lower in professional dancers, with prevalence of low BMD at the lumbar spine ranging from 23% to 40%.[50,51] Prevalence of low BMD in other locations, including the radius (26.7 vs. 15.8%), hip (6.9 vs. 3.9%), and femoral neck (17.8% vs. 16.8%), is also higher in professional dancers versus controls.[52] Additionally, professional dancers who had

been retired on average 25.6 years demonstrated even higher prevalence of low BMD at any site (46.5% of dancers vs. 39.6% of controls).[52]

## THE FEMALE ATHLETE TRIAD AND RELATIVE ENERGY DEFICIENCY IN SPORT

The interrelationship of DE, amenorrhea, and osteoporosis was first noted in the late 1970s and 1980s.[53] In 1992, the American College of Sports Medicine introduced the term Female Athlete Triad (Triad) to describe of the interrelationship of these three entities.[54] Since its introduction, the definition of Triad has become more fluid and reflects an athlete's ability to experience each aspect of the Triad (now defined as EA, menstrual function, and BMD) at various points on three different spectra, depicted in Fig. 13.1.[55]

### Decreased Energy Availability

EA is defined as the energy remaining from dietary energy intake (EI) for physiological functioning after accounting for exercise energy expenditure (EEE).[10] In general, a daily EA ≥45 kcal/kg of fat free mass (FFM) is recommended to maintain healthy physiological functioning, but there are likely individual variations in energy needs.[10,13,14,56] Markers of bone mineralization and protein synthesis have been shown to be disrupted at EA <30 kcal/kg FFM/day.[57] Key micro- and macronutrients required for bone development can also be diminished, such as vitamin D, calcium, phosphorus, and protein.[58] Additionally, markers of other metabolic and reproductive changes can become apparent below 30 kcal/kg FFM/day.[10]

Both adolescent and professional dancers have been observed to consume less than 85% of the recommended daily allowance of calories.[59,60] This state of low EA may be inadvertent, or it can be due to ED/DE. In some cases, acute bouts of exercise stimulate hormones, such as peptide YY (PYY) and glucagon-like peptide 1 (GLP-1), involved in satiety and appetite regulation.[61] The resulting effect is a transient decrease in appetite that may lead to inadequate EI for the amount of energy expended.[61] Additionally, many athletes are unaware of their body's nutritional needs following vigorous training and unknowingly consume insufficient calories for refueling.

Dancers are at an increased risk for developing ED/DE due to the sport's emphasis on aesthetics and leanness.[62] Ballet dancers consistently weigh 10%–12% below ideal body weight.[63] Dancers can be affected by many types of EDs, including anorexia nervosa, bulimia

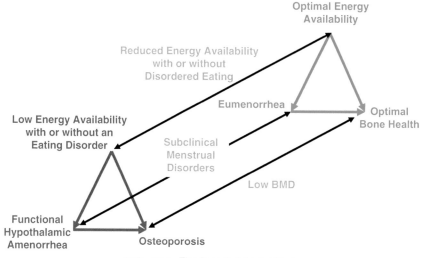

FIG. 13.1 The Female Athlete Triad.

nervosa, and other types of eating disorders listed in the Diagnostic and Statistical Manual of Mental Disorders, Fifth Edition (DSM-5).[64] Combined results from multiple dance studies have shown the prevalence of EDs to be approximately 12% of all dancers; ballet dancers have a slightly higher prevalence at 16.4%.[4] The pooled results from one meta-analysis found that dancers were three times more likely to suffer from EDs than non-dancers.[4] A study by Ringham, et al. found that 83% of professional dancers had a lifetime history of anorexia nervosa, bulimia nervosa, and/or other types of ED.[65]

## Amenorrhea

With persistently low EA, there is insufficient caloric and nutrient intake to maintain healthy physiological function. As the body allocates resources to the most vital systems needed for survival, the reproductive system becomes inhibited, leading to menstrual dysfunction. This is referred to as functional hypothalamic amenorrhea (FHA). FHA is caused by an interruption to the hypothalamic-pituitary-ovarian (HPO) axis and the hormones involved in the normal reproductive cycle.[66] When EA is inadequate, gonadotropin releasing hormone (GnRH) pulsatility is disrupted, inhibiting gonadotropin (FSH and LH) release. This minimizes the release of gonadal steroids, such as estrogen and progesterone.[66]

Menstrual dysfunction is common among dancers, with as many as 70% of professional dancers reporting some form of menstrual irregularity during their lifetime.[67] In one study, 36% of dancers stopped menstruating during times of increased activity with 30% of the same population experiencing a loss of menstruation for >3 months (secondary amenorrhea).[68] Delayed menarche (primary amenorrhea) is also common in dancers. A study examining menstrual patterns in 89 young professional dancer's reported 12% had not achieved menarche by $14.3 \pm 0.4$ years.[69] A negative correlation between body mass index and age of menarche has been strongly demonstrated in adolescent dancers.[68]

## Bone Effects of Low Energy Availability and Amenorrhea

Low EA and decreased estrogen have independent and interrelated negative effects on bone. Loucks et al. found that manipulating EA to < 30 kcal/kg FFM/day in normally menstruating women led to decreased protein synthesis and mineralization, decreased insulin (thus inhibiting amino acid uptake), decreased insulin-like growth factor 1 (IGF-1), and decreased triiodothyronine (T3), all within 5 days of the onset of energy deficiency and before a decrease in estrogen occurred.[10] Hormones associated with menstruation are extremely important to bone. Estrogen, in particular, is an important antiresorptive agent, especially at trabecular-rich bone, such as the lumbar spine. Higher mean estradiol levels in the first year postmenarche have been associated with stronger bones at skeletal maturity in young women while delayed menarche has been correlated with a lower BMD in adulthood.[17]

Devlin et al. applied hip structural analysis (HSA) to DXA results in a study of 84, healthy, 17 year-old girls, to estimate bone strength. Controlling for physical activity, girls with the highest tertile of estradiol levels during the first year after menarche had 5%–14% greater strength in the hip's femoral neck and intertrochanteric regions.[39]

Amenorrhea in athletes in the setting of low EA is also a marker for the disruption of many hormonal axes important for bone. In comparison to their eumenorrheic counterparts, such amenorrheic athletes have lower levels of leptin, T3, glucose, FSH, estradiol, progesterone, insulin, and a lower IGF-1/IGFBP-1 ratio (therefore less bioavailable IGF-1). They also have higher ghrelin and cortisol levels.[58]

Studies in exercisers, including dancers, have used DXA to measure BMD; peripheral quantitative CT (pQCT) and high resolution pQCT (HRpQCT) to measure bone cortical/trabecular geometry and microarchitecture, respectively; HSA and finite elemental analysis to assess bone strength; and bone markers to assess bone turnover. Such work has demonstrated independent and interactive negative effects of low EA, decreased estrogen status, and perturbations of various hormones and bone markers on bone density, quality, and strength.[70–72]

Importantly, later menarche and oligo/amenorrhea during adolescence are consistently associated with higher stress fracture incidence and lower lumbar spine BMD in dancers.[5,73,74] Such findings place dancers at high risk for career-altering injuries and severe, osteoporotic-related fractures later in life.

## Relative Energy Deficiency in Sport

In 2014, with continued research on energy deficiency in athletes, the International Olympic Committee defined a new syndrome, Relative Energy Deficiency in Sport (RED-S).[14] RED-S expands upon the Triad, suggesting other health and performance decrements associated with inadequate energy and also recognizes that male athletes can be affected. For example, using suppressed resting metabolic rate (RMR) as a surrogate for low EA, Staal et al. found that 25%–80% of male dancers have RED-S, depending on predicted RMR calculation methodology.[75] The RED-S model highlights various health and performance risks of low EA in various populations, while still incorporating the Triad concept. See Fig. 13.2.[14]

Both Triad and RED-S are highly prevalent in those who participate in sports where it is believed that having a low BMI improves performance, leanness is emphasized, or there are weight limits to participate.[13,14] Due to the high intensity activity associated with dance, as well as a desire and pressure to meet "body ideals," dancers often suffer from Triad/RED-S. Identifying when a dancer may be at risk for Triad or

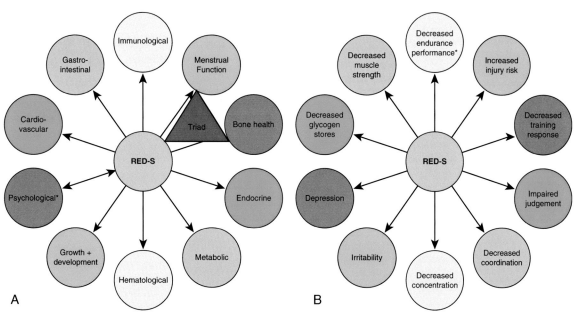

A

B

FIG. 13.2 Health and performance consequences of relative energy deficiency in sport. **(A)** Health consequences. **(B)** Performance consequences.

RED-S is critical to mitigate the long-term effects on bone, reproductive, and other aspects of health.

## DIAGNOSIS

Dancers should be screened for Triad/RED-S during their preparticipation physicals or annual health screens.[13] A dancer's height and weight should be measured at such medical appointments, and individual growth curves should be closely monitored for signs of abnormality. For those younger than 20, weight status should be determined by calculating expected body weight; otherwise, BMI for age cutoffs can be used.[55] If the dancer's growth no longer correlates with his/her prior growth trajectory, there should be a suspicion low EA.[15] Standardized growth charts for children and adolescents are provided by the CDC.[76]

Because aspects of both Triad and RED-S can present along a continuum, it is important to evaluate dancers further even if only one component is initially noted. Warning signs include a variety of musculoskeletal, cardiovascular, gastrointestinal, renal, and neuropsychiatric symptoms.[14] Clinical manifestations include, but are not limited to, ED, FHA, and low BMD.[55,77]

Obtaining a good medical history helps screen dancers for risk factors pertaining to low BMD and determine when interventions may be necessary. Fracture history—including both bone stress injuries (BSI) and traumatic fractures—is an important component of this history.[55,77] The site and cause of the BSI, as well as the age it occurred, aid in understanding the risk of the injury. Bone stress injuries of trabecular-rich bones, such as the femoral neck, have been associated with lower BMD.[78,79] This is potentially caused by the signaling effects of gonadal hormones, as estrogen has antiresorptive effects, particularly at trabecular-rich sites, that are diminished in instances of low EA.[79] If a stress injury occurs in a bone that is more trabecular-rich, such as the femoral neck, pelvis, or calcaneus, there may be increased concern that the dancer may have low BMD for age.[80] Additionally, amenorrheic athletes with a history of at least two BSI may have low BMD, and this clinical status may serve as a biomarker for bone health.[74]

A dancer may have other medical conditions that affect bone health. These conditions include celiac disease, hypothyroidism, delayed puberty (with sufficient nutrition), and gonadal failure. Even if a condition does not directly modulate bone health, the dancer could be treating the condition with a medication that affects bone. Chemotherapeutics, systemic glucocorticoids, and anticonvulsants can all be deleterious to bone.[81]

Reviewing the dancer's training volume and dietary history is essential in determining the dancer's energy requirements. Consultation with a sports dietitian to determine the dancer's energy needs is very helpful, especially if the dancer is a vegan, a vegetarian, or has any other dietary restrictions. Dietary restrictions place the dancer at a higher risk of energy deficiency. Medications, vitamins, and supplements should also be carefully reviewed as part of the comprehensive history, including calcium and vitamin D intake. Based on the dancer's intake, their calcium and vitamin D supplementation can be altered to maximize bone health.

Menstrual history is an important component of diagnosing Triad/RED-S. Age of menarche, number of menses in a year, and history of irregularity all contribute to understanding the ways an athlete's menstrual history could affect bone.[14,55] Combined oral contraceptive (COC) pills can result in menstruation even in the presence of energy deficiency. Despite the osteoprotective effects of *endogenous* estrogen, COCs do not have the same protective effect and are *not* recommended for bone protection in the case of FHA/Triad/RED-S.[66] Because COCs can cause normal menses, dancers with other signs of Triad/RED-S should be investigated for energy deficiency. Dancers using COCs and suspected of energy deficiency can stop taking the medication to determine if they will menstruate naturally. Importantly, other forms of contraception, such as hormone-containing intrauterine devices (IUD), can cause menstrual dysfunction in otherwise healthy dancers.

As previously mentioned, bone health is significantly determined by genetics. Thus, family history should also be considered when treating a dancer for poor bone health. Family history of osteoporosis, ED/DE, thyroid disorders, and malabsorption disorders can all be relevant to the practitioner. Armed with this history, the clinician can better investigate other possible causes of low bone density, such as hypothyroidism or celiac disease.

## MEDICAL TESTING
### Bone Density Measurement

DXA is recognized as the gold standard for measuring BMD.[74] DXA scans analyze different areas of the body, such as the hip, spine, radius, and whole body, and measure BMD and body composition.[82] In patients 19 years or younger, the total body less head and lumbar spine are the recommended sites for measuring bone density.[7] In patients over the age of 19, the lumbar spine, total hip, and femoral neck are the recommended sites of BMD measurement.[7] DXA reports include BMC, BMD, Z-scores, and T-scores (only in older populations) as measures of bone health. The standards for use of each measure in different populations are reviewed in the **Definitions** section.

## Lab Testing

Depending on the indications, laboratory testing may vary. Serum 25-OH vitamin D is a useful measure for those with poor bone health, particularly because vitamin D supplementation is cheap and effective. A complete blood count (CBC), total iron binding capacity (TIBC), serum ferritin, and total iron measurements collectively inform iron deficiency or anemia status. If vitamin D or iron levels are low, screening for malabsorptive disorders, such as celiac disease, may be indicated. A comprehensive metabolic panel (CMP), which includes calcium and liver function tests, should be ordered to evaluate for electrolyte and liver abnormalities. Adding phosphorus, magnesium, and parathyroid hormone levels will also inform the practitioner about bone metabolism. Thyroid pathology can be assessed by measuring TSH levels (along with free T4 only if there is concern for a pituitary abnormality). ESR and CRP may be added to rule out inflammatory processes. If a dancer has low bone density, spot urine calcium and creatinine or a 24-h urine calcium and creatinine collection can determine if the dancer is excreting excess calcium in the urine and also screen for familial hypocalciuric hypercalcemia.[66,83]

Given the importance of estrogen on bone, immediately testing reproductive hormone levels is tempting. However, if the dancer is low weight and amenorrheic, she should be somewhat weight-restored and have not used COCs for at least 6 weeks before measuring hormone levels. At that point, lab measurements to determine the cause of amenorrhea are more useful. A urine pregnancy test, FSH, LH, estradiol, and prolactin can all help to assess a brain (hypothalamus/pituitary) versus ovarian process. If the prolactin level comes back high, a thorough review of the patient's medications should be undertaken, as many increase prolactin. After this, a repeat prolactin and possibly a pituitary-dedicated brain MRI should be ordered to evaluate for a pituitary tumor (e.g., prolactinoma). If a growth abnormality is suspected, in addition to the amenorrhea, IGF-1 levels help to screen for acromegaly and growth hormone deficiency.[66,83]

Athletes are not less susceptible to polycystic ovary syndrome (PCOS) than nonathletes. Often menstrual dysfunction in athletes of normal weight can be explained by PCOS rather than hypothalamic amenorrhea.[81] If PCOS is suspected, total testosterone, free testosterone, sex hormone binding globulin, DHEAS, and 8 a.m. 17-OH progesterone should be measured. A pelvic ultrasound or other abdominal imaging may be useful depending on results.[66,83]

Significant weight loss or low BMI can cause stress on the heart. If a dancer has a very low BMI for age, it is important to further assess for medical stability.[66] The practitioner should obtain orthostatic vital signs in the office. If the dancer is bradycardic or orthostatic on examination, an electrocardiogram should be performed and a higher level of care (e.g., hospital admission) should be strongly considered.

## TREATMENT

There are different approaches to treating bone health in dancers depending on the etiology.

Treatment for Triad/RED-S is best approached using an interdisciplinary team.[84] This team should include a physician, dietitian, and for those dancers struggling with an ED or significant DE, a mental health professional.[13] Increasing the dancer's BMI and EA to restore normal gonadal steroids and other hormone levels are the principle goals when treating Triad/RED-S. This can be achieved by increasing energy intake through dietary changes, decreasing the caloric expenditure from physical activity (dance and other activities), or a combination. A dietitian may lead this intervention and nutritional counseling and monitoring may be enough to increase EA. Often, minor changes, such as increasing caloric intake by 20%–30% over baseline energy requirements or decreasing exercise by 10%–20%, are sufficient to increase EA.[55] When this intervention fails, such as in the setting of severe ED, counseling with a mental health professional, abstinence from dance to undergo more intensive treatment, close medical monitoring, and possible inpatient treatment may be required.

In addition to increasing EA, optimization of calcium and vitamin D (and other micronutrient) intake is important for bone health. Many adolescents do not consume enough calcium to support healthy bones. Children and adolescents ≤18 years should consume 1300 mg of calcium per day and adults 19 years old to menopause (or until age 50 in men) should consume 1000 mg of calcium per day.[85] Calcium intake should be divided throughout the day because only 500 mg of calcium can be absorbed at a time.[86] Although it is best for adolescents to get calcium through their diet, supplementation may be required to reach the recommended daily allowance, particularly in the setting of lactose intolerance.

Daily vitamin D intake should be at least 600—800 IU, although keeping blood levels of 25(OH) vitamin D $\geq$ 30 ng/mL (a level considered to optimize PTH levels and calcium absorption) frequently requires higher maintenance therapy (e.g., 1000 + IU/day).[87] Vitamin D consumption is often inadequate in the diet and may require supplementation. If the dancer is vitamin D deficient on diagnostic testing, much higher vitamin D intake may temporarily be needed. Such a regimen includes a prescription dose of 50,000 IU of vitamin D to be taken once weekly for 6 weeks followed by daily maintenance therapy.[87]

Normalization of menses may lag several months behind energy repletion. Menstrual function typically will not be restored until weight is maintained at a BMI of greater than 18.5.[55,88] Athletes often require an even higher weight to restore menstrual function due to differences in body composition, including more lean mass, than nonathletes.

If a patient is normal weight but not menstruating regularly, a progesterone challenge test can be administered to induce withdrawal bleeding and confirm that the outflow tract is patent. Such regimens include 10 mg of medroxyprogesterone daily for 10 days.

Patients with a healthy BMI who have undergone nutritional and psychological counseling, but still do not have a return of spontaneous menstruation, may benefit from short-term use of transdermal estrogen therapy with cyclic oral progesterone for bone health.[66] Studies involving adolescents with anorexia nervosa and young athletes with oligo-amenorrhea have demonstrated that transdermal estrogen + cyclic oral progesterone improves BMD at 6 months, with continued gains at 12 or more months.[89,90] Such a delivery method of estrogen has also proven superior to COC treatment for bone health.[90] This may be due to the differing effect of transdermal estrogen and COCs on IGF-1. IGF-1 is important for bone formation and remodeling. Oral contraceptive pills decrease IGF-1 systemically while transdermal estrogen maintains and may even increase levels of IGF-1, further promoting bone mineralization.[89,90]

The use of bisphosphonates is not recommended to increase BMD in premenopausal women due to the potential teratogenicity of the medication.[55] Bisphosphonates can be used with caution under the strict supervision of an endocrinologist, although this is not typical practice. Bisphosphonates have a prolonged terminal half-life of 10 years, with teratogenic risk therefore lasting a decade following use.[91]

Bone density interventions require long-term follow-up. The bone remodeling process takes approximately 3—6 months.[92] For this reason, any treatment for low BMD is typically conducted for at least 6—12 months with DXA monitoring no sooner than 6 months.[13]

## PROGNOSIS

Dancers who have low BMD for their age during adolescence are still able to improve BMD if caught early. Small changes in BMD translate into large reductions in fracture risk.[92] If dancers with Triad/RED-S continue to exhibit ED/DE behaviors and do not increase their EA until their mid-20s or beyond, then they are unlikely to ever reach optimal peak bone mass and will be at an increased risk of osteoporosis as adults. The dancers will be at a significantly higher risk of developing BSI and osteoporotic-related fractures that may significantly curtail their dancing career.[74] Thus, early education and behavior modification are critical.

## PREVENTION

The best strategy to optimize bone health is to take preventative measures against the development of conditions that reduce BMD. Maximizing bone accrual in adolescence and young adulthood sets the dancer on the path to a lifetime of healthy bones. Many of the conditions that are harmful to bone, such as amenorrhea, are born from a mismatch between energy intake and exercise energy expenditure. Prevention of low EA is a team effort involving coaches, trainers, parents, and athletes. Dancers should be educated on the risks of inadequate EA and meet with sports dietitians to ensure their dietary habits can support their training programs. Should a problem be detected, swift treatment can allow the dancer to miss minimal time, and dancers should be encouraged to share their medical concerns and seek treatment.

## CONCLUSIONS

Although dancers participate in a significant amount of weight-bearing exercise, other modifiable risk factors associated with dance increase their susceptibility for impaired bone health. Preventing Triad/RED-S, including avoiding a delay in menarche, maintaining normal menstrual function, and optimizing EA, enhances bone growth potential during adolescence. Education on the importance of developing strong bones through adequate nutrition and awareness of Triad/RED-S warning signs should be provided to dancers, their families, and instructors. Additionally, emphasis should be placed on promoting healthy ideals about body image to further prevent the development of Triad/RED-S. Healthy habits need to be started at the beginning of a dancer's training and maintained throughout the dancer's career to optimize bone health during the performing years and beyond.

# REFERENCES

1. Burge R, Dawson-Hughes B, Solomon DH, Wong JB, King A, Tosteson A. Incidence and economic burden of osteoporosis-related fractures in the United States, 2005-2025. *J Bone Miner Res.* 2007;22(3):465−475.
2. Bone Health, Osteoporosis: A Report of the Surgeon General. Reports of the Surgeon General. Rockville, MD; 2004.
3. Behringer M, Gruetzner S, McCourt M, Mester J. Effects of weight-bearing activities on bone mineral content and density in children and adolescents: a meta-analysis. *J Bone Miner Res.* 2014;29(2):467−478.
4. Arcelus J, Witcomb GL, Mitchell A. Prevalence of eating disorders amongst dancers: a systemic review and meta-analysis. *Eur Eat Disord Rev.* 2014;22(2):92−101.
5. Warren MP, Brooks-Gunn J, Fox RP, Holderness CC, Hyle EP, Hamilton WG. Osteopenia in exercise-associated amenorrhea using ballet dancers as a model: a longitudinal study. *J Clin Endocrinol Metab.* 2002;87(7):3162−3168.
6. Laskey MA. Dual-energy X-ray absorptiometry and body composition. *Nutrition.* 1996;12(1):45−51.
7. 2013 ISCD Combined Official Positions. *International Society for Clinical Densitometry.* 2014.
8. Nattiv A, Loucks AB, Manore MM, Sanborn CF, Sundgot-Borgen J, Warren MP. The female athlete triad position stand American Collegue of sports medicine. *Med Sci Sport Exerc.* 2007;39(10):1867−1882.
9. Weaver CM, Gordon CM, Janz KF, et al. The National Osteoporosis Foundation's position statement on peak bone mass development and lifestyle factors: a systematic review and implementation recommendations. *Osteoporos Int.* 2016;27(4):1281−1386.
10. Loucks AB, Kiens B, Wright HH. Energy availability in athletes. *J Sports Sci.* 2011;29(suppl 1):S7−S15.
11. Practice Committee of American Society for Reproductive Medicine. Current evaluation of amenorrhea. *Fertil Steril.* 2008;90(suppl 5):S219−S225.
12. Longe JL. The Gale Encyclopedia of Medicine. 5th ed. 9 volumes p.
13. Nattiv A, Loucks AB, Manore MM, et al. American College of Sports Medicine position stand. The female athlete triad. *Med Sci Sports Exerc.* 2007;39(10):1867−1882.
14. Mountjoy M, Sundgot-Borgen J, Burke L, et al. The IOC consensus statement: beyond the female athlete triad−relative energy deficiency in sport (RED-S). *Br J Sports Med.* 2014;48(7):491−497.
15. Mountjoy M, Sundgot-Borgen JK, Burke LM, et al. IOC author consensus statement update 2018: relative Energy Deficiency in Sport (RED-S). *Br J Sports Med.* 2018; 52(11):687−697.
16. Golden NH, Abrams SA, Co N. Optimizing bone health in children and adolescents. *Pediatrics.* 2014;134(4): e1229−e1243.
17. Baxter-Jones AD, Faulkner RA, Forwood MR, Mirwald RL, Bailey DA. Bone mineral accrual from 8 to 30 years of age: an estimation of peak bone mass. *J Bone Miner Res.* 2011;26(8):1729−1739.
18. Bailey DA. The saskatchewan pediatric bone mineral accrual study: bone mineral acquisition during the growing years. *Int J Sports Med.* 1997;18(suppl 3): S191−S194.
19. Faulkner RA, Bailey DA, Drinkwater DT, Wilkinson AA, Houston CS, McKay HA. Regional and total body bone mineral content, bone mineral density, and total body tissue composition in children 8-16 years of age. *Calcif Tissue Int.* 1993;53(1):7−12.
20. Tanner JM, Davies PS. Clinical longitudinal standards for height and height velocity for North American children. *J Pediatr.* 1985;107(3):317−329.
21. Khosla S, Melton 3rd LJ, Dekutoski MB, Achenbach SJ, Oberg AL, Riggs BL. Incidence of childhood distal forearm fractures over 30 years: a population-based study. *JAMA.* 2003;290(11):1479−1485.
22. Faulkner RA, Davison KS, Bailey DA, Mirwald RL, Baxter-Jones AD. Size-corrected BMD decreases during peak linear growth: implications for fracture incidence during adolescence. *J Bone Miner Res.* 2006;21(12): 1864−1870.
23. Hedstrom EM, Svensson O, Bergstrom U, Michno P. Epidemiology of fractures in children and adolescents. *Acta Orthop.* 2010;81(1):148−153.
24. Bachrach LK. Acquisition of optimal bone mass in childhood and adolescence. *Trends Endocrinol Metab TEM.* 2001;12(1):22−28.
25. Clarke B. Normal bone anatomy and physiology. *Clin J Am Soc Nephrol.* 2008;3(suppl 3):S131−S139.
26. Finkelstein JS, Brockwell SE, Mehta V, et al. Bone mineral density changes during the menopause transition in a multiethnic cohort of women. *J Clin Endocrinol Metab.* 2008;93(3):861−868.
27. Khosla S, Riggs BL. Pathophysiology of age-related bone loss and osteoporosis. *Endocrinol Metab Clin North Am.* 2005;34(4):1015−1030.
28. Ensrud KE. Epidemiology of fracture risk with advancing age. *J Gerontol A Biol Sci Med Sci.* 2013;68(10):1236−1242.
29. Wright NC, Looker AC, Saag KG, et al. The recent prevalence of osteoporosis and low bone mass in the United States based on bone mineral density at the femoral neck or lumbar spine. *J Bone Miner Res.* 2014;29(11):2520−2526.
30. Black DM, Cummings SR, Genant HK, Nevitt MC, Palermo L, Browner W. Axial and appendicular bone density predict fractures in older women. *J Bone Miner Res.* 1992;7(6):633−638.
31. Cummings SR, Black DM, Nevitt MC, et al. Bone density at various sites for prediction of hip fractures. The Study

Osteoporotic Fractures Res Group. *Lancet.* 1993; 341(8837):72–75.

32. Karasik D, Hsu YH, Zhou Y, Cupples LA, Kiel DP, Demissie S. Genome-wide pleiotropy of osteoporosis-related phenotypes: the Framingham study. *J Bone Miner Res.* 2010;25(7):1555–1563.

33. Seeman E, Tsalamandris C, Formica C, Hopper JL, McKay J. Reduced femoral neck bone density in the daughters of women with hip fractures: the role of low peak bone density in the pathogenesis of osteoporosis. *J Bone Miner Res.* 1994;9(5):739–743.

34. Evans RA, Marel GM, Lancaster EK, Kos S, Evans M, Wong SY. Bone mass is low in relatives of osteoporotic patients. *Ann Intern Med.* 1988;109(11):870–873.

35. Nieves JW, Formica C, Ruffing J, et al. Males have larger skeletal size and bone mass than females, despite comparable body size. *J Bone Miner Res.* 2005;20(3):529–535.

36. Zengin A, Prentice A, Ward KA. Ethnic differences in bone health. *Front Endocrinol.* 2015;6:24.

37. Courteix D, Lespessailles E, Peres SL, Obert P, Germain P, Benhamou CL. Effect of physical training on bone mineral density in prepubertal girls: a comparative study between impact-loading and non-impact-loading sports. *Osteoporos Int.* 1998;8(2):152–158.

38. Hind K, Burrows M. Weight-bearing exercise and bone mineral accrual in children and adolescents: a review of controlled trials. *Bone.* 2007;40(1):14–27.

39. Devlin MJ, Stetter CM, Lin HM, et al. Peripubertal estrogen levels and physical activity affect femur geometry in young adult women. *Osteoporos Int.* 2010;21(4):609–617.

40. Lorentzon M, Mellstrom D, Ohlsson C. Association of amount of physical activity with cortical bone size and trabecular volumetric BMD in young adult men: the GOOD study. *J Bone Miner Res.* 2005;20(11):1936–1943.

41. Nichols DL, Bonnick SL, Sanborn CF. Bone health and osteoporosis. *Clin Sports Med.* 2000;19(2):233–249.

42. Johnston Jr CC, Slemenda CW. Peak bone mass, bone loss and risk of fracture. *Osteoporos Int.* 1994;4(suppl 1):43–45.

43. Tenforde AS, Fredericson M. Influence of sports participation on bone health in the young athlete: a review of the literature. *PM R.* 2011;3(9):861–867.

44. Bass S, Pearce G, Bradney M, et al. Exercise before puberty may confer residual benefits in bone density in adulthood: studies in active prepubertal and retired female gymnasts. *J Bone Miner Res.* 1998;13(3):500–507.

45. Gunter K, Baxter-Jones AD, Mirwald RL, et al. Jump starting skeletal health: a 4-year longitudinal study assessing the effects of jumping on skeletal development in pre and circum pubertal children. *Bone.* 2008;42(4):710–718.

46. Nordstrom A, Karlsson C, Nyquist F, Olsson T, Nordstrom P, Karlsson M. Bone loss and fracture risk after reduced physical activity. *J Bone Miner Res.* 2005;20(2): 202–207.

47. Hewett E, Tufano J. *Bone Health in Female Ballet Dancers: A Review.* 2015.

48. Matthews BL, Bennell KL, McKay HA, et al. Dancing for bone health: a 3-year longitudinal study of bone mineral accrual across puberty in female non-elite dancers and controls. *Osteoporos Int.* 2006;17(7):1043–1054.

49. Burckhardt P, Wynn E, Krieg MA, Bagutti C, Faouzi M. The effects of nutrition, puberty and dancing on bone density in adolescent ballet dancers. *J Dance Med Sci.* 2011; 15(2):51–60.

50. Armann SA. *Bone Mass, Menstrual Abnormalities, Dietary Intake, and Body Composition in Classical Ballerinas.* Arizona State University; 1986.

51. Hoch AZ, Papanek P, Szabo A, Widlansky ME, Schimke JE, Gutterman DD. Association between the female athlete triad and endothelial dysfunction in dancers. *Clin J Sport Med.* 2011;21(2):119–125.

52. Khan KM, Green RM, Saul A, et al. Retired elite female ballet dancers and nonathletic controls have similar bone mineral density at weightbearing sites. *J Bone Miner Res.* 1996;11(10):1566–1574.

53. Drinkwater BL, Nilson K, Chesnut III CH, Bremner WJ, Shainholtz S, Southworth MB. Bone mineral content of amenorrheic and eumenorrheic athletes. *N Engl J Med.* 1984;311(5):277–281.

54. Yeager KK, Agostini R, Nattiv A, Drinkwater B. The female athlete triad: disordered eating, amenorrhea, osteoporosis. *Med Sci Sports Exerc.* 1993;25(7):775–777.

55. De Souza MJ, Nattiv A, Joy E, et al. 2014 Female athlete triad coalition consensus statement on treatment and return to play of the female athlete triad: 1st International Conference Held in San Francisco, California, May 2012 and 2nd International Conference Held in Indianapolis, Indiana, May 2013. *Br J Sports Med.* 2014;48(4):289.

56. Melin A, Lundy B. Commentary 3: measuring energy availability. In: Burke L, Deakin V, eds. *Clinical Sports Nutrition.* 5th ed. Sydney: McGraw Hill; 2015:146–157.

57. Ihle R, Loucks AB. Dose-response relationships between energy availability and bone turnover in young exercising women. *J Bone Miner Res.* 2004;19(8):1231–1240.

58. Ackerman KE, Misra M. Bone health and the female athlete triad in adolescent athletes. *Phys Sportsmed.* 2011;39(1): 131–141.

59. Frusztajer NT, Dhuper S, Warren MP, Brooks-Gunn J, Fox RP. Nutrition and the incidence of stress fractures in ballet dancers. *Am J Clin Nutr.* 1990;51(5):779–783.

60. Benson JE, Geiger CJ, Eiserman PA, Wardlaw GM. Relationship between nutrient intake, body mass index, menstrual function, and ballet injury. *J Am Diet Assoc.* 1989; 89(1):58–63.

61. King NA, Burley VJ, Blundell JE. Exercise-induced suppression of appetite: effects on food intake and implications for energy balance. *Eur J Clin Nutr.* 1994;48(10): 715–724.

62. Smolak L, Murnen SK, Ruble AE. Female athletes and eating problems: a meta-analysis. *Int J Eat Disord.* 2000; 27(4):371–380.

63. Kaufman BA, Warren MP, Dominguez JE, Wang J, Heymsfield SB, Pierson RN. Bone density and amenorrhea in ballet dancers are related to a decreased resting

metabolic rate and lower leptin levels. *J Clin Endocrinol Metab.* 2002;87(6):2777–2783.

64. American Psychiatric Association. *American Psychiatric Association. DSM-5 Task Force. Diagnostic and Statistical Manual of Mental Disorders: DSM-5.* 5th ed. Washington, DC: American Psychiatric Association; 2013:947.

65. Ringham R, Klump K, Kaye W, et al. Eating disorder symptomatology among ballet dancers. *Int J Eat Disord.* 2006; 39(6):503–508.

66. Gordon CM, Ackerman KE, Berga SL, et al. Functional hypothalamic amenorrhea: an endocrine society clinical practice guideline. *J Clin Endocrinol Metab.* 2017;102(5): 1413–1439.

67. Hincapie CA, Cassidy JD. Disordered eating, menstrual disturbances, and low bone mineral density in dancers: a systematic review. *Arch Phys Med Rehabil.* 2010;91(11): 1777–1789.e1.

68. Stracciolini A, Quinn BJ, Geminiani E, et al. Body mass index and menstrual patterns in dancers. *Clin Pediatr.* 2016; 56(1):49–54.

69. Frisch RE, Wyshak G, Vincent L. Delayed menarche and amenorrhea in ballet dancers. *N Engl J Med.* 1980; 303(1):17–19.

70. Ackerman KE, Misra M. Neuroendocrine abnormalities in female athletes. In: Gordon CM, LeBoff M, eds. *The Female Athlete Triad: A Clinical Guide.* Springer US; 2015:85–109.

71. Papageorgiou M, Elliott-Sale KJ, Parsons A, et al. Effects of reduced energy availability on bone metabolism in women and men. *Bone.* 2017;105:191–199.

72. Southmayd EA, Mallinson RJ, Williams NI, Mallinson DJ, De Souza MJ. Unique effects of energy versus estrogen deficiency on multiple components of bone strength in exercising women. *Osteoporos Int.* 2017;28(4):1365–1376.

73. Keay N, Fogelman I, Blake G. Bone mineral density in professional female dancers. *Br J Sports Med.* 1997;31(2): 143–147.

74. Ackerman KE, Cano Sokoloff N, DENM G, Clarke HM, Lee H, Misra M. Fractures in relation to menstrual status and bone parameters in young athletes. *Med Sci Sports Exerc.* 2015;47(8):1577–1586.

75. Staal S, Sjodin A, Fahrenholtz I, Bonnesen K, Melin A. Low RMRratio as a surrogate marker for energy deficiency, the choice of predictive equation vital for correctly identifying male and female ballet dancers at risk. *Int J Sport Nutr Exerc Metab.* 2018:1–24.

76. Statistics NCfH. CDC Growth Charts: United States; 2000.

77. Mountjoy M, Sundgot-Borgen J, Burke L, et al. RED-S CAT. Relative energy deficiency in sport (RED-S) clinical Assessment Tool (CAT). *Br J Sports Med.* 2015;49(7):421–423.

78. Tenforde AS, Parziale AL, Popp KL, Ackerman KE. Low bone mineral density in male athletes is associated with bone stress injuries at anatomic sites with greater trabecular composition. *Am J Sports Med.* 2018, 0363546517730584.

79. Marx RG, Saint-Phard D, Callahan LR, Chu J, Hannafin JA. Stress fracture sites related to underlying bone health in athletic females. *Clin J Sport Med.* 2001;11(2):73–76.

80. Ackerman KE, Nazem T, Chapko D, et al. Bone microarchitecture is impaired in adolescent amenorrheic athletes compared with eumenorrheic athletes and nonathletic controls. *J Clin Endocrinol Metab.* 2011;96(10):3123–3133.

81. Hagmar M, Berglund B, Brismar K, Hirschberg AL. Hyperandrogenism may explain reproductive dysfunction in olympic athletes. *Med Sci Sports Exerc.* 2009;41(6): 1241–1248.

82. Gunter KB, Almstedt HC, Janz KF. Physical activity in childhood may be the key to optimizing lifespan skeletal health. *Exerc Sport Sci Rev.* 2012;40(1):13–21.

83. Shangold M, Rebar RW, Wentz AC, Schiff I. Evaluation and management of menstrual dysfunction in athletes. *JAMA.* 1990;263(12):1665–1669.

84. Nazem TG, Ackerman KE. The female athlete triad. *Sports Health.* 2012;4(4):302–311.

85. Atkinson SA, McCabe GP, Weaver CM, Abrams SA, O'Brien KO. Are current calcium recommendations for adolescents higher than needed to achieve optimal peak bone mass? The Controversy. *J Nutr.* 2008;138(6): 1182–1186.

86. Harvey JA, Zobitz MM, Pak CY. Dose dependency of calcium absorption: a comparison of calcium carbonate and calcium citrate. *J Bone Miner Res.* 1988;3(3):253–258.

87. Holick MF, Binkley NC, Bischoff-Ferrari HA, et al. Evaluation, treatment, and prevention of vitamin D deficiency: an Endocrine Society clinical practice guideline. *J Clin Endocrinol Metab.* 2011;96(7):1911–1930.

88. Arends JC, Cheung MY, Barrack MT, Nattiv A. Restoration of menses with nonpharmacologic therapy in college athletes with menstrual disturbances: a 5-year retrospective study. *Int J Sport Nutr Exerc Metab.* 2012;22(2):98–108.

89. Misra M, Katzman D, Miller KK, et al. Physiologic estrogen replacement increases bone density in adolescent girls with anorexia nervosa. *J Bone Miner Res.* 2011;26(10): 2430–2438.

90. Ackerman KE, Slattery M, Singhal V, et al. Transdermal 17-β estradiol has a beneficial effect on bone parameters assessed using HRpQCT compared to oral ethinyl estradiol-progesterone combination pills in oligoamenorrheic athletes: a randomized controlled trial. *J Bone Miner Res.* 2018;32(suppl 1). Available from: http://wwwasbmrorg/education/2017-abstracts [Internet].

91. Franchimont N, Canalis E. Management of glucocorticoid induced osteoporosis in premenopausal women with autoimmune disease. *Autoimmun Rev.* 2003;2(4): 224–228.

92. Bauer JJ, Snow CM. What is the prescription for healthy bones? *J Musculoskeletal Neuronal Interact.* 2003;3(4): 352–355. discussion 6.

## CHAPTER 14

# Cross-Training for the Dancer

MATTHEW WYON, PHD, MSC

## INTRODUCTION

All performing artists use their body in the expression of their art form, although dance probably requires the greatest physical demand. The term "artistic athlete" has been applied to professional dancers to reflect this physical demand[1] while recognizing the different outcome goals of athletes and artists. Dance is the generic term that covers a diversity of genres that through their differing techniques and choreography place differing physiological stresses on the body. Break dancing requires greater upper body strength, ballet requires more flexibility, tap dancing requires better ankle flexibility, whereas others are required to dance and sing at the same time while wearing complex costumes.

For a long time, technique class and rehearsal were the fundamental training environments to prepare the dancer for performance. Recent studies have suggested that classes and rehearsals might prepare the dancer technically to perform but physiologically there is a big difference between these training settings and performance.[2] In fact, dancers became significantly physically fitter during performance periods.[3] Dance performance can cover a wide diversity of physical demands even within a single genre[4] that can further complicate performance preparation. There have been suggestions that class and rehearsal should be adapted to make up for these shortfalls; Krasnow and Chatfield[5] noted that trying to achieve technical excellence and optimal physical conditioning in dance class and rehearsal is impossible without compromising one or the other. In addition, it also means that the teacher or rehearsal director has to be a master of technique and supplemental training. Similar to the multi-team approach implemented in sport,[6] it is important that teachers, dance masters/mistress, and support staff (medical and science) are doing the role that they are trained for and not overstepping their education and training as this optimizes training exposure and performance while reducing injury risk.

Dancers who are physiologically stronger, both in muscular strength and cardiorespiratory conditioning, dance better and are less prone to injury.[7–9] Consequently, supplemental training needs to become an integral aspect of a dancer's life whether during preprofessional training or their professional careers. Our bodies are reactive organisms that respond to new stresses by adapting. This is why supplemental training is essential aspect of a dancer's training as the physical stress imposed by class and rehearsals may often plateau until performance periods when there is a sudden increase in load.[3] Presently, somatic practices are the main form of supplemental training although there is little published evidence of their benefits.[10]

Fundamentally, any exercise form that places a physical stress on the body enough to cause adaptation is beneficial, although there are other criteria that need to be considered as well and these will be covered later. The worry that supplemental training will alter the aesthetic lines of a dancer or their flexibility is without scientific justification. For individuals to change their muscle size to the point of being aesthetically wrong for dance, they would have done the "wrong" type of strength training for a long time and would have consumed a huge amount of calories. This is something that rarely happens in dance where dancers' caloric intake is often below recommended levels. Similarly, the myth about flexibility is indirectly connected with the myth of muscle size; however, there is no scientific evidence that strength training can have a negative effect on flexibility. On the contrary, there is evidence that shows increases in flexibility due to strength training, especially developpé height.[11,12] Gymnasts provide a good example: they are significantly stronger than dancers and have the same range of movement.[13]

The amount of training that a dancer is exposed, whether it is class, rehearsal, rehabilitation, or supplemental training, needs to be monitored as this is linked to overtraining, underperformance, and injury.[14,15] Training load can be measured in a number of ways

Performing Arts Medicine. https://doi.org/10.1016/B978-0-323-58182-0.00014-6

and should include dance and nondance stresses,[16] but fundamentally it provides an indicator of how much exercise is being done (*time × intensity*). Our bodies can only cope with a certain increase in stress a week, approximately 5%[17]; recent studies have suggested using the acute:chronic workload as a means of preventing overload. This ratio is calculated by the current weeks training load (acute) against a 4-week average (chronic); a very high acute:chronic workload ratio has been linked to increased injury risk.[18] During a single session a dancer is exposed to a series of stimuli (metabolic, neuromuscular, mental, and hormonal) that alter their physiological status. The greater the volume, intensity, and duration of training sessions, the greater the physiological responses the body has to cope with. The immediate response to a session is fatigue as well as a reduction in muscle glycogen levels, lactate accumulation and ultimately a dancer's performance capacity. The magnitude of these effects is dependent on the intensity and duration of the session, the number of sessions that day, and the dancers underlying physiological conditioning. The same session carried out immediately after a holiday and then later in the term will have greatly different physiological and psychological effects, with the former feeling much harder and taking longer to physically recover from compared to the later session when the dancer's conditioning has improved.

If the load increases above this bar for a period of time, the body is continually in a state of breakdown and more prone to injury. Rest is a vital component and has often been ignored by dance, where there is always the tendency to add to class, rehearsal, and performances to the schedule rather than to take one away. Dance injury surveys nearly always report that fatigue, tiredness, or overtraining is the most often self-reported causes of injury.[19,20] Therefore, before the implementation of a supplemental training program into a dancer's schedule; their current training load, rest periods, and performance schedule needs to be reviewed to make sure the increased training has a beneficial and not a detrimental effect. When a dancer has an injury and is off dance or has restricted dance schedules, supplemental training can stimulate the body with a different focus. This has been shown to have a number of benefits from improving psychological well-being to maintaining/improving present conditioning. Resistance training is possible by splitting muscle groups (upper/lower body) or main/auxiliary exercises; and cardiorespiratory training by unloading the body, such as aqua jogging.

Although the focus of supplemental training for the dancer is on performance enhancement/preparation, the actual starting point of training can range from injured to injury-free. Accordingly, the endpoint is also dependent on the physical demands of the forthcoming performance. This stance also encompasses injury prevention and rehabilitation training and puts a positive spin on this training. As mentioned previously, the training program needs to be integrated into the dancer's schedule, as it is supplemental to their dance training (class, rehearsals, and performance). Dance training often requires high levels of skill, thus moderate levels of fatigue can have major detrimental impacts on fine motor control. Therefore, the scheduling of supplemental training has to be carefully planned to not affect dancers' primary training goals. The fatigue is short term and affects the neuromuscular system,[21] hence the subsequent effect on the fine motor control; strength and power training causes a greater neuromuscular fatigue than cardiorespiratory interventions. Ideally a 2-h recovery period is needed after strength training and an hour after cardiorespiratory training, before uncompromised dance movement can be performed. Preferably, supplemental training should be scheduled at the end of the training day to avoid these potential negative consequences.

Professional dancers are often scheduled to do approximately 38 h of class, rehearsals, and performances a week and adolescent dancers in preprofessional training between 12 and 30 h depending on their age. Thus, dancers are already undertaking considerable training, especially in comparison to their sporting counterparts, and consequently beneficial effects can be achieved with relatively little intervention. Two studies reported beneficial improvements in physical fitness and dance performance with only one[9] or two[7] 60-min physical training sessions a week. Therefore, supplemental training needs to be quality-focused, rather than quantity of training sessions, and based on the requirements of the individual. Developing training programs for adolescent dancers has the added complexity, as adolescents cannot just be considered small adults due to growth spurts and hormonal adjustments during puberty.[22]

A dancer's *training age* is also very important; this age is not their chronological age, but the number of years they have participated in a specific activity. So a dancer who is 25 years old, and has been dancing since the age of 8, has a dance training age of 17. The same rule applies in supplemental training. The same dancer of 18 years old that has no experience in supplemental training has a training age of 0 years. This is very important when working with dancers; because they can pick up new movements very quickly, it is easy to increase the load-stress placed on them too fast. This can increase injury risk, as the physiological support structure (muscle, tendon, and ligament strength) cannot develop rapidly.

## SCREENING

Screening is a vital aspect of intervention training as it ascertains the base from which the program is developed; it also provides base line data for return to dance for injured dancers. The more comprehensive the screen, the better the information available to the strength and conditioning coach. Screening is often time, equipment, and tester-skill dependent, and it is recognized in an ideal world each dancer would have a medical, physiotherapy, physiology, and psychology screens but few companies or schools have the time or money to carry all these out. This chapter is focused on supplemental training, and therefore the screening protocols discussed are focused on these variables. Specific physiological testing guidelines have been developed for dancers[23] but in summary the areas that need to be covered are anthropometric, cardiorespiratory, muscle function, balance/stability, and flexibility. The tests selected need to be scientifically reliable and valid for dancers and sensitive enough to monitor change.[24] The utilization of general population tests, such as handgrip dynamometer (upper body strength) or step test (cardiorespiratory fitness), is not sufficient in validity or sensitivity to provide the information required for intervention.

The use of an adapted Performance Profile[25] is beneficial as it allows the trainer to understand what the dancer perceives as relevant as well as its comparative importance to their dance genre. The dancer is asked to write down all the physical attributes they think are important as a dancer and for dance performance before, first, rating each one between 1 and 10 (little importance—extremely important) and, second, their aptitude at the attribute 1 (poor) to 10 (excellent). This provides important information on the dancer's understanding of the physical demands of dance and their own physical fitness, by comparing it to the screening test results. Discrepancies will potentially require an education intervention alongside training programs to help with training compliance. For example, if a male ballet dancer scores muscular strength attribute at 4 and himself at 7 and the screening test records an isometric pull force of 67 kg, then prior to a strength training intervention a discussion is needed to understand his views on muscular strength and why it could be more beneficial than he thinks

and what normal isometric pull force scores are for dancers. Training programs need to be developed in conjunction with the individual dancer, as this has been shown to help with training compliance; it also needs to be emphasized that the training program is not for life but as the dancer adapts to the training and/or has new choreography then the program also needs to be modified.

## BASIC PRINCIPLES OF SUPPLEMENTAL TRAINING

Our body, especially muscles, is reactive, learning entities that require changing stressors to improve or maintain their current ability.[26] If an absolute training stress is just maintained (e.g., 20 min running at 8 km/h) then the body learns to cope with it more efficiency (economy of movement) by adapting and the benefits diminish over time.[27] Muscles therefore need to be challenged or overloaded by increasing the stress placed on them by either increasing the load or changing the movement. As mentioned earlier the body can cope with approximately a 5% increase in load a week[17]; this can be measured by the number of jumps, total weight lifted (repetitions $\times$ weight), distance covered, etc. It is important to monitor the increase in training stress as a total of all training the dancer is exposed to, including dance (class, rehearsal, and performances) and supplemental training, so that the later increases do not coincide with increased dancing hours.

Post-exercise recovery time is another important aspect of training; at a cellular level, it has been shown that it takes approximately 48-h to recover from a strength training session and 12−18 h from a cardiorespiratory training session.[28,29] There is a similar acute neuromuscular effect from strenuous strength training resulting in reduced force production and voluntary neural activity 1−2 h posttraining.[21] Research has also shown the benefits of reducing training load for a week every 4−6 weeks, a process referred to as *supercompensation*, as this allows the body to fully recover with subsequent increases in fitness parameters.[30]

At a basic physiological level, supplemental training affects the neuromuscular, endocrine, and bioenergetic systems. Therefore, care needs to be taken in exercise selection and its application. As the weight/load a muscle moves increases muscle fiber, motor unit recruitment changes from small to large and muscle fibers from type I to type II.[31] During eccentric and fast movements, type II fibers are recruited before type I irrespective of load.[32,33] The work-to-rest ratio of both strength and cardiorespiratory training will develop specific energy pathways and their accompanying enzymes and metabolites.[34] The time a muscle is under tension affects the release of hormones related to protein resynthesize and growth.[35]

The following sections of this chapter will provide more specific information on cardiorespiratory, muscle, and flexibility development.

## CARDIORESPIRATORY TRAINING

The data from work-to-rest ratio from video performance analysis,[4] cardiorespiratory fitness tests, and self-reported causes of injury all indicate that fatigue is an issue. Dance has been classified as high-intensity intermittent exercise that utilizes all the energy systems.[13] Aerobic power research on dancers has indicated that professional males are generally between 40 and 60 mL/kg per minute and females between 30 and 50 mL/kg per minute[13,36,37] compared to 44 mL/kg per minute (males) and 35 mL/kg per minute (females) in the general population and anaerobic thresholds between 75% and 85% (general population 50%−60%). Rather than such a wide range, ideally male dancers should have aerobic capacities between 50 and 60 mL/kg per minute and females 45−55 mL/kg per minute, as this will provide the necessary aerobic foundation and recovery capabilities for the majority of dance activity. The limited data on dance performance indicated that dancers were performing close to the maximum capacities,[8] but more importantly an analysis of oxygen uptake data suggest that there is a discrepancy between the stresses placed on the dancer during training (class and rehearsal) and performance[2] that could account for the reported underdeveloped anaerobic threshold. Time spent in this anaerobic or lactate zone is minimal during training but accounts for approximately 35% of performance time.[2]

Glycolysis (aerobic) and anaerobic (glycolytic, phosphate) production systems are focused on replenishing the energy used during muscle contraction[38] and should be viewed as a continuum. The increase in the by-products of adenine triphosphate (ATP) breakdown (adenine diphosphate (ADP), phosphate (Pi), adenine monophosphate (AMP)) stimulates these systems to maintain resting ATP levels. At any one time, all energy systems are in use but the percentage use of each energy system is determined by the rate of demand. During a 6-s maximal effort the glycolytic contribution is estimated to be 49%; at 30 s the aerobic contribution is approximately 16%, the glycolytic 56%, and the phosphate 28%.[39] As the maximum exercise period increases, the percentage of energy derived from anaerobic metabolism decreases; at approximately 2 min the demand is equal between the aerobic and anaerobic systems and at 4 min the aerobic system largely dominates energy replenishment.[39] The change in dominance of the energy systems results in a decrease in available ATP, which in turn causes a reduction in muscle contraction force. Training causes central and peripheral adaptations; at a cellular level, aerobically trained individuals have been shown to have higher concentrations of mitochondria, glycogen, creatine phosphokinase, phosphofructokinase, myokinase, etc., while anaerobic stimulus sees increases in sodium-potassium ATPase and possibly lactate dehydrogenase. Therefore, care needs to be taken with the prescription of supplemental training so that performance is not inadvertently compromised.

### Training Intensity

Prescribing cardiorespiratory training can be either specific or generic to the individual and depends on the fitness test undertaken. The use of gas analysis with a graded exercise test will highlight specific break points that provide accurate training zones[40] for aerobic and anaerobic training. The most important of these is the ventilatory breakpoint or aerobic threshold; above this intensity the anaerobic energy systems start to produce a significant part of energy production with an accompanying increase in lactate production. This breakpoint generally occurs around 85% of aerobic capacity ($VO_2$max) or 90% of maximum heart rate (220−age) or 75%−85% of your heart rate reserve (220−age−resting HR = HR reserve) but can vary with training exposure. Using estimated data means that the prescribed training intensities can be less than optimal or detrimental to the intended goals.

Aerobic conditioning forms the foundation of the cardiorespiratory systems and training can either be continuous or interval in nature. Continuous training is often steady state and the intensity needs to be under the aerobic threshold; the length of the session does not need to be more than 20 min. Interval training implements a 1:1 ratio, the high−moderate intensity periods (1−3 min) are followed by lower intensity recovery periods (Table 14.1). The high−moderate periods need to be at the aerobic threshold that corresponds to an intensity that the high−moderate interval period can only just complete.

Glycolytic (lactate) training uses intervals with a 1:3 ratio; the "work" periods should last between 60 and 90 s followed by a low intensity recovery period; a good target is 10 intervals. The heart rate during the

**TABLE 14.1**
**Cardiorespiratory Training Interventions**

| Variable | TRAINING GOAL | | | | |
|---|---|---|---|---|---|
| | Aerobic | Aerobic | Glycolytic | Phosphate | LSD |
| Intensity (% $HR_{max}$) | 70–90 | 85–90 | 90–95 | 100+ | 60–70 |
| Work to rest ratio | | 1:1 | 1:3 | 1:5 | |
| Work time | 20 min | 1–3 min | 60–90 s | 10–20 s | 30–60 min |
| Number of sets | 1 | 10 | 6–10 | 10–20 | 1 |
| Number of sessions/week | 1–2 | 1–2 | 1–2 | 1–2 | 1 |

work periods needs to be above the aerobic threshold and will generate high levels of lactate. This is mentally tough training and requires a good aerobic foundation to aid recovery between the work bouts. If this aerobic fitness has not been developed sufficiently, then few interval bouts can be achieved before fatigue negatively affects the work bouts with a loss of training intensity.

Similar to glycolytic training, phosphate (ATP-CP) training employs intervals with a 1:5 ratio. The increased rest periods allow for greater intensity during the exercise bouts (10–20 s), often referred to as supramaximal intensity. A target of 10–20 bouts should be achievable.

Long, slow distance (LSD) training can be a beneficial addition as a recovery mechanism but also as foundation training prior to the start of school/season to get the body used to longer periods of exercise. The intensity is low–moderate around 60%–70% of HR maximum or just above the lower ventilatory breakpoint (Table 14.1).[40]

### Exercise Mode

Because the physiological adaptations are both central and peripheral[41] the exercise mode needs to resemble dance movement; therefore running or a cross-trainer is better than cycling, which is better than swimming. Dance movement can be used but the emphasis needs to be on the training effect rather than movement accuracy and use big whole-body movements.

### Training Frequency

The number of training sessions that need to be incorporated into a week is obviously dependent on the individual dancer's cardiorespiratory profile and the forthcoming demands of their season. In the development phase, four sessions a week are required, dropping to two during maintenance periods (heavy rehearsal and performance periods).

## MUSCULAR RESISTANCE TRAINING

Resistance training is often hard to implement, as dancers perceive that it causes large and inflexible muscles. If correctly prescribed neither of these outcomes will occur: to increase muscle mass, large amounts of calories need to be eaten with specific type of strength training over a long period of time; loss of flexibility is due to a lack of stretching. There is more evidence of beneficial effects of resistance training from increased jump height, reduced incidence of injury, and increased *developpé* height (Table 14.2).[42] Resistance training can be split into five areas: preparation, strength, hypertrophic, power, and endurance training that have different effects on muscular adaptation. At a muscular level, resistance training causes reactive adaptation with initial catabolic followed by anabolic processes that last between 12 and 48 h depending on the type of loading; strength training has a longer recovery time than endurance training,[29] and can result in localized pain.[43] There is also a neuromuscular adaptation aspect to training that have been shown to account for most of initial muscle function improvements, especially in untrained people, and this can be applicable to dancers due to their, often young, training age. All types of resistance training increase intramuscular coordination but strength interventions have been shown to have increased benefit for intramuscular recruitment but limited effects on intermuscular coordination compared to endurance training.[44] The different training interventions cause differing endocrine responses with hypertrophic training promoting the release of testosterone, growth hormone (GH), cortisol, and insulin-like growth factor-1 (IGF-1), while strength training causes increased release of luteinizing hormone, cortisol, and growth hormone.[45] It is the training that promotes GH and IGF-1 release, because of its tissue-remodeling role, that is linked to hypertrophy.[46]

**TABLE 14.2**
**Resistance Training: Sets, Reps, and Rest According to Training Goal**

| Variable | Strength | TRAINING GOAL | | |
| | | Power | Hypertrophy | Endurance |
| --- | --- | --- | --- | --- |
| Load (% 1 Rep$_{max}$) | 80–90 | 70–90 | 60–80 | 40–60 |
| Reps per set | 1–5 | 1–5 | 6–12 | 15–60 |
| Sets per exercise | 4–7 | 3–5 | 4–8 | 2–4 |
| Rest between sets (min) | 2–6 | 2–6 | 2–5 | 1–2 |
| Speed of reps | Slow–moderate | Fast | Moderate | Slow–moderate |

At its most basic level, all human movement, including dance, can be broken down into the following patterns: squat, lunge, twist, push/pull, gait (walking/running), and balance.[47] The exercise choices should be made based on screening data, injury history, and performance demands. Preparation training should be implemented after holiday periods and injury; it is often conducted in conjunction with a physiotherapist/athletic trainer and focuses on joint stability, mobility, and rectifying muscle imbalances. It is then recommended that a period of anatomic adaptation training occurs, which can take the form of circuit training, and builds a good foundation for more specific interventions: strength, power, and/or endurance. Training load is calculated by the load, number of repetitions per set, number of sets per exercise, number of exercises, and number of training sessions per week. As mentioned previously, too rapid an increase in training load or not enough recovery time can lead to overtraining and increased risk of injury.[16]

## Exercise Selection

Exercises can be grouped as either *"core"* or *"assistance"* based on the amount of muscle involved and its applicability/mimickery of dance movement, the specific adaptation to imposed demands (SAID) principle. Core exercises utilize one or more large muscle groups over multiple joints; while assistance exercises are usually single-joint exercises and use smaller muscles. Assistance exercises are often incorporated for injury prevention or rehabilitation purposes and allow the conditioning of isolated muscles that are specific to the dance form, for example, standing calf raises for ballet. Core exercises that place a load on the spine can also be categorized as *"structural"* as they require stabilization, either static or dynamic, of the torso during the movement. The deadlift and back squat are good

examples of *core structural* exercises while a forward step lunge incorporating a torso twist adds a dynamic aspect to a core structural movement. Exercise selection also should promote muscular balance across joints, between opposing muscles, and bilaterally. Although there is little published evidence of muscular imbalances in dance literature, clinical experience has highlighted imbalances between the anterior/posterior chains, internal/external hip rotators, and left/right leg strength and balance. The posterior chain is often weaker than the anterior, and exercises such as the deadlift would help to rectify this imbalance. The external rotators are often stronger than the internal due to the time dancers spend in turnout. Carrying out exercises such as forward lunges in parallel provides a core exercise that challenges this imbalance. Bilateral differences are often a product of dance training with the left leg having greater dynamic balance (less travel during turns) and concentric power (split leg jump take off), while the right leg is eccentrically stronger (landing from split leg jumps). It must be emphasized that muscle balance does not necessarily mean equal strength but just the appropriate ratio between one muscle group and another; though often-cited research suggests that the imbalance should not be more than 10%.[48]

Exercise selection is also determined by access to equipment and training experience. Resistance machines are often used for beginners; free weight exercises are often more beneficial as they engage more muscles, especially stabilizers, but they require greater technique experience. It is often beneficial to develop these techniques during preadolescence with body weight or little/no resistance in anticipation of postadolescent supplemental training. The time available for supplemental training will also determine exercise selection as some are more time efficient than others. Within a training session the order exercises are carried out generally moves from core to assistance, multi-joint to single-joint, large muscle mass to small; though preexhaustion, alternated, superset, and compound set exercise routines can be introduced as the training experience of the dancer increases.[47]

### Plyometric Training

Dancers, particularly male ballet dancers, are often considered to have big jumps but published data indicate that their vertical jump height is considerably lower than comparable sports people and in some instances the general population. Fundamental to this is that dancers are told to jump but not how to jump, and coach queuing is focused on aesthetic aspects rather than the correct muscles to engage. This has led to a lot of dancers perceiving that the feet and quadriceps are the main determinants of jump height and do not engage the posterior chain (hamstrings and gluteals), maximize the stretch-shortening cycle, or minimize the amortization time. The focus of plyometric training is to enable a muscle to reach maximal force as quickly as possible and involves the stretch-shortening cycle. The exercises utilize the elastic components of muscles and tendons to increase power by decreasing amortization time, the time between a muscle's stretch and subsequent contraction. Plyometric training places huge forces on the body and should be carried out when the dancer is rested and not fatigued, even so it can cause muscle soreness if not introduced gradually and therefore needs to be carefully scheduled. The training load is monitored by the number of (foot) contacts, height of fall, and horizontal velocity that is made during a session (beginners 80−100, intermediate 100−120, and advanced 120−140) and the work to rest ratio should be the same as phosphate training (1:5). The exercises chosen again should reflect the movement patterns in the dance genre but typical lower body plyometric drills include jumps in place, multiple hops and jumps, depth jumps, and box drills.[49]

## FUNCTIONAL CORE TRAINING

It is often hard to transfer isolated core training to functional movement, and therefore there has been a movement toward incorporating the two by engaging the core muscles during dynamic whole-body movements.[50] Ideally, this can be achieved during all supplemental and dance training, although specific training is often required.[51,52]

## FLEXIBILITY

Dancers often have extremely good range of movement (ROM), and there are a higher proportion of hypermobile individuals than seen within other sports.[53] Published data suggest that there are more hypermobile dancers during preprofessional training than in professional dance. Moreover, this could be due to the higher injury incidence in this population.[54] Both hyperflexible and hypermobile dancers require supplemental training that focuses on joint stability and active ROM. The later training concentrates on developing muscular strength in the agonist muscle thereby reducing the difference between active and passive ROM, and anecdotal data suggest that the bigger the difference between these two measures increases injury risk. Training should focus on end-of-range training that incorporates the entire kinetic chain, and when working on developpé height the exercises should be carried out standing in the center.[12]

Research in athletes has suggested that passive stretching has a negative effect on muscle function potentially due to either neuromuscular or series elastic component impairment[55]; though this has not been reported in dance, possibly due to the different performance requirements.[56] A mixture of passive and dynamic stretching is probably ideal as warm up/preparation training. Recent research into passive stretch intensity has highlighted an increase in inflammatory markers at high intensities (9/10),[57] therefore postexercise recovery stretching should be at a low to moderate intensity (4−6/10)[58] with the stretched muscle not being under tension, for example, hamstring stretches to be done while lying on the back rather than standing.

Supplemental training needs to be an integral part of a dancer's training to support their technical prowess; ideally, this should be incorporated into their existing schedules. Physical training needs to start during adolescence and be an integral part of a professional dancer's timetable, carefully planned so as not to compromise rehearsals and performances. The focus should be on performance enhancement, working on areas of weakness and preparing the body for forthcoming rep. The mantra must be "quality not quantity," so that the supplemental training provides enough stimuli to cause adaptation but not so much that it risks overtraining.

## REFERENCES

1. Koutedakis Y, Sharp NCC. *The Fit and Healthy Dancer*. Chichester: John Wiley and Sons; 1999.
2. Wyon M, Abt G, Redding E, Head A, Sharp N. Oxygen uptake during of modern dance class, rehearsal and performance. *J Strength Cond Res*. 2004;18(3):646−649. https://doi.org/10.1519/13082.1.

3. Wyon M, Redding E. The physiological monitoring of cardiorespiratory adaptations during rehearsal and performance of contemporary dance. *J Strength Cond Res.* 2005; 19(3):611−614.

4. Wyon M, Twitchett E, Angioi M, Clarke F, Metsios G, Koutedakis Y. Time motion and video analysis of classical ballet and contemporary dance performance. *Int J Sports Med.* 2011;32(11):851−855. https://doi.org/10.1055/s-0031-1279718.

5. Krasnow DH, Chatfield SJ. Dance science and the dance technique class. *Impulse.* 1996;4:162−172.

6. Dijkstra HP, Pollock N, Chakraverty R, Alonso JM. Managing the health of the elite athlete: a new integrated performance health management and coaching model. *Br J Sports Med.* 2014;48(7):523−531. https://doi.org/10.1136/bjsports-2013-093222.

7. Angioi M, Metsios G, Twitchett E, Koutedakis Y, Wyon M. Effects of supplemental training on fitness and aesthetic competence parameters in contemporary dance: a randomised controlled trial. *Med Probl Perform Art.* 2012;27(1): 3−8.

8. Beck S, Wyon M, Redding E. Changes in energy demand of dance activity and cardiorespiratory fitness during one year of vocational contemporary dance training. *J Strength Cond Res.* 2018;32(3):841−848.

9. Twitchett E, Angioi M, Koutedakis Y, Wyon M. Do increases in selected fitness parameters affect the aesthetic aspects of classical ballet performance. *Med Probl Perform Art.* 2011;26(1):35−38.

10. Bergeron C, Greenwood M, Smith T, Wyon M. Pilates training for dancers: a systematic review. *Natl Dance Soc J.* 2017;2(1).

11. Marshall L, Wyon M. The effect of whole body vibration on jump height and active range of movement in female dancers. *J Strength Cond Res.* 2012;26(3):789−793.

12. Wyon M, Smith A, Koutedakis Y. A comparison of strength and stretch interventions on active and passive ranges of movement in dancers: a randomised controlled trial. *J Strength Cond Res.* 2013;27(11):3053−3059. https://doi.org/10.1519/JSC.0b013e31828a4842.

13. Koutedakis Y, Jamurtas A. The dancer as a performing athlete: physiological considerations. *Sports Med.* 2004; 34(10):651−661. https://doi.org/10.2165/00007256-200434100-00003.

14. Kellman M. Preventing overtraining in athletes in high-intensity sports and stress/recovery monitoring. *Scand J Med Sci Sports.* 2010;20:95−102.

15. Koutedakis Y, Sharp NC. Seasonal variations of injury and overtraining in elite athletes. *Clin J Sport Med.* 1998;8(1): 18−21.

16. Drew MK, Finch CF. The relationship between training load and injury, illness and soreness: a systematic and literature review. *Sports Med.* 2016;46(6):861−883.

17. Stone M. Overtraining: a review of the signs, symptoms and possible causes. *J Strength Cond Res.* 1991;5: 35−50.

18. Hulin BT, Gabbett TJ, Lawson DW, Caputi P, Sampson JA. The acute: chronic workload ratio predicts injury: high chronic workload may decrease injury risk in elite rugby league players. *Br J Sports Med.* 2015;50(4): 231−236.

19. Brinson P, Dick F. *Fit to Dance?* London: Calouste Gulbenkian Foundation; 1996.

20. Laws H. *Fit to Dance 2-Report of the Second National Inquiry into Dancers' Health and Injury in the UK.* London: Newgate Press; 2005.

21. Häkkinen K. Neuromuscular fatigue and recovery in male and female athletes during heavy resistance exercise. *Int J Sports Med.* 1993;14(02):53−59.

22. Pfeiffer RD, Francis RS. Effects of strength training on muscle development in prepubescent, pubescent, and postpubescent males. *Phys Sportsmed.* 1986;14(9):134−143.

23. Wyon M. Testing the aesthetic athlete. In: Winter E, Jones A, Davison R, Bromley P, Mercer T, eds. *Sport and Exercise Physiology Testing Guidelines: British Association of Sport and Exercise Science Testing Guidelines.* Vol. 2. London and New York: Routledge, Taylor and Francis Group; 2007: 249−262.

24. Atkinson G, Nevill A. Method agreement and measurement error in the physiology of exercise. In: Winter E, Jones A, Davidson R, Bromley P, Mercer T, eds. *Sport and Exercise Physiology Testing.* Vol. 1. Abingdon, UK: Routledge; 2007:41−48.

25. Butler RJ, Hardy L. The performance profile: theory and application. *Sport Psychol.* 1992;6:253−264.

26. Koutedakis Y, Clarke F, Wyon M, Aways D, Owolabi EO. Muscular strength: applications for dancers. *Med Probl Perform Art.* 2009;24(4):157−165.

27. Sparrow W, Newell K. Metabolic energy expenditure and the regulation of movement economy. *Psychon Bull Rev.* 1998;5(2):173−196.

28. Bangsbo J, Saltin B. Recovery of muscle from exercise - its importance for subsequent performance. In: Macleod M, Williams M, Sharp N, EFN SPON, eds. *Intermittent High Intensity Exercise: Preparation, Stresses and Damage Limitations.* 1993:49−69.

29. Rogozkin VA. The effect of the number of daily training sessions on skeletal muscle protein synthesis. *Med Sci Sports.* 1976;8(4):223−225.

30. Lehmann M, Foster C, Gastmann U, Keizer H, Steinacker JM. Definition, types, symptoms, findings, underlying mechanisms, and frequency of overtraining and overtraining syndrome. In: *Overload, Performance Incompetence, and Regeneration in Sport.* Springer; 1999: 1−6.

31. Bottinelli R, Pellegrino M, Canepari M, Rossi R, Reggiani C. Specific contributions of various muscle fibre types to human muscle performance: an in vitro study. *J Electromyogr Kinesiol.* 1999;9(2):87−95.

32. Buchthal F, Schmalbruch H. Contraction times and fibre types in intact human muscle. *Acta Physiol Scand.* 1970; 79(4):435−452.

33. Takekura H, Fujinami N, Nishizawa T, Ogasawara H, Kasuga N. Eccentric exercise induced morphological changes in the membrane systems involved in excitation-contraction coupling in rate skeletal muscle. *J Physiol (Camb)*. 2001;93:571−583.

34. Wyon M. Cardiorespiratory training for dancers. *J Dance Med Sci*. 2005;9(1):7−12.

35. Yarasheski KE, Campbell JA, Smith K, Rennie M, Hollosy J, Bier D. Effect of growth hormone and resistance exercise on muscle growth in young men. *Am J Physiol*. 1992;262(3):E261−E267.

36. Liiv H, Wyon M, Jurimae T, Saar M, Maest J, Jurimae J. Anthropometry, somatotypes and aerobic power in ballet, contemporary dance and DanceSport. *Med Probl Perform Art*. 2013;28(4):207−211.

37. Wyon M, Allen N, Cloak R, Beck S, Davies P, Clarke F. Assessment of maximum aerobic capacity and anaerobic threshold of elite ballet dancers. *Med Probl Perform Art*. 2016;31(3):145−149.

38. Newsholme E. Basic aspects of metabolic regulation and their application to provision of energy in exercise. In: Poortmans J, ed. *Principles of Exercise Biochemistry*. 2nd ed. Basel: Karger; 1993:51−88.

39. Hultman E, Bergstrom M, Spriet LL, Soderlund K. Energy metabolism and fatigue. In: Taylor AW, ed. *Biochemistry of Exercise VII*. Illinios: Human Kinetics Books; 1990.

40. Wasserman K, Hansen J, Sue D, Whipp B, Casaburi R. *Principles of Exercise Testing and Interpretation*. 2nd ed. Philadelphia: Lea & Febiger; 1994.

41. Saltin B, Strange S. Maximal oxygen uptake: "old" and "new" arguments for a cardiovascular limitation. *Med Sci Sports Exerc*. 1992;24(1):30−37.

42. Koutedakis Y, Stavropoulos-Kalinoglou A, Metsios G. The significance of muscular strength in dance. *J Dance Med Sci*. 2005;9(1):29−34.

43. Cheung K, Hume PA, Maxwell L. Delayed onset muscle soreness. *Sports Med*. 2003;33(2):145−164.

44. Hakkinen K. Neuromuscular and hormonal adaptations during strength and power training: a review. *J Sports Med Phys Fitness*. 1989;29:9−26.

45. Kraemer WJ, Ratamess NA. Hormonal responses and adaptations to resistance exercise and training. *Sports Med*. 2005;35(4):339−361.

46. McCall GE, Byrnes WC, Fleck SJ, Dickinson A, Kraemer WJ. Acute and chronic hormonal responses to resistance training designed to promote muscle hypertrophy. *Can J Appl Physiol*. 1999;24(1):96−107.

47. Bompa T, Cornacchia L. *Serious Strength Training*. Champaign, IL: Human Kinetics; 1998.

48. Grace TG. Muscle imbalance and extremity injury. *Sports Med*. 1985;2(2):77−82.

49. Radcliffe J, Farentinos R. *High-powered Plyometrics*. Champaign, IL: Human Kinetics; 1999.

50. Faries MD, Greenwood M. Core training: stabilizing the confusion. *Strength Cond J*. 2007;29(2):10.

51. Akuthota V, Ferreiro A, Moore T, Fredericson M. Core stability exercise principles. *Curr Sports Med Rep*. 2008;7(1):39−44.

52. Boyle M. *New Functional Training for Sports*. 2nd ed. Champaign, IL: Human Kinetics; 2003.

53. Day H, Koutedakis Y, Wyon M. Hypermobility and dance: a review. *Int J Sports Med*. 2011;32:485−489.

54. McCormack M, Briggs J, Hakim A, Grahame R. Joint laxity and the benign joint hypermobility syndrome in student and professional ballet dancers. *J Rheumatol*. 2004;31(1):173−178.

55. Behm DG, Bambury A, Cahill F, Power K. Effect of acute static stretching on force, balance, reaction time, and movement time. *Med Sci Sport Exerc*. 2004;36(8):1397−1402.

56. Morrin N, Redding E. Acute effects of warm-up stretch protocols on balance, vertical jump height, and range of motion in dancers. *J Dance Med Sci*. 2013;17(1):34−40.

57. Apostolopoulos N, Metsios G, Tauton J, Koutedakis Y, Wyon M. Acute inflammation response to stretching: a randomised trial. *Ital J Sports Rehabil Posturology*. 2015;2(4):368−381.

58. Apostolopoulos N. Microstretching®: a new recovery regeneration technique. *New Stud Athl*. 2004;19(4):47−56.

## CHAPTER 15

# Return-to-Dance Strategies and Guidelines for the Dancer

MELODY HRUBES, MD

## INTRODUCTION

The annual incidence of injury in professional dancers ranges from 67% to 95%.[1] The goal of dance rehabilitation is to address the cause of injury, and prepare the dancer for a successful return to previous level of function while minimizing reinjury. Often, an injured dancer can fully recover with improved skills and a decreased injury risk. Dance-specific rehabilitation is of paramount importance to achieving the best possible outcome.[2]

Addressing physical function, while extremely important, does not take all of the distinct demands on a dancer into consideration. For this reason, a team-based approach to rehabilitation is appropriate. Each injured dancer wants to maximize the likelihood of returning to their specific ability level, but has unique needs for how this might be achieved. A holistic approach to recovery is necessary.

Rehabilitation of a dance injury should be led by a medical practitioner with experience in both musculoskeletal medicine and the specific demands placed on a dancer's body and psyche. Dance requires a sport-specific vocabulary that should be utilized by the members of the team with the dancer to ensure optimal communication. Depending on the injury type, the rehabilitation team may include physicians, physical or occupational therapists, athletic trainers, massage therapists, nutritionists and/or dieticians, psychiatrists or psychologists, chiropractors, podiatrists, acupuncturists, and other somatic practitioners. Dance teachers or artistic directors may also be involved. When available, the in-house medical team provides valuable insight into the demands of the company and the dancer's premorbid function, and is involved in the transition of care when formal rehabilitation is complete. A young dancer might not have access to an onsite medical team, so the dance teacher and physician may communicate directly regarding appropriate activity level. The composition of the rehabilitation team shifts to best address the injury and the contributing factors. For example, a nutritionist will not play as large a role when a dancer is determined to have adequate nutrition, but will be crucial to the team when a dancer is dealing with an eating disorder, disordered eating, or relative energy deficiency in sport (RED-S).

With any injury in dance, the rehabilitation process must address both the intrinsic and extrinsic contributions to the injury to maximize the potential for successful return to dance. Dancers more commonly suffer from overuse injuries (65%), but traumatic injuries are a significant issue 35%.[3] The majority of dance injuries are due to a combination of multiple intrinsic and extrinsic variables. Intrinsic risk factors for injury, such as strength imbalance, inadequate flexibility, malalignment, or incorrect biomechanics and technique, can often lead to overuse injuries or contribute to traumatic dance injuries. Extrinsic risk factors for injury include the dancer's environment and can lead to traumatic injuries, such as a poorly lit staircase causing a dancer to fall down the stairs, loose costuming causing a dropped lift, or slippery shoe soles causing a fall. These extrinsic factors are important to identify, as they remain a recurrent injury risk for that dancer and a new injury risk to other dancers.

## DANCE MEDICINE REHABILITATION PROGRESSION PROTOCOL

Dance injuries require a multifactorial approach to management. This rehabilitation progression protocol for dance medicine (Table 15.1) integrates the multiple aspects that should be addressed. As every injury is unique, the different stages may blend into one another as some aspects progress faster than others. This provides a generalized tool that can be tailored to develop each individual rehabilitation plan. Throughout the

*Performing Arts Medicine.* https://doi.org/10.1016/B978-0-323-58182-0.00015-8

| | | | IV: Dance-Specific Movement | V: Return to Rehearsal | VI: Independence |
|---|---|---|---|---|---|
| **I: Initial Assessment** | **II: Injury Management** | **III: Progression** | | | |
| Dance-specific history | Pain management | Strengthening | Balance and proprioception | Involve Artistic Director, teacher | Training regimen |
| Establish diagnosis and injury-specific protocols | Swelling and inflammation management | Stability | Rhythm and cadence progression | Dynamic warm-up, active cool-down | Transition to maintenance program |
| Musculoskeletal evaluation | Support and stabilization | Flexibility | Turn progression | Dance-specific environment | Continuous monitoring |
| Dance-specific special tests and considerations | Manual therapy | Range of motion | Jump progression | | |
| Mental health | Fitness maintenance | | Partnering and lifting | | |
| Nutrition | Home exercise program | | | | |

**TABLE 15.1**
**Dance Medicine Rehabilitation Progression Protocol**

rehabilitation process, it is critical to keep the dancer dancing and integrated into the company or class as allowed by the limitations of the injury. In dance, as with other sports, simply ceasing all activity for a week or two without addressing the underlying cause of the injury is seldom successful and can create distrust between the athlete and the medical profession.

**Set Expectations:** It is important to share with the dancer a typical timeframe for return to dance after their specific injury, with the understanding that each injury is unique. Be prepared for questions regarding the possible outcome after the injury. This allows the dancer and their company to realistically plan for the short-term and long-term future. Always overestimate the amount of time it will take to return. It is easier to return to dance earlier than to push back a return date. In addition, discuss the goals with the dancer, specifically their previous level of function, upcoming performances or auditions, and future expectation of function. A young dancer who plans to be a professional has different requirements than the young dancer who wishes to be able to attend class a few times per week. This step is necessary early in the rehabilitation process, as inaccurate expectations are associated with decreased satisfaction and pain after injury.[4]

Create an understanding that proper participation in their rehabilitation involves more than the dancer arriving on time for physical or occupational therapy appointments. Mental preparation, showing up well-rested and mentally prepared for sessions, ensuring proper and adequate nutrition for healing, and complying with the home exercises are also integral to a successful rehabilitation program. Although some dancers might not be compliant with the home exercises assigned, other dancers will do far more than requested (if 10 is good, 100 is better), which can also be counterproductive. Specific instructions on following through with the home exercise program and not doing too little or too much should be addressed. Understanding why the rehabilitation is important helps the dancer to find motivation and gain perspective on the process.[5] Educating the dancer throughout the rehabilitation process on health and prevention increases their confidence, and improves their body awareness and ability to successfully return to their previous level of dance.

The dancer should be aware that progression will occur, as specific targets are met. In some aspects, foundational work that can be perceived as basic and boring by the dancer should be conducted. Isolating and activating the hip abductors might be frustrating for an active individual, but must be accomplished to do multijoint dance movements correctly and safely. Injuries happen when athletes skip steps and jump to levels of function for which their body has not been properly prepared. One must walk before running. Alternatively, in this case, properly perform a plié prior to attempting a sauté (or petit jete).

Communication throughout the rehabilitation process between the patient and team members will also be important. Educate the dancer to talk about diagnostic test results, activity progression, and new pain or uncertainty with their providers. Encourage the dancer to engage in dialogue when something is not made clear. This establishes the dancer as an integral part of the medical team and teaches them to start listening to their body and to communicate their thoughts or concerns with the team.

## PHASE I: INITIAL ASSESSMENT

The initial evaluation is critical to establishing a comprehensive rehabilitation plan. For this reason, the injury is only one aspect addressed in this phase. The initial evaluation should also include a dance-specific history as well as general musculoskeletal and neurologic exams.

### Dance-Specific History

Exacerbating or alleviating positions and activities are an important component of the history, as well as any interventions, appointments, or imaging they have undergone. Ask about activities outside of dance and use this information to plan the rehabilitation schedule. Many dancers are students, teachers, or workers who work to supplement their income. Consequently, how they use their bodies outside of dance might impact their injury.

### Establish Diagnosis and Injury-Specific Protocols

The first priority during an initial exam is to make a diagnosis, or confirm the ongoing diagnosis is accurate and specific enough to guide the rehabilitation process. This encounter could be the dancer's first medical assessment, or they may have been referred to obtain a dance-specific plan of care. Establish the mechanism of injury if it is known. Document any restrictions or progression protocols if present, such as flexion or neutral-based core strengthening in a spondylolisthesis, or focusing on regaining full range of motion while avoiding open chain exercises after an anterior cruciate ligament reconstruction.

### Musculoskeletal Evaluation

The musculoskeletal exam addresses both neurological and musculoskeletal components of injury in addition to posture, alignment, joint range of motion, flexibility, strength, and conditioning. Even when the injury seems localized, the musculoskeletal evaluation must be generalized and the practitioner must be aware of regional interdependence. Frequently, dancers will dance injured or partially injured prior to realizing that medical intervention is necessary. This leads to secondary injury or pain due to compensatory mechanics that the dancer developed in an attempt to continue their baseline function. Sometimes secondary injuries occur, or secondary pain sites develop due to these altered arthrokinematics. It is important to try to "peel away" the layers of compensatory strategies to isolate and treat the initial injury.

**Posture and Alignment:** Baseline posture is different among dance styles due to aesthetic differences; it is important to evaluate for correct postural muscle activation as well as compensations due to muscle tightness, weakness, or joint hypermobility.

**Joint Range of Motion:** The range of motion of the lumbar spine and bilateral hips, knees, ankle, and great toe is assessed. If a dancer is trained in classical ballet, passive hip ROM is compared to total active turnout.[6] Classical ballet turnout is well researched, but debate continues on the determinants of range of motion in professional dancers, and how it should be measured. Dance style will determine how much range of motion is necessary at each joint. During injury, loss of ROM at one joint leads to an increased requirement for ROM at an adjacent joint, either proximal or distal due to the multijoint contributions of dance movement. Hypermobile dancers require education to avoid weight bearing at the end range of motion such as standing in genu recurvatum, and to promote correct muscle activation. This can be achieved through proprioception and stability training.

**Flexibility:** Asymmetries in flexibility may be an early sign of injury. Dancers are more flexible than nonperformance athletes.[7] For this reason, what may seem like adequate flexibility might actually be inadequate for their needs. Inexperience with the unique requirements of dancers may lead to an erroneous conclusion that a dancer has adequate flexibility when, in reality, dancers require much greater range of motion for their sport.

**Cardio-Conditioning:** Endurance and strength are important for dancers. Adequate conditioning[8] decreases the rate of fatigue, and fatigue is associated with increased injury.[9] Dance class or rehearsal does not adequately train the dancer for dance performance,[8,10,11] Performance demands vary widely[8] depending on the type of dance, choreography, and role.

**Strength:** Adequate strength to support the movements of the dancer throughout the range of motion they are utilizing is a necessity.

## Dance-Specific Special Tests and Considerations

**Joint Hypermobility:** Dancers may be screened for hypermobility using the Beighton Assessment of Hypermobility Scale, discussed in detail in Chapter 12, Role of Screening in the Professional Dance Company. Although hypermobility can be an occupational advantage for some dancers, it may increase the risk of injury.[12-14] In generalized ligamentous laxity, one of the main static stabilizers of the joint (the ligaments) are loose, leading to increased reliance on the other static stabilizers (capsule, cartilage) and dynamic stabilizers (muscles that cross the joint). This increases the risk of cartilage tears and muscle tightness. Hypermobility is associated with an increase in recovery time when compared to dancers with nonjoint hypermobility syndrome.[15]

**Balance and Proprioception:** Always assess a dancer's balance and proprioception, as both are key to the most fundamental movements of dance. Even a dancer with excellent balance and proprioception might need to be reassessed and retrained. Balance, for example, can be compromised after concussion. This can be evaluated with single and double limb stance with eyes open and closed, with progression to releve and dance-specific dynamic balance if performing well.

**Dance Movements:** Dancers who study ballet should have genre-specific evaluation of the biomechanics of common movements. First, ask them to demonstrate first, second, and fifth positions to gain a general understanding of how the dancer moves, and have them add in arms to assess scapular movement. Plié may be performed in each of these positions. There should be even weight bearing with the calcaneus remaining on the ground throughout the movement. In addition, confirm symmetric knee flexion aligned over the second toe with symmetrical turnout. Look for improper biomechanics including toe curling, pronation, or anterior tibialis recruitment. Assess spinal mobility with cambré and port de bras forward, monitoring for segmental movement without hinging at a specific level, or excessive lateral lean or rotation. Watch the dancer jump from the front and from the side to ensure the knees, hips, and core contribute to the movement and their heels make contact with the floor in a controlled manner. Improper mechanics include lumbar hyperlordosis, or landing on entire foot instead of on the forefoot. For single leg jump, the pelvis should not drop and the knee should not have a valgus moment. If a dancer has an injury it may preclude them from participating in the full exam.

**Turnout:** Functional turn out should be assessed by looking for signs of forced turnout, such as increased anterior pelvic tilt, "screwing" into the knees with excessive external tibial rotation, or excessive pronation at the subtalar joint. Turnout discs can be used to accurately determine functional turnout (Fig. 15.1). It is difficult to use improper mechanics while using the functional turnout discs. Traditionally, the range of motion necessary for proper turnout has been accepted as 70 degrees from the femoral-acetabular joint.[16] However, many recent studies have suggested that the actual range of motion in the typical ballet dancer hip is between 39.7 and 52.0 degrees.[17-19] This suggests that there is more range of motion than the traditional understanding of 5 degrees from the tibial external rotation at the knee and 15 degrees from the ankle and foot.

## Mental Health

The subject of mental health in dancers is covered in detail in a previous chapter. However, psychological variables are known to affect the outcome of dance injuries in both student and professional dancers,[20] so must also be addressed when treating a dancer with a physical injury. Times of stress, such as an injury, can exacerbate preexisting conditions or prolong the

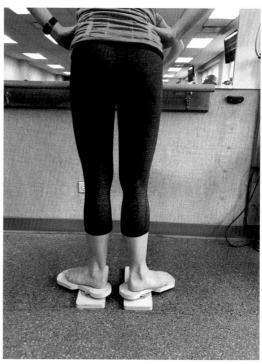

FIG. 15.1 Functional footprints

length of recovery. Injury recovery time for ballet students with a history of self-induced vomiting was significantly longer (median of 22.8 days) than recovery time for students who did not self-induce vomiting.[21] These symptoms might not have surfaced during the initial injury, but may come to light with the mental and physical challenges of rehabilitation. The level of fear a dancer experiences after an injury is consistently associated with poor injury recovery outcomes and should be addressed throughout the recovery and rehabilitation process.[22] For professional dancers, an injury increases the likelihood of losing a company position.[23]

Mental fatigue is also of concern for dancers. Understanding the influence psychological factors have on the injured dancer and encouraging the dancer to address them can positively influence the duration and outcome of injury rehabilitation.[24,25]

### Nutrition

Nutrition needs to be optimized for recovery from any injury. If low bone mineral density, or fatigue due to inadequate energy intake or anemia contributed to the injury, then involve a nutritionist in the treatment plan. If inadequate energy intake was intentional, then also involve a psychologist or psychiatrist.

## PHASE II: INJURY MANAGEMENT

After the initial assessment, focus shifts from injury diagnosis to managing the early symptoms of the injury with modalities to decrease pain, swelling, and inflammation, protection of the injured structure, manual therapy, and relative rest.

### Pain Management

Dancer comfort is a priority in rehabilitation. If necessary, medications should be used. Understanding physician expectations for prescription medications is important. If an antibiotic is prescribed due to concern for infection, that prescription should be completed. Pain medications are often to be taken as needed, but may be prescribed considering a dancer's medical condition or other medications. Sometimes a nonsteroidal anti-inflammatory drug is given at a high dose to prevent heterotopic ossification, or is avoided to promote wound healing. When the reasoning for prescribing or withholding medication is unclear, encourage the dancer to ask follow-up questions for clarification from the prescribing provider. They may also ask about supplementing with over the counter medications, oral or topical. Although pain medications might be

necessary early in an injury, they must be stopped prior to initiating return to dance. Pain or discomfort provide important warning signals that something is not right, allowing minor issues to be addressed as part of the rehabilitation process.

Modalities provide multiple options for pain management. Possibilities include thermal modalities (dry heat, hydrocollator, and cryotherapy), ultrasound, phonophoresis, intermittent pneumatic compression therapy, and electrotherapeutics (transcutaneous electrical nerve stimulation, iontophoresis, neuromuscular electrical stimulation). Injury type and dancer preference influence the modalities utilized.

### Swelling and Inflammation Management

Swelling is common after an injury but can lead to muscle inhibition and slow rehabilitation progression. An ankle joint effusion decreases peroneous longus activity,[26] and it only takes 20 mL of excess fluid in the knee joint for arthrogenic inhibition of the vastus medialis muscle to occur.[27] Compression can reduce posttraumatic edema, inflammatory response, and soft tissue scarring while improving proprioceptive feedback.[28] This can be done with taping, wrapping, or bracing. A short course of antiinflammatory medication may be appropriate if swelling limits range of motion or causes compensatory movement patterns. When utilizing antiinflammatory medication, consider a purposeful approach, such as a prescription strength dose, with a time limit of 1 week to progress through this stage more quickly.

### Support and Stabilization

Support for injured muscles, ligaments, and joints is important to prevent further injury and compensatory behaviors. Stabilization should be prioritized after a ligament tear, joint subluxation, or dislocation, and can be helpful in dancers with hypermobility syndrome. If the dancer is able to perform during the rehabilitation process, bracing is often not possible due to aesthetics. Taping is less bulky and commonly used, with 27.6% of surveyed dance medicine physical therapists[5] utilizing a variety of tape types for injured dancers. Taping can be used for support and stability,[29] compression, proprioception,[30] facilitation of muscle concentric contraction,[31] promotion of muscle inhibition in hypertonic muscles,[32] or even to promote dancer confidence.[33] Orthotics can also be used to promote proper biomechanics, particularly in dancers with hyperpronation,[34] and can be fashioned to fit in ballet slippers or stage shoes. If stability cannot be achieved through the above techniques, surgery might be necessary.

## Manual Therapy

Manual therapy can be used to mobilize soft tissue, improve joint range of motion, and decrease edema. After injury, tissue mobilization is necessary to avoid scarring and contractures. When releasing tight and spasmed muscles, care must be taken to assess for joint instability as the tightness may be in response to joint instability, and releasing the muscle could lead to recurrence of injury. Joint contracture can occur after prolonged immobilization, and joint malalignment may be premorbid or in response to injury. Obtaining proper alignment and maintaining functional range of motion during the recovery phase can decrease overall rehabilitation duration. Manual therapy can include myofascial release with hands or tools, joint mobilization or manipulation, massage, or manual traction.

Dry needling, trigger point injections, acupuncture, and cupping can provide a deeper muscle tissue myofascial release. Practitioner experience, patient education, and expectations heavily influence whether or not these options are be considered.

## Fitness Maintenance

Instead of ceasing all activity after injury, provide the dancer with alternative activities that are safe to perform with their injury while maintaining cardiovascular fitness. This also provides the dancer with an alternative outlet for their energy and use of their time that they would typically fill with dance class, rehearsals, and performances. Seldom does an injury require complete rest, which leads to deconditioning and loss of muscle elasticity. It is critical to keep the dancer dancing, even if activity must be significantly modified to protect the injury or prevent future injury. When possible, integrate dance participation into the rehabilitation plan early after injury, creating a space that allows the dancer to maintain their identity as a dancer. Modify daily class to include work at the barre without moving to the center, or restrict activity to the noninjured limb or partial weight bearing. When regular dance class participation is not safe, consider Floor Barre, which modifies the basic movements of ballet to nonweight bearing prone, sidelying and supine positions, or Aqua Barre, which substitutes a pool noodle for the barre and utilizes isometric contractions and water resistance to promote strength and stability. Pilates and Gyrotonics can often be modified to accommodate injury restrictions.

Use terms with positive connotations such as cross-training or fitness maintenance instead of negative connotations such as stop or shut down. Depending on the injury type, swimming or cycling is a low-impact workout than running or dancing. If injury is due to or concurrent with disordered eating or RED-S, careful consideration of energy availability and its relation to bone health is vital prior to integrating cardiovascular maintenance into the rehabilitation process.

## Home Exercise Program

Starting a home exercise program early in the rehabilitation process establishes it as an important and integral part of return to dance. Initial exercises given to the patient can focus on preserving joint range of motion and muscle strength.

## PHASE III: PROGRESSION

During this phase, deficits found during the initial assessment are addressed, and a solid foundation for successful rehabilitation can be established. Treatment of the initial injury and compensatory behaviors continue. Multiple aspects of the rehabilitation process can be addressed simultaneously (mobilizing tight soft tissue while strengthening weak muscles and realigning or stabilizing joints), while others must occur in a stepwise fashion (gluteus medius isolation and activation prior to single leg squat). Skipping steps risks missing important developments. Injuries in dance provide an opportunity to address underlying issues that might have been keeping the dancer from realizing their full potential or highest skill level.

As mentioned at the beginning of this chapter, the importance of keeping a dancer dancing cannot be overstressed. Modifications that were necessary in previous rehabilitation phases can now be reassessed. Throughout this phase, imagery and somatic practice can be introduced as methods to improve motor learning.[35] Imagery, or visualizing movement, enhances the coping skills of injured athletes and promotes rehabilitation adherence.[36] Mental imagery focusing on healing and relaxation is associated with improved pain tolerance.[37] Somatic practices such as The Feldenkrais Method for mindful movement or Alexander Technique improve awareness of movement patterns.

### Strengthening

Strengthening may be due to preinjury weakness or weakness acquired after injury. Dancers might not have true weakness, and instead have a strength imbalance,[38] or simply an inability to coordinate specific muscles, causing maladaptive compensation techniques. A perceived loss of strength by the dancer is associated with significantly increased recovery time[22]; and strength imbalances increase injury risk.[39]

Initiate strengthening with controlled, isolated movements to minimize compensation by other muscles, providing neuromuscular reeducation when necessary to encourage proper form and movement patterns. Control and coordination is important as dancers can learn maladaptive recruitment patterns, so those movements need to be broken down to their parts and retrained to ensure correct biomechanics. Begin with isometric movements, progressing to isotonic, and then isokinetic as appropriate.[28] Create strengthening exercises from functional movement whenever possible, such as working on hip external rotators with arabesque-type movements. Gradually increase movement complexity with a goal of integrating the activation of multiple muscles at increasing velocity. Mamie Air and Dr. Rietveld developed a dance-specific graded rehabilitation schedule plan that progresses the dancer through increasing impact exercises. Phase 1 is without impact and begins at the barre, progressing to center and excludes jumps or turns. Phase 2 allows small, controlled, and assisted jumps such as sauté, progressing from petit allegro to eventually grand allegro.[40]

Reassure the injured dancer that muscle strength can be gained without increased muscle bulk or loss or flexibility. Some dancers avoid strength training under the impression that their muscles will hypertrophy, which negatively affects the aesthetic appearance.[41] Others avoid strength training due to concern for loss of flexibility, when in fact strength training is positively associated with flexibility scores.[42]

## Stability

Stabilization after injury is important. Proper stability is a combination of neural (proprioception, reflexes, muscular reaction time), muscular (strength, power, and endurance), and mechanical (ligaments) factors.[43] Deficits in proprioception have been demonstrated after ankle sprains,[44] but high school athletes who participated in a balance training program significantly reduced the risk of an ankle sprain,[45] and high-level male athletes who participated in neuromuscular training significantly decreased the incidence of anterior cruciate ligament injury.[46]

As ligaments are integral to stability, proprioceptive training is of particular importance for dancers with hypermobility syndrome. Emphasis deep core control, isometric cocontraction when appropriate, and eccentric stabilization, especially at end-range of motion, is imperative. Initiate stability training with weight shifting, and then single leg balance on a stable surface. As stability improves, integrate an unstable surface such as a thick mat,

Balance Board, or Bosu Ball into single leg balance and add squats and jumps in multiple directions. Functional neuromuscular and proprioceptive training provides a dancer with a dynamically stable joint that improves function and reduces risk of reinjury.[47]

## Flexibility

Flexibility is crucial in many styles of dance, and is a product of muscle extensibility and joint mobility,[48] so stretching is fundamental to dancers. Stretching increases tendon unit compliance, increasing the amount of energy absorbed by a tendon when the muscle is activated which reduces muscle fiber trauma.[49] In dance, this would be beneficial in changements, which requires landing in a demi-plie position with an elongated achilles immediately after the gastro-soleus complex concentrically contracted to initiate the jump.

There are many types of stretches, with varying benefit and risk of injury. Proprioceptive neuromuscular facilitation is a more effective form of stretching than static or ballistic,[50] and it also improves muscle strength after 8 weeks.[51] In static stretching, 30 s in duration is the most effective, as it is more effective than shorter duration stretches but as effective as holding a stretch for a longer amount of time.[52] Static stretching should not be done prior to class, rehearsal, or performance, as it reduces muscle strength at slow contraction velocities for the next 1−2 h.[53] It should also be done with care. One survey of ballet students (age 17−25) found that 88% of rear thigh injuries occurred during slow activities such as flexibility training with splits in sagittal plan or warm-up/cool-down, while only 12% of the injuries occurred during powerful movements such as grande jete.[54]

## Range of Motion

Dancers are significantly more likely to change their level of dance after injury if they felt they had limited range of motion.[22] Any discrepancy between total passive turnout and total active turnout should be addressed. Muscle weakness or tightness, tissue restriction, or poor motor control[55] can lead to forced turnout. Dancers can improve active turnout by strengthening the hip external rotators.[56] Tools to assist in proper measurement and strengthening include a goniometer, rotator discs, or functional footprints (Fig. 15.1). Functional footprints have the degrees of rotation marked, and tilt to stop rotation if the weight is not evenly distributed (Fig. 15.2).

Educate dancers on safe joint range of motion, as they might feel the sensation of a muscle stretch due to generalized ligamentous laxity or previous injury.

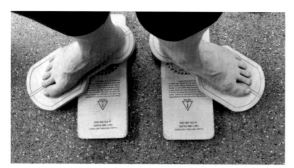

FIG. 15.2 Functional footprints - measuring turnout

In these situations, visual cues can be given and proprioceptive exercises utilized to encourage safe joint range of motion.

## PHASE IV: DANCE-SPECIFIC MOVEMENT

When the injury has healed and a firm foundation for recovery is in place, progression to the more difficult and complex maneuvers required of dance is appropriate to prepare the dancer for return to the demands of class, rehearsal, and performances. Similar to a distance runner whose first run back from an injury should not be 26.2 miles, a dancer who has been restricted from full activity cannot simply be dropped back into class or rehearsal and assume continued success. Even when all contributing factors of an injury, both intrinsic and extrinsic, have been addressed, the dancer must progress toward the goal in a step-wise fashion. When progressing through increasingly difficult physical demands, it will be important to teach the dancers to listen to their body. As mentioned previously in this chapter, pain is the body's way of communicating that something is wrong, so should not be muted by medications. Delayed pain can also be an indication of progression that is advancing too quickly. Soreness can be a positive indication that the muscles are being appropriately challenged. This can be an opportunity to have a dialogue with the dancer on the difference between pain and soreness, and the importance of knowing the difference to prevent future injuries.

Regular status checks should be built into the rehabilitation process as an opportunity to assess progress, goal achievement, and estimated return to dance. Response with necessary modifications can be done in a timely fashion. To help keep the dancer focused, there may need to be adjustments to the home exercise, correction of previous assumptions, and reminders of the overall goals. A dancer might overcorrect certain cues given early in rehabilitation, with a tucked pelvis becoming a swayback or an overpronator beginning to hang on to their lateral ligaments, necessitating updated cueing and correction. The home exercise program should be advanced as appropriate to ensure that it is functional and engaging.

### Balance and Proprioception

Dance-specific stability should prepare them for movements common in the studio and for the demands of their goals. Progress can be made from double-limb to single limb stance on a stable surface to an unstable surface, and jazz shoe or barefoot to en pointe when appropriate and applicable. Assess weight shift from double to single leg stance into passé. The dancer should maintain neutral pelvic alignment without trendelenberg, modified trendelenberg, or hip hiking, and should use their deep hip rotators to maintain hip external rotation. In ballet, start the dancer at the barre before moving to the center, with petite allegro prior to grand allegro.

### Rhythm and Cadence Progression

Use a metronome to slowly increase speed while maintaining proper technique and alignment to help the dancer prepare for various tempos and situations.

### Turn Progression

When it is appropriate to integrate turns into the rehabilitation process, start with turn preparations. Have the dancer hold balance in the fourth position, perform, and hold a plié prior to moving to passé, also controlling that position. This ensures that the dancer can begin turning upright, in proper position, instead of throwing themselves into the turn from the fourth position, never achieving correct body positioning. Start with single turns, and then multiple turns and traveling turns. Have the dancer use different shoes, eventually progressing to pointe shoes if applicable.

### Jump Progression

Jumping is an area of high risk for injury. It requires endurance, adequate range of motion, and strength. The Harkness Center for Dance Injuries developed an elegant progression for jumps[57] that suggests starting with a minimum load phase equivalent to walking, such as plié relevé and prances. Monitor alignment of the hip flexors, knee flexors, and dorsiflexors in the sagittal plane, and knee alignment in the frontal plane. Start with three sessions of 10−30 s at a jump speed of 80−90 beats per minute. Toe to heel landing must be controlled. When integrating jumps into a rehabilitation schedule, allow 48−72 h of recovery after each session, monitoring for joint irritation or delayed onset muscle soreness. When a particular load phase is tolerated with correct technique over two or three sessions, a higher load phase can be attempted. A moderate load phase, equivalent to running, includes jumps in the first position (jumping with two feet and landing on two feet) or chasse. A maximum load phase, when jumping from two feet and landing with one, incorporates sissone assemble or horizontal jumping.[57]

### Partnering and Lifting

Throughout rehabilitation, be aware of the partner's weight and lift expectations. When the dancer is ready, have the partner attend sessions to address typical lifts.

## PHASE V: RETURN TO REHEARSAL

Promotion occurs when transitioning away from formal rehabilitation and returning to full participation in class and rehearsal. During this time, continue formal rehabilitation to address any difficulties or concerns that arise, working toward mastery of the skills addressed during the previous phases.

### Involve Artistic Director or Teacher

With the dancers permission, communicate with the dancer's artistic director, staff, or teacher throughout rehabilitation. They may be essential to successful transition back to the company, particularly after a prolonged absence due to injury or when the company does not have an in-house medical staff. During the Promotion phase, ask if they will take the dancer through a modified class as they often identify areas of concern that might limit the dancer's return, from biomechanics to aesthetics or timidity. They are also aware of upcoming choreography demands, allowing rehabilitation to prepare for specific choreography styles or demands (multiple high jumps or turns, modern or en pointe) allowing the dancer to better prepare physically and mentally. This also applies to cardiorespiratory training, which can be tailored for the demands of the choreography or classes that will be rejoined.

### Dynamic Warm-Up, Active Recovery Cool Down

Educate the dancer on the importance of preparing the mind and body for class, rehearsal, and performance as well as a cool down afterward. A light cardiovascular warm up such as walking, marching, body swing, and step-hops around the room, followed by 30 s of static stretches and then 30 s of dynamic stretches can improve balance, jump height, and hamstring range of motion.[58] Encourage easy mobilization at the ankles, knees, hips, and shoulders to activate muscles and gradually increase heart rate and body temperature. Discourage aggressive static stretching as it can increase injury risk[59] and lead to muscle inhibition.[53] Tailor the warm-up to address areas of tightness or muscles the dancer has difficulty activating, and consider performance-specific choreography such as leaps or turns. The cool down allows for a gradual decrease in body temperature and heart rate, and is the appropriate time for soft tissue stretching and mobilization. If the resources are available, cryotherapy or compression boots can assist with recovery.

### Dance-Specific Environment

Simulate the environment the dancer will return to as much as possible, including flooring material such as a sprung floor, wood slats, steel, or tile. Stages can be raked (at an incline) or flat; consequently, it may be appropriate to perform some of the rehabilitation on a raked surface. Footwear type, such as tap shoes, pointe shoes, or ghillies in Irish dance, greatly affect the way a dancer interacts with the floor. The rehabilitation practitioner should ensure good fit and biomechanics while the dancer is shod. Costumes that involve heavy headdresses or restrictive corsets change the center of gravity and breathing technique. These may be utilized during practice. Dancers should be able to concentrate despite bright or flashing lights, audience chatter, and other performers walking in front or behind them. Face the dancer away from mirror so that they do not rely on watching themselves for technique or balance. Vary lighting, using a bright light to simulate a spotlight, or require eyes closed to simulate a blackout, when all the lights are turned off onstage.

## PHASE VI: INDEPENDENCE

When the formal rehabilitation process is complete, and the dancer has successfully returned to their previous level of function, the dancer is not finished with the rehabilitation program but has simply transitioned to an independent maintenance program. This program is integrated into warm-up, class, rehearsals, and performances, with the goal of minimizing reinjury and preventing new injury. In cases of prolonged recovery, consider scheduling a reassessment within a few weeks after promotion to self-sufficiency. This provides an opportunity to address any pain or dysfunction issues that arise, correct exercise biomechanics, revisit issues the dancer struggled with throughout rehab, address new choreography concerns, and adjust the maintenance plan accordingly.

## REFERENCES

1. Ojofeitimi S, Bronner S. Injuries in a modern dance company: effect of comprehensive management on injury incidence and cost. *J Dance Med Sci.* 2011;15:116–122.
2. Ekegren C, Quested R, Brodnick A. Injuries in pre-professional ballet dancers: incidence, characteristics and consequences. *J Sci Med Sport.* 2014;17:271–275.
3. Solomon R, Micheli L, Solomon J. The "cost" of injuries in a professional ballet company. *Med Probl Perform Art.* 1995;10:3–10.
4. Anakwe R, Jenkins P, Moran M. Predicting dissatisfaction after total hip arthroplasty: a study of 850 patients. *J Arthroplasty.* 2011;26:209–213.
5. Sabo M. Physical therapy rehabilitation strategies for dancers: a qualitative study. *J Dance Med Sci.* 2013;17:11–17.
6. Liederbach M. Screening for functional capacity in dancers. *J Dance Med Sci.* 1997;1:93–106.
7. DiTullio M, Wilczek L, Paulus D, et al. Comparison of hip rotation in female classical ballet dancers versus female nondancers. *Med Probl Perform Art.* 1999;4:154–158.
8. Wyon M. Cardiorespiratory training for dancers. *J Dance Med Sci.* 2005;9:7–12.
9. Liederbach M, Gleim G, Nicholas J. Physiologic and psychological measurement of performance stress and onset of injuries in professional ballet dancers. *Med Probl Perform Art.* 1994;9:10–14.
10. Cohen J, Segal K, McARdle W. Heart rate response to ballet state performance. *Phys Sportsmed.* 1982;10:120–133.
11. Schantz P, Astrand P. Physiologic characteristics classical ballet. *Med Sci Sports Exerc.* 1984;16:472–476.
12. McCormack M, Briggs J, Grahame R. Joint laxity and the benign joint hypermobility syndrome in student and professional ballet dancers. *J Rheumatol.* 2004;31:173–178.
13. Hamilton W, Hamilton L, Marshall P. A profile of the musculoskeletal characteristics of elite professional ballet dancers. *Am J Sports Med.* 1992;20:267–273.
14. Micheli L, Gillespie W, Walaszek A. Physiologic profiles of female professional ballerinas. *Clin Sports Med.* 1984;3:199–209.
15. Briggs J, McCormack M, Hakim A, Grahame R. Injury and joint hypermobility syndrome in ballet dancers—a 5-year follow-up. *J Rheumatol.* 2009;48:1613–1614.
16. Thomasen E. *Diseases and Injuries of Ballet Dancers.* Arjus, Denmark: Arhus Universitetsforlaget I (English translation); 1982.
17. Bauman P, Singson R, Hamilton W. Femoral neck anteversion in ballerinas. *Clin Orthop.* 1994:57–63.
18. Gilbert C, Gross M, Klug K. Relationship between hip external rotation and turnout angle for the five classical ballet positions. *J Orthop Sports Phys Ther.* 1998;27:339–347.
19. Khan K, Roberts P, Nattrass C, et al. Hip and ankle range of motion in elite classical ballet dancer and controls. *Clin J Sport Med.* 1997;7:174–179.
20. Mainwaring L, Finney C. Psychological risk factors and outcomes of dance injury, a systematic review. *J Dance Med Sci.* 2017;21:87–96.
21. Thomas J, Keel P, Heatherton T. Disordered eating and injuries among adolescent ballet dancers. *Eat Weight Disord.* 2011;16:e216–222.
22. Junck E, Richardson M, Dilgen F, et al. A retrospective assessment of return to function in dance after physical therapy for common dance injuries. *J Dance Med Sci.* 2017;21:156–167.
23. Garrick J, Requa R. Ballet injuries: an analysis of epidemiological and financial outcome. *Am J Sports Med.* 1993;12:586–590.
24. Mainwaring L, Krasnow D, Kerr G. And the dance goes on: psychological impact of injury. *J Dance Med Sci.* 2001;5:105–115.
25. Noh Y, Morris T, Anderses M. Psychological intervention programs for reduction of injury in ballet dancers. *Res Sports Med.* 2007;15:13–32.
26. Hopkin J, Palmieri R. Effects of ankle joint effusion on lower leg function. *Clin J Sport Med.* 2004;14:1–7.
27. Spencer J, Hayes K, Alexancer I. Knee joint effusion and quadriceps reflex inhibition in man. *Arch Phys Med Rehabil.* 1984;65:171–177.
28. Clanton T, Coupe K. Hamstring strains in athletes: diagnosis and treatment. *J Am Acad Orthop Surg.* 1998;6:237–248.
29. Ewalt K. Bandaging and taping considerations of the dancer. *J Dance Med Sci.* 2010;14:103–113.
30. Cools A, Witvrouw E, Danneels L, Cambier D. Does taping influence electromyographic muscle activity in the scapular rotators in healthy shoulders? *Man Ther.* 2002;7:154–162.
31. Thelen M, Dauber J, Stoneman P. The clinical efficacy of Kinsio tape for shoulder pain: a randomized, double-blinded, clinical trial. *J Orthop Sports Phys Ther.* 2008;38:389–395.
32. Yasukawa A, Patel P, Sisung C. Pilot study: investigating the effects of Kinesio taping in an acute pediatric rehabilitation setting. *Am J Occup Ther.* 2006;60:104–110.
33. Sawkins K, Refsuage K, Kilbreath S, Raymond J. The placebo effect of ankle taping in ankle instability. *Med Sci Sport Exerc.* 2007;39:781–787.
34. Nowacki R, Air M, Rietveld A. Use and effectiveness of orthotics in hyperpronated dancers. *J Dance Med Sci.* 2013;17:3–10.
35. Baston G. Revisiting overuse injuries in dance in view of motor learning and somatic models of distributed practice. *J Dance Med Sci.* 2007;11:70–75.
36. Wesch N, Hall C, Prapavessis H, Wesch N. Self-efficacy, imagery use, and adherence during injury rehabilitation. *Scand J Med Sci Sports.* 2012;22:695–703.
37. Hamson-Utley J, Martin S, Walters J. Athletic trainer's and physical therapists' perceptions of the effectiveness of psychological skills within sport injury rehabilitation programs. *J Athl Train.* 2008;43:258–264.

38. Liederbach M, Hiebert R. The relationship between eccentric and concentric equinus in classical dancers. *J Dance Med Sci.* 1997;1:55−61.
39. Aagaard P, Simonsen E, Magnusson S, Larsson B, Dyhre-Poulsen P. A new concept for isokinetic hamstring: quadriceps muscle strength ratio. *Am J Sports Med.* 1998;26:231−237.
40. Air M, Rietveld A. Dance-specific, graded rehabilitation: advice, principles, and schedule for the general practitioner. *Med Probl Perform Art.* 2008;23:114−119.
41. Koutedakis Y, Stavropoulos-Kalinoglou A, Metsios G. The significance of muscular strength in dance. *J Dance Med Sci.* 2005;9:29−34.
42. Pratt M. Strength, flexibility, and maturity in adolescent athletes. *Am J Dis Child.* 1989;143:560−563.
43. Konradsen L, Olesen S, Hansen H. Ankle sensorimotor control and eversion strength after acute ankle inversion injuries. *Am J Sports Med.* 1998;26:72−77.
44. Glencross D, Thornton E. Position sense following joint injury. *J Sports Med Phys Fitness.* 1981;21:23−27.
45. McGuine T, Keene J. The effect of a balance training program on the risk of ankle sprains in high school athletes. *Am J Sports Med.* 2006;34:1103−1111.
46. Caraffa A, Cerulli G, Projetti M, et al. Prevention of anterior cruciate ligament injuries in soccer: a prospective controlled study of proprioceptive training. *Knee Surg Sports Traumatol Arthrosc.* 1996;4:19−21.
47. Griffin L, Agel J, Albohm M, et al. Noncontact anterior cruciate ligament injuries: risk factors and prevention strategies. *J Am Acad Orthop Surg.* 2000;8:141−150.
48. Deighan M. Flexibility in dance. *J Dance Med Sci.* 2005;9:13−17.
49. Witvrouw E, Mahieu N, Danneels L, McNair P. Stretching and injury prevention: an obscure relationship. *Sports Med.* 2005;34:443−449.
50. Sady S, Wortman M, Blanke D. Flexibility training: ballistic, static or proprioceptive neuromuscular facilitation. *Arch Phys Med Rehabil.* 1982;63:261−263.
51. Handel M, Horstmann T, Dickhutch H, et al. Effects of contract-relax stretching training on muscle performance in athetes. *Eur J Appl Physiol.* 1997;76:400−408.
52. Roberts J, Wilson K. Effect of stretching duration on the active and passive range of motion in the lower extremity. *Br J Sports Med.* 1999;33:259−263.
53. Power K, Behm D, Cahill F, et al. An acute bout of staic stretching: effects of force and jumping performance. *Med Sci Sports Exerc.* 2004;36:1389−1396.
54. Askling C, Lund H, Saartok T, et al. Self-reported hamstring injuries in student dancers. *Scand J Med Sci Sports.* 2002;12:230−235.
55. Grossman G. Measuring dancer's active and passive turnout. *J Dance Med Sci.* 2003;7:49−55.
56. Pata D, Welsh T, Bailey J, Range V. Improving turnout in university dancers. *J Dance Med Sci.* 2014;18:169−177.
57. Sandow E, Dilgen F. A jump progression protocol for dancers returning to dance after injury. In: *Presented at: International Association for Dance Medicine & Science 2017 Annual Conference, Houston, TX*; October 12−15, 2017. Harkness Jump Progression (IADMS 2017) https://cdn.ymaws.com/www.iadms.org/resource/resmgr/am_pdfs/iadms-2017-schedule.pdf.
58. Morrin N, Redding E. Acute effects of warm-up stretch protocols on balance, vertical jump height, and range of motion in dancers. *J Dance Med Sci.* 2013;17:34−40.
59. Shrier I. When and whom to stretch? Gauging the benefits and drawbacks for individual patients. *Phys Sports Med.* 2004;33:22−26.

## FURTHER READING

1. Liederbach M, Kremenic I, Orishimo K, et al. Comparison of landing biomechanics between male and female dancers and athletes, Part 2. *Am J Sports Med.* 2014;42:1089−1095.
2. Barrack R, Skinner H, Brunet M, et al. Joint laxity and proprioception in the knee. *Phys Sportsmed.* 1983;11:130−135.

## CHAPTER 16

# Managing Psychological Disturbances in Performing Artists

LYNDA MAINWARING, PHD, C. PSYCH • SHULAMIT MOR, PHD, C. PSYCH

## INTRODUCTION

Performing artists experience an intimate and intense long-term relationship with their specific art form. This relationship involves sacrifices, challenges, struggles, victories, defeats, self-improvement, and the interaction with teachers, administrators, colleagues, and most importantly the audience. The nature of the performing arts is that the artist's message is communicated only through the delivered act within the duration of a particular performance. In other words, if a work is not performed, its communicative message is nonexistent. Performance is the final product for all the performing arts; works are completed and revealed only by their performance. Moreover, a performance requires the presence of the audience to come to life. This lifeline between the audience and the performer creates the magic and the risks of the profession. Given the pressures and importance of performance, it is not surprising that psychological distress of various and unique forms are quite high in the performing arts profession. For example, Vaag, Bjorngaard, and Bjerkeset[1] found psychological distress to be more prevalent among musicians when compared to a general work sample whereby musicians scored higher on measures of depression and anxiety. Similarly, Maxwell, Seton, and Szabo[2] reported that actors are vulnerable to depression, anxiety, and stress above levels indicated in the general population. Raeburn, Hipple, Delaney, and Chesky[3] in their review of musicians' health reported that depression and anxiety were among the most frequently cited nonmusculoskeletal problems. Dancers are also prone to psychological distress related to performance pressures, risks, and outcomes of injury.[4,5] As Brandfonbrener[6] highlights, factors such as long working hours, sleep deprivation, lack of help-seeking, and extreme pressure to perform contribute to psychosocial difficulties and stress in performing artists.

Given the extraordinary characteristics of the performing arts professions, it is critical for clinicians to understand the nature and context of the distress. It is not unusual for practitioners to see actors, musicians, or dancers who present with symptoms of major depressive disorder, social anxiety, or eating disorders. Although the symptom clusters are similar to those presented by individuals in the general population, the concerns, stressors, and professional context are quite different. Issues related to treatment adherence, rest, sleep, onset of symptoms, or management of pain and discomfort can be quite different for the performing artist. Therefore, the purpose of this chapter is to highlight the major issues with which performing artists struggle and provide guidelines for their management. We will not describe the specific symptoms and diagnostic criteria of the associated pathologies, but rather provide insight about the specific context by reference to contemporary research, and years of the authors' clinical and personal experience with the performing arts world. Disorders with which clinicians are familiar such as depression, anxiety, sleep disorders, and those relevant but less common in performers (body dysmorphic disorder, trauma-related disorders) are not included in the chapter.

Struggles with stress and anxiety are inevitable experiences faced by all humans. Performers face additional, work-specific stressors not usually experienced by the general population. These include years of practicing and perfecting technical skills, performing in front of audiences regularly, and the insecurity of maintaining a career and sometimes a shortened career trajectory.

Common mental health challenges shared by performers include burnout, disordered eating and eating disorders, coping with and managing injuries, perfectionism, performance anxiety, and managing identity and insecurity related to problems building, sustaining, and terminating a performance career. Each is discussed

Performing Arts Medicine. https://doi.org/10.1016/B978-0-323-58182-0.00016-X

in terms of the presenting problem, the prevalence of the problem when available, management strategies and practical guidelines and recommendations for practitioners.

## PERFORMANCE ANXIETY

By its nature, every performance involves self-presentation and exposure to judgment and criticism. Any negative consequences such as a bad review or poor audition can be deleterious to a career. It is not surprising that performance anxiety (often called stage fright) is a common occurrence in all performing arts.[7–10] It appears from the research literature to be distinct from occupational stress and trait anxiety.[7]

Music performance anxiety (MPA) has been studied extensively for more than 25 years[7,11] and reports of prevalence range from 16% to 75%.[8,12] The latest music and health survey conducted by the International Conference of Symphony and Opera Musicians (ICSOM) found that in a sample of 447 musicians 98% of participants reported experiencing performance anxiety "at one time or another" with the onset age of 11–15 years old.

The Diagnostic and Statistical Manual of Mental Disorders 5th edition (DSM-5) specifies that individuals who are anxious only when performing in front of an audience "appear to represent a distinct subset of social anxiety disorder in terms of etiology, age at onset, physiological response, and treatment response."[13] Females in general experience anxiety more than males,[14,15] and female musicians also experience higher MPA than males.[16,17]

Performance anxiety can be experienced physiologically (e.g., sweaty palms, rapid heartbeat), behaviorally (e.g., immobilization, over rehearsal), and cognitively (e.g., negative self-talk, and impaired concentration). As Hays[18] points out, most performers experience an elevated physiological arousal prior to or during performance, but it is the attention to and interpretation of the arousal that can either enhance or unravel a performance. Mor[19] distinguishes between *Up Performance* (i.e., peak performance), *Stage Fright*, and *Stage Terror* arguing that perceived control (both internal and external) determines the performer's perception of the performance situation. Stage fright appears to be a situation in which the artist loses some control during the performance but is still able to project a reasonable account of the performed piece. Stage terror, on the other hand, represents a complete loss of control resulting in memory block and a dissociative state. This debilitating anxiety reaction shuts the person down with an inability to execute the highly trained skills on command. Such reactions are extremely traumatic for

performers who have been preparing for months or years for a particular audition or performance.

## MANAGEMENT OF PERFORMANCE ANXIETY

Research indicates that the best interventions to manage performance anxiety are a combination of cognitive and behavioral techniques such as cognitive restructuring, relaxation, and mental skills training.[20–25] Virtual reality exposure training has been found to be effective as well.[26] Implementation of these techniques requires the assistance of healthcare providers trained in behavioral management strategies or mental skills consultants who are well versed in sport psychology strategies for management of performance anxiety.

β-Blockers (e.g., propranolol) or antianxiety medication is often prescribed to help manage performance anxiety. The latest ICSOM survey[27] indicated that 70% of ICSOM musicians have tried using β-blockers for performance anxiety for auditions (90%), solo or featured performance (74%), and orchestra performance (36%).

Unfortunately, using pharmaceuticals over one's lifelong career can create dependency or interact adversely with other substances (e.g., caffeine) and cause a cycle of dysfunctional behaviors (e.g., sleep disorders, multiple physician prescriptions, substance abuse). In addition, although they may be beneficial in reducing some physiological reactions, certain medications can increase salivation or dry mouth, which can be detrimental to singers, instrumentalists, or actors. More importantly, depending on external solutions does nothing to teach performers how to handle their performance anxiety and thus is not beneficial in terms of developing a sense of a self-efficacy and competence. A better strategy would be for the clinician to refer to practitioners who can help the artist with nonpharmaceutical strategies. A good referral network of clinicians (psychologists, psychiatrists, psychotherapists, counsellors, and mental skills trainers) with training in managing anxiety disorders specific to performance issues is crucial.

### Guidelines and Recommendation

General practitioners may feel more comfortable to prescribe medication, but as noted, a complete reliance on medication is not psychologically salutary. Recommendations for management include the following:
- Identify the problem and the appropriate course of treatment.
- Communicate the range of options available to the artist. These might include nonmedical approaches

such as psychological intervention, physical exercises, massage, yoga, and Alexander Technique.
- Consider the time frame for treatment relative to the artist's performance schedule.
- Use caution with pharmacological interventions and consider their benefits carefully with the needs of the artist. Make sure that the artist is well informed and aware of the advantages and disadvantages of the medication, in particular using it without medical supervision.
- Refer the performer to a Performing Art clinic if available in his or her geographical location.

## PERFECTIONISM

Perfectionism in the academic literature is defined as the striving for high standards while being overly concerned about mistakes or having doubts about actions.[28] The paradox of perfectionism is that in the general population the unyielding pursuit of being perfect is considered pathological whereas in the performing arts pursuing a perfect performance is inherent to the nature of the profession. Clearly, performers face daunting tasks: each performance is expected to be better than the one before and the elusive goal of the perfect performance is ever present. Furthermore, an added stressor for performers is the awareness that the audience also expects a perfect performance, which essentially is never defined or determined.[9]

Distinguishing between the pursuit of *performance perfection*[29] and perfectionism as pathological is critical when considering the performing arts world and high demand careers.

Dancers and musicians typically manage their perfectionistic tendencies by constantly striving for a higher level of performance and pushing themselves both physically and mentally. If they perceive that they fall short, which is typical because performers are usually dissatisfied with themselves or their performance, anxiety becomes intolerable and they may seek assistance, or maintain an intense training schedule and push themselves incessantly often with deleterious consequences. Perfectionism, injury, and stress are related.[30]

Originally conceptualized as an enduring, multidimensional trait,[31] the more recent conceptualization of perfectionism is that it is domain specific.[32,33] Striving for perfection in one area of life (performance) does not necessarily mean that one will strive for perfection in other areas. Scientists have recognized that professional competence and excellence are prerequisites for success in the performance and athletic world, and there may be adaptive aspects of perfectionism.[34–37]

Clinicians need to consider the high demands for perfection that are associated with the performing arts in any diagnosis consideration of a high-level performer. Often, issues related to perfectionism or high demands in the performing arts will present as anxiety-related disorders, and management of the anxiety with appreciation for the context is essential.

## MANAGEMENT OF PROBLEMS RELATED TO THE PURSUIT OF PERFECTION IN PERFORMANCE

When working with performers, clinicians need to distinguish between perfectionism as a pathologic personality trait that manifests in potentially dysfunctional behavior and anxiety that has its roots in the extraordinary demands originating from the culture. The latter pushes dancers, for example, to perform at the highest standards, setting the bar higher than may be possible to sustain. The astute clinician has to recognize that the high demand for excellence and the pursuit of the flawless performance is built into the culture, and that the pursuit of perfection does not necessarily mean that artists are perfectionists. Rather, they may require assistance to modulate or remove the pursuit of unrealistically high standards.

A good clinical interview with or without completion of a self-report perfectionism scale can identify whether the performer suffers from perfectionism or whether the tendency to strive for exceptionally high standards is within a healthy limit given the context in which the performer works. There are numerous scales available to measure perfectionism (the two most common scales are the Multidimensional Perfectionism Scale: MPS by Frost, Marten, Lahart, & Rosenblate[28]; the Multidimensional Perfectionism Scale: MPS by Flett & Hewitt[31]) but awareness of their limitations is important.

### Guidelines and Recommendations

- Identify the professional demands and how they may be implicated with the artists presenting problem.
- Consider whether perfectionism is present or whether the pursuit of perfect performances is appropriate, and the difficulties are more related to stress, coping, and anxiety.
- Develop realistic mutually agreed upon goals that recognize the pressures of performance.
- Assist with self-confidence and empowerment so that the artist develops perceived control over some aspects of the situation. Often, providing validation

for, and assistance with, the feelings associated with constant criticism and daunting demands are important supportive functions of the clinician. It may not be possible to modify the work situation, but helping the performer to gain perspective and realize that well-being and self-worth are not dependent on the opinions of others is crucial.

- Supportive counseling can be beneficial, and various techniques to assist with perfectionism can be used such as cognitive restructuring, positive affirmation, and visualizations.

## CAREER TRAJECTORY

In addition to issues of performance anxiety, the persistent insecurity of an uncertain career trajectory is perhaps the most anxiety-provoking factor experienced by many performing artists whose lives revolve around the constant search for work opportunities. Even the most successful performers cannot afford to become complacent as each performance is judged and evaluated. The popular saying "you are only as good as your last performance" demonstrates the sense of insecurity experienced by all performers and explains why the constant striving for a better performance is inherent in the profession. Unless they become a part of a theatre, ballet company, or an orchestra, performers wander from one gig to another. Even those who are lucky to obtain a stable job continue to face the noted above job-specific stressors.

An additional complicated factor in some of the performing arts domains is the inherent time limit in one's career. Although instrumentalists can perform well into their 80s, dancers and singers are aware from the onset of their career that when they age, retirement is inevitable regardless of their professional success. It is the tragedy of the performer that achieving mastery in the chosen art requires a complete dedication from a very early age and there is no guarantee that the artist will go on to develop a successful and self-sustaining career. This dedication occurs to the exclusion of other interests and leads to the development of a narrow sense of self. When an obstacle arises to prevent the fulfillment of the performer's goal either due to lack of success or an injury, a severe identify crisis occurs.[38] Moreover, other gifted artists might not even attempt to establish themselves for fear of failure, thus condemning themselves to a life of disappointment and unhappiness. Thus, it is not difficult to see why many performers struggle with symptoms of depression and anxiety throughout their careers.

## MANAGEMENT OF PROBLEMS RELATED TO CAREER ISSUES

There is not much a clinician can do when faced with a patient who continuously struggles with career issues other than be empathic and supportive. A clinical evaluation for severe depression and anxiety is required, and a referral to a performing art psychologist might be needed. If it becomes evident that the patient is facing career-ending issues, scrutiny of self-harm behavior is needed and appropriate measures must be taken. Connecting the artist with a career transition center might be helpful. There are centers in many countries, but they tend to be centrally located in a major city, and not throughout the country.

### Guidelines and Recommendations

- Identify the specific issue with which the artist is struggling.
- Evaluate risk and self-harm behavior.
- If the artist is facing termination of career issues, a frank discussion pertaining to other options is needed and often a referral to a vocational specialist is extremely beneficial and empowering.
- Make recommendations or referrals to available transition centers.

## DISORDERED EATING

Performing artists, especially those whose professional presentations aspire to an aesthetic ideal or body image are particularly vulnerable to disordered eating (e.g., anorexia nervosa, bulimia nervosa, and binge eating disorder). Environmental pressure, the demand for the elusive perfect performance and reliance on external evaluation combine to create an environment conducive to the development of this disorder.

Many performers work in environments in which thinness, overall image, flawless personal presentation, and eating behaviors are strongly influenced by culturally determined ideals of body image. Moreover, they may face great external pressures to conform to traditional professional ideals (e.g., the waif-like ballerina). Research tells us that perfectionism and perceived lack of control is closely associated with, and a risk factor for, disordered eating.[39,40] In dance, especially ballet, dancers learn early that the valued aesthetic ideal is thinness[41] and that it is rewarded.[42] For example, Garner, Garfinkel, Rockert, and Olmsted[43] reported that 25.7% of a sample of ballet dancers had anorexia nervosa. A more recent report by Ringham et al.[44] reported 83% in ballet dancers. Pressures from teachers, choreographers, parents, peers, and directors play a significant role in dancers' disordered eating.[45–48] There is a high incidence of disordered eating in musicians as well.[49]

## MANAGEMENT OF DISORDERED EATING

The many faces of disordered eating as well as the prevalence of this disorder create myriad opportunities for performers to neglect their bodies and hover below the radar of the detection of pathological behavior. Often, the performer is involved in a vicious cycle of disordered eating patterns, and a full-blown disorder is well entrenched before the performer seeks help. Alternatively, performers may not receive appropriate help until they have retired (and present with a significantly damaged body).

Once the performer arrives at the clinician's office, a supportive, nonjudgmental climate is important for helping the artist through the difficult process of self-revival. It is not easy to help individuals toward the road to recovery and go against a system that condones disordered eating. A diagnosis may bring the gravity of the situation to the attention of the performers and encourage participation in treatment, or they may retreat to the depths of denial. Confronting individuals with the truth of the dangers of the situation requires a balancing act of gentle persuasion to comply with treatment, encouraging healthy eating and conveying critical truths about the risks and dangerous health outcomes. Finding an appropriate program or developing a workable treatment plan can be very challenging for the practitioner. Unfortunately, few programs for treatment exist, and those with a specific focus on performing artists are virtually nonexistent.

A good referral network and familiarity with the range of community options is always a good management strategy. One of the challenges, of course, with performers is their rehearsal, performance, and touring schedules. Artists can be away for weeks or months, and access to suitable professionals is typically difficult. Larger dance companies or schools have physicians, psychiatrists, and psychologists available and often treat their members or students in-house. Most performers, however, do not have such resources easily available and do not have the money to engage health providers not covered by insurance systems.

## Guidelines and Recommendations

- Validate feelings and acknowledge the demanding and unique climate in which the performer is working.
- Maintain open and honest communication while providing support and a safe space. Artists will not continue with practitioners who do not provide supportive atmospheres and/or understand the unique circumstances of their profession.
- Often, it is useful to enlist the help of a friend, colleague, or family member to help the performer stay on track with the recommended plan.
- Develop and maintain a referral network that can provide access to counseling and programs that can be used with clients with disordered eating.
- Consult with colleagues who have expertise or experience with clients with disordered eating.
- Refrain from focus on weight or body mass index (BMI) and focus on the establishment of healthy behaviors and a supportive environment.

## INJURIES

Performing artists suffer a range of musculoskeletal injuries. Dancers and musicians tend to present with overuse or repetitive strain injuries related to their discipline.[50] Typically, artists either do not acknowledge their injuries or are reluctant to seek treatment because of fear of losing opportunities.[51] Often, injuries become chronic or recurrent, and they are managed solely by the performer with, at times, irreversible negative consequences. When performers finally do seek treatment, they are often faced with practitioners who either do not understand the nature and complexity of the injury, or the crucial and life sustaining importance of their profession (e.g., "just stop playing"). Many clinicians are unfamiliar with the technical demands of artistic performance, the culture of performance, and the ramifications of an injury. Consequently, artists feel misunderstood and do not trust medical practitioners. Only when the medical professional is sensitive to the specific demands and the unique demands of the profession can a rapport and working alliance be established. There are few specialty clinics for dancers, musicians, and actors; therefore, many injured performers, if they do seek treatment, choose a sports medicine clinic. Sports medicine practitioners are well aware of performance issues related to sports and athletics and the consideration needed in recovery and rehabilitation. Unfortunately, sport psychology consultants are not necessarily well informed of the specific demands of the performing arts professions and might not be able to help the performer.

Each artistic specialty has injury patterns unique to their instrument, genre, or physical demands. For example, professional singers are vulnerable to laryngeal pathologies,[52] ballet dancers to lower limb[53] and back injuries,[54,55] modern dancers to knee injuries,[56] and violinists to neck, shoulder, and temporomandibular joint injuries.[57] Age, posture, experience, and fitness also play a role in injury occurrence. Schafle, Requa, and Garrick[58] reported that in a sample of 3252 dancers, most injuries occurred in ballet, followed by aerobic dance and then modern dance, and most injuries occurred in 13−18 year olds. The majority of dancers, for example, have experienced injury.[56,59] Many suffer from unacknowledged psychological distress associated with injury impact and recovery.[5,51] Each profession has unique aspects related to performance rehearsals, touring, auditions, and performances that have significant bearing on how injuries might manifest and how they might be addressed. As not all companies have access to physicians or therapists to prevent and treat injuries, performers tend to cope with injuries in a personal way and continue to train, rehearse, and perform.[4] Few specialty clinics exist. Self-management strategies create their own issues, and a web of difficulties may arise secondary to the injury (e.g., substance abuse, other injuries, pain management, psychological distress, burnout, or exhaustion).

In addition to musculoskeletal injuries, performing artists are also vulnerable to mild traumatic brain injuries (mTBI) or concussion. Most research, to date, has focused on elite athletes, and we have little knowledge about the concussion prevalence and experience of performing artists. However, Russell and Daniell[60] recently reported that 67% of their sample of actors and theater technicians had experienced concussion. Although management of musculoskeletal injuries vary according to anatomical location and contemporary treatment guidelines, management of sport concussive injuries is currently informed by the most recent consensus statement from the Concussion in Sport Group.[61] The heterogeneity of concussions necessitates that each case is managed individually with reference to the literature on concussion in sport that has emerged in the last 30 years. Guidelines for managing concussion injuries in the performing arts are only just emerging.[60,62]

The physical impact of injury is obvious, but the psychological consequences are usually overlooked.

Despite over 30 years of research that clearly shows significant psychological sequelae, we tend to neglect the emotional and cognitive response to injury. This is especially true with concussion because of its invisible nature. Athletes and performers typically do not report concussions because of fear of being removed from activity. Moreover, psychological sequelae of mTBI are different from those of musculoskeletal injuries.[63]

## MANAGEMENT OF PSYCHOLOGICAL SEQUELAE FROM INJURY

Managing psychological sequelae of injuries requires the consideration of many factors, all of which cannot be addressed by medical practitioners. Practitioners need an awareness of the array of concerns identified by the research and how they play a role in recovery and return to activity, and how they may be managed. Management and treatment take many forms: In some cases, acknowledging the psychological sequelae and validating feelings may be sufficient to facilitate appropriate coping throughout recovery. In others, a referral to a psychologist, psychiatrist, mental health practitioner, or performance or sport psychology consultant may be warranted. The importance of the psychological aspects of injury is emphasized in the consensus statement by the American College of Sport Medicine,[64] and empirical research suggests that emotional sequelae of acute and chronic injuries should be addressed.[65,66] Furthermore, acknowledging and treating psychological sequelae of those who face career-ending injuries are important.[38]

### Guidelines and Recommendations

- Psychological recovery from injury may not coincide with physical recovery.
- Be familiar with and able to recognize the signs and symptoms of stress related to injury.
- Ask patients about or monitor their reactions, feelings and thoughts related to the injury and returning to activity. Fear of reinjury may be an undiagnosed factor in the ability to return to activity.
- Validate patients' feelings if they express them.
- Help the patient understand the injury and the process of recovery. Performers and athletes typically have keen kinesthetic senses, and they like to be informed about the injury and healing process.[67]
- Encourage the use of stress management techniques and make suggestions for either counseling or implementation of a few self-directed stress management strategies.

- In the case of child or youth performers, ensure that parents or guardians are informed about the injury and recovery process.
- Modified and Graduated Activity: Be aware that removing performers from their professional lives with recommendations of complete rest may be contraindicated to psychological well-being. If complete rest of a limb, for example, is required, then exercises for the opposing limb or mental rehearsal is valuable. Find ways to help the patient identify modifications and adaptations to activities to facilitate recovery, and develop a graduated return to activity schedule.[61] Performers and athletes will often ignore suggestions for complete rest and cessation of activity.
- Be cognizant that the social support networks for injured performers are tied to their profession. If artists are removed from activity, they are also estranged from their usual social supports.
- Establish a referral network to mental health practitioners or psychologists with expertise in performance or sport psychology and refer patients when appropriate. It may be important to refer during the course of rehabilitation or upon discharge for continued support in the recovery and reintegration process.

## BURNOUT AND DEPRESSION

Performing artists are particularly vulnerable to burnout. This is due to the demands and context of the work (long hours, years of training, job uncertainty, and lack of control and focus on achievement). Prolonged unresolvable work-related stress and a mismatch between personal resources and the unyielding job demands can lead to burnout.

Burnout is conceptualized as a three-dimensional syndrome comprising emotional exhaustion, cynicism or feelings of depersonalization, and a lack of perceived professional efficacy arising in response to chronic occupational stress.[68-71] Exhaustion involves feeling overextended, lacking energy, and emotionally drained in combination with low mood. Mental and physical fatigue is at the heart of burnout.[72] Cynicism manifests as being demotivated and feeling removed, withdrawn, or alienated from work. A sense of reduced performance, lack in professional efficacy, or diminished sense of accomplishments involves feelings of inadequacy, incompetence, and reduced self-confidence in relation to work achievements and demands.

Burnout has been studied extensively across most occupations except for the performing arts. It is deemed an increasingly serious issue in industrialized societies.[73-75]

The extent to which burnout overlaps with depression and is distinct has been explored recently[76,77] There is evidence, however, that the syndromes are distinct at a biological level. For example,[78,79] proinflammatory markers (high-sensitivity C-reactive protein and fibrinogen) in women were related to burnout and not depression; whereas, in men, the same markers were related to depression but not burnout. Toker et al. also showed that employees scoring the highest in burnout had a 79% increased risk of a coronary heart disease diagnosis over the course of the study.

Burnout affects individuals systemically: evidence is accumulating for neurologic dysfunction and difficulty to modulate emotions.[80] Gray matter volume reductions in the hippocampus, caudate, and putamen as well as cortical thinning of the medial prefrontal cortex are seen.[81] These brain structures serve memory, emotional functioning, and attention.[82] Neuroendocrine dysfunction is evident,[83] and burnout has been classified as a hypercortisolemic disorder.[84]

Burnout is not identified as a DSM-5 classification: It is recognized, however, in the International Classification of Diseases[85] as a factor that influences health and is defined as a *state of vital exhaustion* (coded Z73.0). Consequently, there is no formal recognition of burnout as a disorder.

## MANAGEMENT OF BURNOUT

Individual and group interventions can be beneficial for helping patients manage burnout. Stress management, mindfulness techniques, and support groups can be useful. Also, helping patients with mood and sleep disturbances is important because both are associated with burnout. In some cases, time off or a change in occupation or location may be appropriate. However, these options are not always possible for performers, and such suggestions will be met with resistance. Asking about nutrition is also a good idea because the demands and culture of the occupation, mixed with the exhaustion, often lead to disordered eating. Ensuring that the artist has support through the time it takes to come to terms with an appropriate course of action is critical.

### Guidelines and Recommendations

- Entertain differential diagnosis options given the overlap of burnout with depression. In some cases, it may not be easy or necessary to make the distinction unless a major depressive disorder warrants medication.

- Provide options for treatment, individual, or group-based support.
- Acknowledge and validate the stressors typically facing artists.
- Ask about social supports to ensure social isolation does not exacerbate the problem.
- Ask about eating and sleeping habits and make suggestions for improvement where applicable.
- Manage in similar ways to depressive disorders given the similarities.
- Refer the individual to a healthcare provider that can provide support and strategies to facilitate recovery.

## SUBSTANCE ABUSE

Substance use, misuse, and abuse intertwine in the lives of performing artists. Whether it is a predisposition for sensation seeking or a way of coping, artists can use different substances to manage the "snares and entanglements of their creative lifestyles (such as substance abuse and professional stress)."[86] Alcohol, tobacco, caffeine, cannabis, analgesics, stimulants, sleeping pills, and psychoactive drugs are readily available. Estimates of use vary among studies, but clear patterns emerge. Younger musicians and male musicians compared with older and female musicians[87] and nonclassical musicians compared with classical musicians[3] are more likely to report drug use. Alcohol use is more prevalent in musicians than the general population, and tobacco and marijuana use are also frequent.[88] Overall, alcohol is the most abused substance by musicians, and interestingly, alcohol is the substance most portrayed in television and film productions.[89]

Different patterns by genre and profession exist. Musicians involved in intense/rebellious genres such as heavy metal rock bands are more likely to be male, score high on sensation-seeking behaviors, and engage in substance use than nonperformers[88] and the general population.[90] In a comparative analysis of substance use in ballet, dancer sport, and synchronized swimming, binge drinking, cigarette smoking, appetite suppressants, and analgesics were used by all groups and binge drinking and smoking were positively correlated in the dance and swimmer groups.[91]

Cannabis use is also common among performing artists. In a prospective study using a representative sample of adults 18 years of age or older in the United States, Blanco et al.[92] found that cannabis use predicted incidence of substance use disorders (alcohol, nicotine, and other drugs), but not mood or anxiety disorders. A dose-response relationship showed that an increased frequency of cannabis use reported in an interview was associated with an increased likelihood of having a substance use disorder identified in a follow-up study 3 years after the initial interview. The legalizing of cannabis use across North America poses interesting questions about its use in the general population, and the performance world in the future.

Substance-related disorders include 10 separate classes of drugs according to the DSM-5[13]: alcohol, caffeine, cannabis, hallucinogens, inhalants, opioids, sedatives, hypnotics and anxiolytics, stimulants, and tobacco. Activation of the reward system in the brain is the mechanism by which many of the drugs or behavioral patterns (such as gambling and gaming) trigger reinforcement of behaviors. These substances "produce such an intense activation of the reward system that in normal activities may be neglected." (p. 481)[13] The intensity and stimulation of the performance environment, coupled with the use of drugs post-performance, create a cycle of repetitive behavior that can lead to exhaustion, addiction, and ultimately death.

Kenny and Asher[93] concluded, from their review of death records, that popular musicians had shorter lives than the general population and were more likely to die by suicide, homicide, a violent accident, substance overdose, or liver disease. Bellis, Hennell, Lushey, Hughes, Tocque, and Ashotn[94] reported that both North American and European pop stars, within 2 and 25 years of fame, tend to experience two to three times the risk of mortality expected in an average population matched by age, gender, and, for North America, ethnicity.

## MANAGEMENT OF SUBSTANCE ABUSE

Addressing and managing substance use, misuse, and abuse is challenging for clinicians. The inevitability of working with patients with substance use issues emphasizes the importance of management strategies. Performing artists may not acknowledge the use of substances or their misuse. Often, these behaviors are normalized in the performance subculture, and play a role in weight maintenance, stress management, and coping. Supporting performers in a non-judgmental fashion and providing them with appropriate resources is helpful, but structured persistent assistance is critical. Referrals to appropriate facilities or experts are necessary but sometimes difficult to organize.

Guidelines and recommendations for management follow.

## Guidelines and Recommendations:

- Establish a good rapport and safe environment for sensitive discussions about substance use and misuse.
- Recognize signs and symptoms of substance use and substance use disorder.
- Recognize that there may be multiple substance use and abuse issues at a time.
- Establish a referral network and treatment programs for referral options.
- Be aware that substance use is "normal" for performers and the legalization of alcohol and cannabis makes substance use less difficult and more acceptable.
- Substance use may be an indicator of maladaptive coping.
- Establish clear communication paths about the limits of confidentiality. Performers enjoy public attention related to their art but are quite private about personal issues.
- Develop or acquire educational tools and information (e.g., pamphlets, websites) about substance abuse and treatment options to share with patients.
- Acknowledge that the person needs to be motivated and ready to refrain from substance abuse and will need support.

## SUMMARY AND CONCLUSIONS

This chapter aims to provide the medical professional with insight into the struggles faced by performing artists. Issues such as performance anxiety, perfectionism, multiple career-related issues, substance abuse, disordered eating, coping with injuries, and identity problems are some of the unique challenges seen in the performing arts. Although artists might present with symptoms that warrant the diagnoses of depression and anxiety, it behooves the physician to understand the context and background of the artists' difficulties. Many artists are reluctant to seek medical or psychological help for fear that their difficulties, within the context of their profession, will not be understood. It is strongly recommended that physicians interested in working with this population learn about the profession and its demands if they want to help this uniquely creative and interesting population. Practitioner empathy, understanding, patience, and knowledge are the prerequisites for a successful treatment outcome.

## REFERENCES

1. Vaag J, Bjørngaard JH, Bjerkeset O. Symptoms of anxiety and depression among Norwegian musicians compared to the general workforce. *Psychol Music.* 2016;44(2): 234–248.
2. Maxwell I, Seton M, Szabo M. The Australian actors' well-being study. *About Perform.* 2015;13:69–112.
3. Raeburn SD, Hipple J, Delaney W, Chesky K. Surverying popular musicians' health status using convenience samples. *Med Probl Perform Art.* 2003;18(3):113–119.
4. Mainwaring L, Krasnow D, Kerr G. And the dance goes on: psychological impact of injury. *J Dance Med Sci Special Issue Dance Psychol.* 2001;5(4):105–115.
5. Mainwaring L, Finney C. Psychological risk factors and outcomes of dance injury: a systematic review. *J Dance Med Sci.* 2017;23(3):87–96.
6. Brandfonbrener AG. The forgotten patients. *Med Probl Perform Art.* 1992;7(4):101–102.
7. Kenny DT, Davis P, Oates J. Music performance anxiety and occupational stress among opera chorus artists and their relationship with state and trait anxiety and perfectionism. *J Anxiety Disord.* 2004;18:757–777.
8. Patston T, Osborne MS. The developmental features of music performance anxiety and perfectionism in school age music students. *Perform Enhancement Health.* 2016: 42–49.
9. Mor S, Day H, Flett G, Hewitt P. Perfectionism, control, and components of performance anxiety in professional artists. *Cognit Ther Res.* 1995;19(2):207–225.
10. Marchant-Haycox SE, Wilson GD. Personality and stress in performing artists. *Pers Indiv Diff.* 1992;13(10):1061–1068.
11. Salmon PG. A psychological perspective on musical performance anxiety: a review of the literature. *Med Probl Perform Art.* 1990;5:2–11.
12. Lederman RJ. Medical treatment of performance anxiety: a statement in favor. *Med Probl Perform Art.* 1999;14: 117–121.
13. American Psychiatric Association. *Diagnostic and Statistical Manual of Mental Disorders.* 5th ed. Washington, DC: American Psychiatric Association; 2013.
14. American Psychiatric Association. *Diagnostic and Statistical Manual of Mental Disorders.* 4th ed. Washington, DC: American Psychiatric Association; 1994.
15. Lewinsohn PM, Gotlib IH, Lewinsohn M, Seeley JR, Allen NB. Gender differences in anxiety disorders and anxiety symptoms in adolescents. *J Abnorm Psychol.* 1998; 107(1):109–117.
16. Huston JL. Familial antecedents of musical performance anxiety: a comparison with social anxiety. *Diss Abstr Int Sect B: Sci Eng.* 2001;62(1-B):551.
17. Osborne MS, Franklin J. Cognitive processes in music performance anxiety. *Aust J Psych.* 2002;54(2):86–93.
18. Hays K. *Performance Psychology in Action: A Casebook for Working with Athletes, Performing Artists, Business Leaders, and Professionals in High-risk Occupations.* Washington, DC: American Psychological Association; 2009.

19. Mor S. *On Stage, In Front of All These People: A Qualitative Analysis of Artists' Performance Stress*. 2015. Kyoto: Japan.

20. Clark DB, Agras WS. The assessment and treatment of performance anxiety in musicians. *Am J Psychiatry*. 1991;148: 598−605.

21. Harris SR. Brief cognitive-behavioural group counselling for musical performance anxiety. *Int Soc Study Tens Perform*. 1987;4:3−10.

22. Roland DJ. The development and evaluation of modified cognitive-behavioural treatment for musical performance anxiety. *Diss Abstr Int*. 1993:55.

23. Spahn C, Walther J-C, Nusseck M. The effectiveness of a multimodal concept of audition training for music students in coping with music performance anxiety. *Psychol Music*. 2016;4:893−909.

24. Steyn BJM, Steyn MH, Maree DJF, et al. Psychological skills and mindfulness training effects on the psychological well-being of undergraduate music students: an exploratory study. *J Psychol Africa*. 2016;26:167−171.

25. Thomas JP, Nettelbeck T. Performance anxiety in adolescent musicians. *Psychol Music*. 2014;42:624−634.

26. Bissonnette J, Dube F, Provencher MD, et al. Virtual reality exposure training for musicians: its effect on performance anxiety and quality. *Med Probl Perform Art*. 2015;30: 169−177.

27. Beder J. The 2017 musicians health survey results senza sordino. *Int Conf Symph Opera Music (ICSOM)*. 2017; 55(2).

28. Frost R, Marten P, Lahart C, Rosenblate R. The dimensions of perfectionism. *Cognit Ther Res*. 1990;14:449−468.

29. Mainwaring LM. *Performance Psychology in Action: A Casebook for Working with Athletes, Performing Artists, Business Leaders, and Professionals in High-risk Occupations*. Washington, DC: American Psychological Association; 2009:139−159.

30. Krasnow D, Mainwaring L, Kerr G. Injury, stress, and perfectionism in young dancers and gymnasts. *J Dance Med Sci*. 1999;3(2):51−58.

31. Hewitt PL, Flett GL. Dimensions of perfectionism in unipolar depression. *J Abnorm Psychol*. 1991;100:98−101.

32. Dunn JGH, Gotwals JK, Dunn JC. An examination of the domain speciflcity of perfectionism among intercollegiate student−athletes. *Pers Indiv Diff*. 2005;38(6): 1439−1448.

33. Dunn JGH, Craft JM, Causgrove Dunn J, Gotwals JK. Comparing a domain-specific and global measure of perfectionism in competitive female figure skaters. *J Sport Behav*. 2011;34(1):25−46.

34. Gotwals JK, Stoeber J, Dunn JGH, Stoll O. Are perfectionistic strivings in sport adaptive? A systematic review of confirmatory, contradictory, and mixed evidence. *Can Psychol*. 2012; 53:263−279. https://doi.org/10.1037/a0030288.

35. Nordin-Bates SM, Cumming J, Aways D, Sharp L. Imagining yourself dancing to perfection? Correlates of perfectionism among ballet and contemporary dancers. *J Clin Sport Psychol*. 2011;5(1):58−76.

36. Flett GL, Hewitt PL. The perils of perfectionism in sports and exercise. *Curr Dir Psychol Sci*. 2005;14(1):14−18.

37. Hill A. *The Psychology of Perfectionism in Sport, Dance and Exercise*. New York, NY: Routledge; 2016.

38. Mor S. Life after performance: the subjective experience of musicians who undergo career transition. *Proc Int Symp Perform Sci*. 2013:237−242.

39. Drusco R, Silverman J. Body image and perfectionism of ballerinas. *Gen Hosp Psych*. 1979;7:115−121.

40. Tyrka AR, Waldron I, Graber JA, Brooks-Gunn J. Prospective predictors of the onset of anorexic and bulimic syndromes. *Int J Eat Dis*. 2002;32(3):282−290.

41. Annus A, Smith GT. Learning experiences in dance class predict adult eating disturbance. *Eur Eat Dis Rev*. 2009; 17(1):50−60.

42. Benn T, Walters D. Between scylla and charybdis. Nutritional education versus body culture and the ballet aesthetic: the effects on the lives of female dancers. *Res Dance Edc*. 2001;2(2):139−154.

43. Garner DM, Garfinkel PE, Rockert W, Olmsted MP. A prospective study of eating disturbances in the ballet. *Psychother Psychosom*. 1987;48:170−175.

44. Ringham R, Klump K, Kaye W, et al. Eating disorder symptomatology among ballet dancers. *Int J Eat Dis*. 2006; 39(6):503−508.

45. Berry T, Howe H. Risk factors for disordered eating in female university athletes. *J Sport Behav*. 2000;23(3): 207−218.

46. de Bruin APK, Oudejans RRD, Bakker FC. Dieting and body image in aesthetic sports: a comparison of Dutch female gymnasts and non-aesthetic sport participants. *Psychol Sport Ex*. 2007;8(4):507−520.

47. Garner DM, Garfinkel PE. Socio-cultural factors in the development of anorexia nervosa. *Psychol Med*. 1980; 10(4):647−656.

48. Reel JJ, Jamieson KM, SooHoo S, Gill DL. Femininity to the extreme: body image concerns among college female dancers. *Women Sport Phys Act*. 2005;14(1):39−51.

49. Kaplinski ME, Easmon C. Eating disorders in musicians: a survey investigating self reported eating disorders of musicians. *Eat Weight Disord*. 2017:1−9.

50. Hincapié CA, Morton EJ, Cassidy JD. Musculoskeletal injuries and pain in dancers: a systematic review. *Arch Phys Med Rehabil*. 2008;89(1):819−829.

51. Mainwaring L, Kerr G, Krasnow D. Psychological correlates of dance injuries. *Med Probl Perform Art*. 1993;8(1):3−6.

52. Kwok M, Eslick GD. The impact of vocal and laryngeal pathologies among professional singers: a meta-analysis. *J Voice*. 2018. https://doi.org/10.1016/j.jvoice.2017.09.002.

53. Clanin DR, Davison DM, Plastino JG. *Injury Patterns in University Dance Students*. Champaign, IL: Human Kinetics; 1984.

54. Capel A, Medina FS, Medina D, Gómez S. Magnetic resonance study of lumbar disks in female dancers. *Am J Sports Med*. 2009;37:1208−1213.

55. Garrick JG, Requa RK. An analysis of epidemiology and financial outcome. *Am J Sports Med.* 1993;21(4):586—590.
56. Kerr G, Krasnow D, Mainwaring L. The nature of dance injuries. *Med Probl Perform Art.* 1992;7(1):25.
57. Moraes GFS, Antunes AP. Musculoskeletal disorders in professional violinists and violists. Systematic review. *Acta Ortop Bras.* 2012;20(1):43—47.
58. Schafle M, Requa R, Garrick J. *A Comparison of Patterns of Injury in Ballet, Modern, and Aerobic Dance.* Reston, VA: American Alliance for Health, Physical Education, Recreation and Dance; 1990:1—14.
59. Macchi R, Crossman J. After the fall: reflections of injured classical ballet dancers. *J Sport Behav.* 1996;19(3): 221—234.
60. Russell J, Daniell B. Concussion in theater: a cross-sectional survey of prevalence and management in actors and theater technicians. *J Occup Environ Med.* 2018; 60(3):205—210.
61. McCrory P, Meeuwisse W, Dvorak J, et al. Consensus statement on concussion in sport - the 5 th international conference on concussion in sport held in Berlin, October 2016. *Br J Sports Med.* 2017;51.
62. Senthinathan A, Mainwaring L. Concussion consequences and steps to recovery for dancers. In: *Poster Presented at 24th International Association for Dance Medicine & Science Annual Conference, Basel, Switzerland.* 2014.
63. Mainwaring L, Hutchison M, Bisschop S, Comper P, Richards D. Athletes' emotional response to sport concussion compared to ACL injury. *Brain Inj.* 2010;24(4): 589—597.
64. American College of Sports Medicine. Psychological issues related to injury in athletes and the team physician: a consensus statement—2016 update. *Curr Sports Med Rep.* 2017;16(3):189—201.
65. Mainwaring L, Comper P, Hutchison M, Richards D. Examining emotional sequelae of sport concussion. *J Clin Sport Psychol Spec Ed.* 2012;6(3):247—274.
66. Mainwaring L. Psychological factors and sport related concussion. In: Echemendia R, Iverson GL, eds. *The Oxford Handbook of Sport-related Concussion.* New York: Oxford University Press; 2017 [chapter 27].
67. Mainwaring LM. Restoration of self: a model for the psychological response of athletes to knee injuries. *Can J Rehabil.* 1999;12(3):145—156.
68. Maslach C, Jackson SE. The measurement of experienced burnout. *J Org Behav.* 1981;2(2):99—113.
69. Maslach C, Jackson SE. *Maslach Burnout Inventorymanual.* 2nd ed. Palo Alto, CA: Consulting Psychologists Press; 1986.
70. Maslach C, Jackson SE, Leiter MP. *Maslach Burnout Inventory Manual.* 3rd ed. Palo Alto, CA: Consulting Psychologists Press; 1996.
71. Maslach C, Schaufeli WB, Leiter MP. Job burnout. *Ann Rev Psychol.* 2001;52(1):397—422.
72. Cox T, Tisserand M, Taris T. The conceptualization and measurement of burnout: questions and directions. *Work Stress.* 2005;19(3):187—191.
73. Canadian Institute for Health Information. *Canada's Health Care Providers.* Ottawa, Canada: Publisher; 2002.
74. Jamal M, Baba VV. Job stress and burnout among Canadian managers and nurses: an empirical examination. *Can J Public Health.* 2000;91(6):454.
75. West M, Dawson J. Employee engagement and NHS performance. *King's Fund.* 2012;1:23.
76. Bianchi R, Schonfeld IS, Laurent E. Is burnout a depressive disorder? A re-examination with special focus on atypical depression. *Int J Stress Manage.* 2014;21(4):307—324.
77. Bianchi R, Schonfeld IS, Laurent E. Burnout-depression overall: a review. *Clin Psychol Rev.* 2015;36:28—41.
78. Toker S, Shapira I, Berliner S, Melamed S, Shirom A. The association between burnout, depression, anxiety, and inflammation biomarkers: C-reactive protein and fibrinogen in men and women. *J Occup Health Psychol.* 2005; 10(4):344—362.
79. Toker S, Melamed S, Berliner S, Zeltser D, Shapira I. Burnout and risk of coronary heart disease: a prospective study of 8838 employees. *Psychol Med.* 2012;74(8): 840—847.
80. Golkar A, Johansson E, Kasahara M, Osika W, Perski A, Savic I. The influence of work-related chronic stress on the regulation of emotion and on functional connectivity in the brain. *PLoS One.* 2014;9(9):e104550.
81. Savic I. Structural changes of the brain in relation to occupational stress. *Cereb Cortex.* 2015;25(6):1554—1564.
82. Deligkaris P, Panagopoulou E, Montgomery AJ, Masoura E. Job burnout and cognitive functioning: a systematic review. *Work Stress.* 2014;28:107—123.
83. Oosterholt BG, Maes JH, Van der Linden D, Verbraak MJ, Kompier MA. Burnout and cortison: evidence for a lower cortisol awakening response in both clinical and nonclinical burnout. *J Psychol Res.* 2015;78:445—451.
84. Chida Y, Steptoe A. Cortisol awakening response and psychosocial factors: a systematic review and meta-analysis. *Biol Psychol.* 2009;80:265—278.
85. World Health Organization. *The ICD-10 Classification of Mental and Behavioural Disorders: Clinical Descriptions and Diagnostic Guidelines.* 1992.
86. Egan V, Beech A, Burrow L. *Psychotherapy, Literature and the Visual and Performing Arts, Palgrave Studies in Creativity and Culture.* 2018.
87. Chesky K, Hipple J. Musicians' perceptions of widespread drug use among muscians. *Med Probl Perform Art.* 1999; 14(4):187—195.
88. Miller KE, Quigley BM. Sensaton-seeking, performance genres and substance use among musicians. *Psychol Music.* 2011;40(4):389—410.
89. Roberts DF, Christenson PG. *"Here's Looking at You, Kid": Alcohol, Drugs, and Tobacco in Entertainment Media. A Literature Review Prepared for the National Center on Addiction and Substance Abuse a T Columbia University.* New York: National Center on Addiction and Substance Abuse; 2000.
90. Butkovic A, Dopudj DR. Personality traits and alcohol consumption of classical and heavy metal musicians. *Psychol Music.* 2017;45(2):246—256.

91. Zenic N, Peric M, Zubcevic NG, Ostojic Z, Ostojic L. Comparitive analysis of substance use in ballet, dance sport, and synchronized swimming: results of a longitudinal study. *Med Probl Perform Art.* 2010;25(2):75–81.

92. Blanco C, Hasin DS, Wall MM, et al. Cannabis use and risk of psychiatric disorders prospective evidence from a US national longitudinal Study. *JAMA Psychol.* 2016;73(4):388–395.

93. Kenny DT, Asher A. Life expectancy and cause of death in popular musicians: is the popular musician lifestyle the road to ruin? *Med Probl Perform Art.* 2016;31(1):37–44.

94. Bellis MA, Hennell T, Lushey C, Hughes K, Tocque K, Ashton JR. Elvis to eminem: quantifying the price of fame through early mortality of european and North American rock and pop stars. *J Epidemiol Community Health.* 2007;61(10):896–901.

CHAPTER 17

# Healthcare for the Vocal Performing Artist

JAYME ROSE DOWDALL, MD

## INTRODUCTION

There is increasing interest in the care of the vocalist in the popular press. News of concert cancellations or tour postponement is becoming more frequent.[1] Despite the increased public awareness of vocal health concerns, the understanding of the total health needs of the vocal athlete is still evolving. Despite this evolution, there is great demand for clinical services, as 46% of singers experience self-reported dysphonia over their careers according to a recent meta-analysis.[2] This chapter will serve as an overview and include additional resources.

A recent survey was designed to assess the vocal health needs of performing artists. This study was consistent with prior manuscripts as upwards of 55% of performers surveyed noted voice complaints over the prior year. Weekly et al. found that 24% of performers with a vocal complaint did not seek medical attention when this occurred. The most common reason for abstaining from medical attention was that the concern was self-limited. For those that did seek care, over 50% of the vocalists surveyed sought care within 2 weeks (Fig. 17.1).[3] In a study that included both vocal performers (approximately 1/3) and nonperformers with voice complaints (approximately 2/3) the patients waited on average of 3 months from the onset of symptoms to initial evaluation.[4] This suggests future work is necessary to elucidate the unique needs that performers may have for timely access to healthcare providers for evaluation.

## EVALUATION OF THE VOCAL PERFORMING ARTIST

Weekly et al. noted that in addition to singing, many of the professional voice users used their voice

professionally in other ways within their roles as voice teachers, actors, vocal coaches, and music directors.[3] In addition to assessing the vocal load when singing, practitioners must inquire about other professional responsibilities and social responsibilities. The patient history form in Dr. Sataloff's text *Professional Voice, Fourth Edition: The Science and Art of Clinical Care, 3-Volume Set* includes a detailed template for the assessment of the vocal performer.[5] When performing vocalists do access healthcare, the initial diagnosis for a voice disorder is often incorrect in a nonspecialty setting.[4] It is theorized that this is due to a lack of state-of-the-art equipment such as videostroboscopy and/or the absence of subspecialty expertise. Common

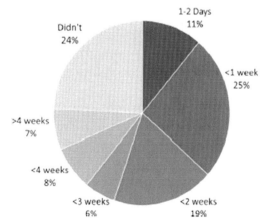

FIG. 17.1 Length of time until vocal performing artists sought medical care. (Reproduced from Weekly EM, Carroll LM, Korovin GS, Fleming R. A vocal health survey among amateur and professional voice users. *J Voice*. 2017. doi: 10.1016/j.jvoice.2017.07.012.)

Performing Arts Medicine. https://doi.org/10.1016/B978-0-323-58182-0.00017-1

**163**

symptoms prompting a vocalist to seek care include voice change accompanied by pain or vocal strain, a decrease in vocal range, an increase in vocal effort. The diagnosis of a voice disorder is made by history, vocal quality findings on physical exam, and endoscopic evaluation of the larynx. Stroboscopic examination yields information about the vibratory properties of the vocal folds. In the healthcare setting, the vocal performing artist is at the center of the team. The team may include many members including voice teacher, director, speech-language pathologist, and laryngologist (Figs. 17.2 and 17.3).[6] Dr. Rubin's book *The Vocal Pitstop: Keeping Your Voice on Track* serves as an excellent guide for artists navigating the healthcare system when vocal difficulty occurs.

Although performing arts medicine has emerged as a subspecialty of clinical practice over the past two decades, there are few clinicians who are familiar with the unique needs of the performer.[7] The knowledge gaps of healthcare providers serving performing vocalists in a college health setting are just now starting to be understood. Many performing singers identify as a student or a teacher. For example, in Massachusetts alone, 31 colleges and universities offer music as a major. In addition to formal coursework, there are numerous productions and an estimated 53 collegiate *a capella* choirs in the Boston area alone. In

a web-based survey of college health providers to identify their clinical approach to vocal performers, we found that 36% of respondents incorrectly identified appropriate vocal hygiene measures, 56% failed to identify symptoms suggestive of a vocal hemorrhage, and 84% failed to identify indications for referral to a voice specialist.[8] This pilot study suggests that there are educational opportunities for healthcare providers who may encounter vocal performers to lead to appropriate referral to facilitate correct diagnosis and team-based treatment. These knowledge gaps may account for the change in diagnosis once vocalists are able to obtain specialty care. Indeed, even when students do not note vocal difficulty, a high percentage of organic lesions are noted on baseline examinations.[9] Students may be a particularly vulnerable patient population in which many choose to seek care from a voice teacher rather than an otolaryngologist.[3] More research into the healthcare needs of vocal performers is needed.

The vocal evaluation in the clinical setting is not limited to the larynx. Providers assess the sound and quality of the singing and speaking voices and posture. Providers also integrate patient history, potential medication side-effects, and evaluate the entire unified airway. The voice is powered by the lungs, the larynx serves as the vibratory source, and the sound is filtered through the vocal tract above the larynx. For additional reading on the anatomy and physiology of vocal mechanics, Dr. Sataloff's text provides detail.[5] Therefore, pathology can occur in many other parts of the body outside the larynx and result in voice disturbance. Indeed, common causes of respiratory illness such as infections, allergies, and irritant exposures are common causes of dysphonia. The repetitive stress of repeated vocalization can lead to dysphonia in hours, even in trained singers.[10] A wonderful overview of occupational considerations for vocalists can be found in the "voice" section of the article entitled *Occupational Health and the Performing Arts: An Introduction* by Hinkamp et al.[10]

For the evaluation of vocal fold vibration, visualizing the laryngeal mucosal wave with a stroboscopic examination is the gold standard. This is performed with or without topical anesthesia. This can also be performed via ridged transoral examination or flexible transnasal evaluation. Both techniques may be used as they each add unique diagnostic information to arrive at the correct diagnosis.[11] Vocal fold lesions in vocalists are most often benign and relate to phonotrauma, the repetitive stress of vocalizing. Vocal fold edema may arise from many causes that impact the entire upper

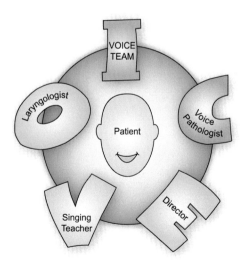

FIG. 17.2 Team approach to vocal health. (Reproduced from Rubin AD, Errico M, Livingston R. *The Vocal Pitstop: Keeping Your Voice on Track.* Compton Publishing Ltd; 2014.)

aerodigestive tract including throat clearing from laryngopharyngeal reflux and allergies or coughing with laryngitis from viral, fungal, or bacterial infections. This is further complicated by the impact of these conditions on the pulmonary drive as well as the constriction of the nasal passages. Mucosal inflammation often occurs along the course of the entire unified airway that disrupts the ability of the nose to properly humidify and condition the air and also disrupts mucocilliary transport.

Vocal emergencies in performing artists are particularly concerning. Voice change, particularly one that is sudden in onset and occurs while phonating, is a symptom that can be a sign of vocal fold hemorrhage or mucosal tear. Other signs and symptoms prompting evaluation include voice change accompanied by discomfort, increased vocal effort, or decrease in the top end of the range when singing softly. A delay in onset when vocalizing can indicate swelling or the development of a vocal lesion.[12] The optimal healthcare of a vocal performer in this situation includes a full vocal evaluation with videostroboscopic examination.[12] Vocal fold hemorrhage is the primary concern when vocal trouble presents prior to a performance. In addition to blood within the vocal fold, the mucosa can tear. Different from a vocal fold hemorrhage, this is not as easily visualized on an examination and can be quite difficult to diagnose. Laryngitis/vocal fold edema can be attributed to many causes of inflammation in the upper aero-digestive tract. As vocal production is driven by the lungs, the vibration is produced by the larynx and is shaped by the pharynx and sinonasal cavity, and the treatment paradigms are holistic and address not only the laryngeal pathology but also treat the upper aero-digestive tract (Fig. 17.3).[12] Acute vocal change can also occur with a background of preexisting benign vocal fold lesions that were present when the singer was in good voice. Due to the high baseline presence of vocal fold findings, determining the appropriate diagnosis in the acute or emergent setting can be challenging. Other variables on a tour or during a show include sleep disruption, dietary changes, travel, new costumes, dust, and irritant exposure from special effects and the addition of choreography and footwear. All of these factors may impact the vocal mechanism. Increased speaking voice commitments such as press obligations, speaking with fans after performances, or cast parties can also increase the speaking voice vocal load. Many vocalists also play instruments, dance, have acting roles, and perform in various venues with acoustical properties that differ from rehearsal or studio spaces. In addition to vocal fold edema, other findings

| Vocal fold hemorrhage |
| Vocal fold mucosal tear |
| Acute laryngitis |
|     Viral |
|     Bacterial |
|     Fungal |
|     Phonotraumatic edema |
| Acute edema on chronic fibrovascular (subepithelial) change/preexisting lesions |
| Asthma exacerbation |
| Upper respiratory tract infection |
|     Pharyngitis, viral/bacterial |
|     Rhinosinusitis, viral/bacterial |
|     Bronchitis, viral/bacterial |
| Allergic rhinitis |
| LPR exacerbation |
| Hormonal/endocrine changes |

FIG. 17.3 Differential diagnosis of vocal emergencies in performers. (Reproduced from Klein AM, Johns MM. Vocal emergencies. *Otolaryngol Clin North Am*. 2007;40: 1063–1080.)

at baseline and in the acute setting commonly found in vocal performers include nodules, polyps, vocal fold cysts, varices, and scar tissue. Stage performances themselves have been observed to cause reduction in vocal quality over time that was not overcome by voice hygiene measures.[13]

## TREATMENT OF DYSPHONIA IN PERFORMING ARTISTS

Thankfully, surgery for benign vocal fold lesions in performers is now seen as a last result. Medical management includes treatment of the underlying source of inflammation with either medical management, dietary, and lifestyle changes or medication. For example, laryngopharyngeal reflux can be treated with dietary changes alone or in combination with H2-blocker and proton pump inhibitors. Allergic symptoms can be treated by avoidance of the allergen, topical nasal steroids, oral antihistamines, or immunotherapy. Special consideration is given to the side-effect profile of the proposed medication. The side-effects are not often systemically dangerous but will produce changes vocal performers note impact their vocal effort, range, and muscle tension. The common medication side effect of dryness can have a large impact on a singer. A comprehensive list of medications and their impact on the voice is provided by the National Center for Voice & Speech and is readily accessible on their website for easy reference.[14] Voice rest is also recommended at times. A specific diagnosis is recommended prior to vocal rest greater than 48 hours due to the negative impact voice rest can have in many domains. Voice rest is commonly used to treat vocal fold edema and to decrease mechanical strain on the vocal folds in the setting of a resolving vocal fold hemorrhage. Although most of the recent studies on vocal rest are in the postoperative setting, there are many shared challenges when voice

rest is recommended without surgical management. It is important to note that during voice rest, patients consistently report a negative quality of life, changes in social interaction, communication difficulties, and inability to work.[15] Patients generally also face challenges that result in decreased compliance with

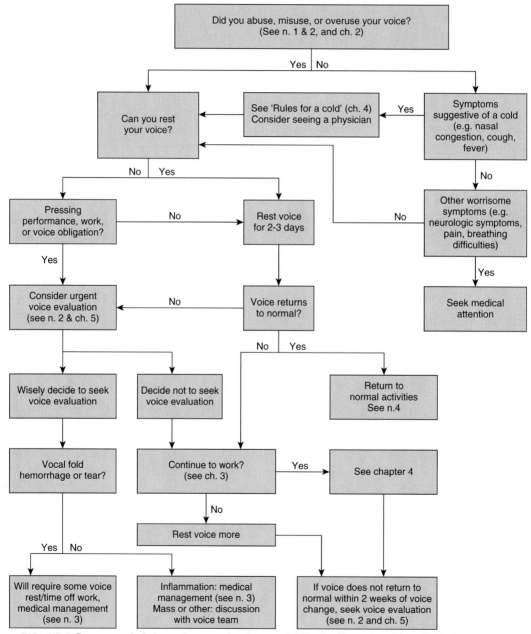

FIG. 17.4 Recommended steps when experiencing vocal difficulty. (Reproduced from Rubin AD, Errico M, Livingston R. *The Vocal Pitstop: Keeping Your Voice on Track*. Compton Publishing Ltd; 2014.)

recommended voice rest. The average duration of recommended voice rest is on the order of a week in the postoperative setting. In a study by Rousseau et al., the mean duration of voice rest was 8.8 days.[15] Vocal rest or restraint may also result in dysphonia due to deconditioning or pathology due to a change in vocal mechanics. Singing voice therapy has been demonstrated to benefit singers, the duration of treatment and the criteria for a handoff between speech-language pathologists in the rehabilitative setting and singing voice specialists or singing teachers in the habilitative setting is evolving.[16] Organizations such as American Speech-Language-Hearing Association (ASHA)[17] and Pan-American Vocology Association (PAVA)[18] are providing additional guidance as we learn more. A paradigm for seeking care when experiencing voice difficulty is found in The Vocal Pitstop: Keeping your Voice on Track (Fig. 17.4).

The mainstay of treatment for vocal fold nodules and polyps is behavioral modification with voice therapy. If patients do not respond to voice therapy, surgery can be considered in conjunction with medical optimization, postoperative vocal rest, and continued postoperative voice therapy.[19–21]

In conclusion, the needs of a vocal performer are unique in the healthcare setting. Several common conditions and best practices have been well described in the literature. Due to the increased prevalence of dysphonia in vocal performers compared to the general population, additional investigation is warranted. Many factors including barriers to seeking healthcare, knowledge gaps in providers who encounter vocal performing artists, and optimal treatment paradigms are evolving. It is encouraging that many researchers and organizations are striving to improve our shared understanding of how to meet the needs of this patient population.

## REFERENCES

1. Warner B. *Why Do Stars like Adele Keep Losing Their Voice?* The Guardian; 2017.
2. Pestana PM, Vaz-Freitas S, Manso MC. Prevalence of voice disorders in singers: systematic review and meta-analysis. *J Voice*. 2017;31:722−727.
3. Weekly EM, Carroll LM, Korovin GS, Fleming R. A vocal health survey among amateur and professional voice users. *J Voice*. 2017. https://doi.org/10.1016/j.jvoice.2017.07.012.
4. Keesecker SE, Murry T, Sulica L. Patterns in the evaluation of hoarseness: time to presentation, laryngeal visualization, and diagnostic accuracy. *Laryngoscope*. 2015;125:666−673.
5. Sataloff RT. *Professional Voice, Fourth Edition: The Science and Art of Clinical Care, 3-Volume Set*. Plural Publishing; 2017.
6. Rubin AD, Errico M, Livingston R. *The Vocal Pitstop: Keeping Your Voice on Track*. Compton Publishing Ltd; 2014.
7. Petty BE. Health information-seeking behaviors among classically trained singers. *J Voice*. 2012;26:330−335.
8. McKinnon-Howe L, Dowdall J. Identifying knowledge gaps in clinicians who evaluate and treat vocal performing artists in college health settings. *J Voice*. 2018;32:385.e7−385.e15.
9. D'haeseleer E, Claeys S, Meerschman I, et al. Vocal characteristics and laryngoscopic findings in future musical theater performers. *J Voice*. 2017;31:462−469.
10. Hinkamp D, Morton J, Krasnow DH, et al. Occupational health and the performing arts: an introduction. *J Occup Environ Med*. 2017;59:843−858.
11. Paul BC, Chen S, Sridharan S, Fang Y, Amin MR, Branski RC. Diagnostic accuracy of history, laryngoscopy, and stroboscopy. *Laryngoscope*. 2013;123:215−219.
12. Klein AM, Johns MM. Vocal emergencies. *Otolaryngol Clin North Am*. 2007;40:1063−1080.
13. Rangarathnam B, Paramby T, McCullough GH. "Prologues to a bad voice": effect of vocal hygiene knowledge and training on voice quality following stage performance. *J Voice*. 2018;32:300−306.
14. NCVS: Giving Voice to America. Available from: http://www.ncvs.org/rx.html. (Accessed: 1st June 2018)
15. Rousseau B, Cohen SM, Zeller AS, Scearce L, Tritter AG, Garrett CG. Compliance and quality of life in patients on prescribed voice rest. *Otolaryngol Head Neck Surg*. 2011;144:104−107.
16. Dastolfo-Hromack C, Thomas TL, Rosen CA, Gartner-Schmidt J. Singing voice outcomes following singing voice therapy. *Laryngoscope*. 2016;126:2546−2551.
17. Stadelman-Cohen T, Burns J, Zeitels S, Hillman R. Team management of voice disorders in singers. *ASHA Lead*. 2009;14:12−15.
18. Pan-american Vocology Association: https://pava24.wildapricot.org/About-Us—About Us.
19. Johns MM. Update on the etiology, diagnosis, and treatment of vocal fold nodules, polyps, and cysts. *Curr Opin Otolaryngol Head Neck Surg*. 2003;11:456−461.
20. Jeong W-J, Lee SJ, Lee WY, Chang H, Ahn S-H. Conservative management for vocal fold polyps. *JAMA Otolaryngol Neck Surg*. 2014;140:448.
21. Bohlender J. Diagnostic and therapeutic pitfalls in benign vocal fold diseases. *GMS Curr Top Otorhinolaryngol Head Neck Surg*. 2013;12.

# Index

*Note:* Page numbers followed by "f" indicate figures, "t" indicate tables.

Radial-sided wrist pain, 22
Radiocarpal or wrist arthritis, 22
Range of motion, 145–146
  range of motion/flexibility, 109–110
Range of movement (ROM), 90, 135
RD. *See* Registered dietician (RD)
Rectus femoris, 79–80
RED-S. *See* Relative Energy Deficiency
  in Sport (RED-S)
Regenerative medicine techniques,
  93
Registered dietician (RD), 15–17
Rehabilitation, 102
Relative Energy Deficiency in Sport
  (RED-S), 17, 77, 100, 117,
  119–122, 139
  amenorrhea, 120
  bone effects of low EA and
    amenorrhea, 120–121
  decreased EA, 119–120
  health and performance
    consequences, 121f
Repetitive motion/overuse, 2
Resistance training, 102
Respiratory sinus arrhythmia (RSA),
  36–37
Resting metabolic rate (RMR), 121
Return-to-dance strategies and
  guidelines
  dance medicine rehabilitation
    progression protocol, 139–141,
    140t
  dance-specific movement, 146–147
  independence, 147–148
  initial assessment, 141–143
    dance-specific history, 141
    dance-specific special tests and
      considerations, 142
    establishing diagnosis and injury-
      specific protocols, 141
    mental health, 142–143
    musculoskeletal evaluation, 141
    nutrition, 143
  injury management, 143–144
  progression, 144–146
    flexibility, 145
    range of motion, 145–146
    stability, 145
    strengthening, 144–145
  return to rehearsal, 147
    dance-specific environment, 147
    dynamic warm-up, active recovery
      cool down, 147
    involving artistic director or
      teacher, 147
Return-to-play program, 28
Rheumatoid arthritis, 21–22
Rhythm and cadence progression, 146
Riverdance production, 10
RMR. *See* Resting metabolic rate
  (RMR)
ROM. *See* Range of movement (ROM)
Rotator cuff dysfunction, 23–24
Royal Academy of Dance, 9

RSA. *See* Respiratory sinus arrhythmia
  (RSA)
Rupture
  achilles tendon, 68
  distal biceps tendon, 23
  hamstring tendons, 81
  ligament, 28
  STT arthritis, 22
  tendon, 22

**S**
Sacroiliac joint, 93
Sagittal band insufficiency, 21–22
Sartorius, 79–80
Scapular region, 23–24
Scapulothoracic dyskinesis, 59
Scoliosis, 91
Screening, 101–102, 131
Screening professional dancers
  benefits of screening, 106
  factors significant to success, 106
  health, 107–108
  location of screening assessments,
    106–107
  objectives of screening, 105–106
  physical assessment, 108–112
    alignment and posture, 108
    balance, 111
    cardiovascular fitness, 108–109
    functional testing, 111–112
    height, weight, and BMI, 108
    hypermobility, 110
    range of motion/flexibility,
      109–110
    strength, 110–111
    technique, 112
  recommendations, 112–114
  screening potential for research, 114
  standardizing screening tool, 107
Sedentary behaviors and sleep,
  99–100
sEMG. *See* Surface electromyography
  (sEMG)
Serum 25-OH vitamin D, 123
Sesamoid injuries, 71–72
Sever's disease, 68–69
Shoulder, 23–24
Show bands. *See* Traditional style
  marching bands
Sleep, sedentary behaviors and,
  99–100
"Snapping hip", 80
SNS. *See* Sympathetic nervous system
  (SNS)
Somatosensory system, 111
SoundSport, 55–56
Spondylolysis, 91–93
Sports hernia. *See* Athletic pubalgia
Sports medicine
  AATA, 4–6, 4t
  issue, 1–3
  practice and performance in
    perspective, 3–4
Star Excursion Test, 111

Steida process, 65–66
Strength
  physical assessment, 110–111
  training, 102
Stress, 36
  fractures, 69–70, 77–78
  "Stress–Portrait of Killer", 36
Subluxation, 22
Subspine impingement, 79
Substance abuse, 158
  guidelines and recommendations,
    159
Supercompensation process, 131
Supramaximal intensity, 133
Surface electromyography (sEMG),
  38–39
Swan neck deformity, 21–22
Swelling management, 143
Sympathetic nervous system (SNS),
  37

**T**
T3. *See* Triiodothyronine (T3)
Tap, 10
Tears
  of anterior band of ulnar collateral
    ligament, 23
  of lateral collateral ligament complex,
    22–23
Temporary threshold shift (TTS),
  45–46
  to discussing in two time periods,
    46–47
Tennis elbow. *See* Lateral epicondylitis
Tension-sided stress fractures, 77–78
Tensor fascia lata (TFL), 81
TFCC sprain, 22
TFL. *See* Tensor fascia lata (TFL)
Theater, background on, 10
Thomasen test, 67
Thoracic outlet syndrome,
  symptomatic, 24–25
Thumb, 21
Thyroid problems, 105–106
TIBC. *See* Total iron binding capacity
  (TIBC)
Tibio-femoral rotation, 13
"Tight hypermobile", 90
Tinnitus retraining therapy (TRT),
  49–50
Tobacco and substance use, 101
Total iron binding capacity (TIBC),
  123
Traditional style marching bands,
  57–58
Triceps tendonitis, 23
Trigger thumb, 21
Triggering, 21–22
Triiodothyronine (T3), 120–121
Trombone, 27
Trombonists, female, 27
TRT. *See* Tinnitus retraining therapy
  (TRT)
Trumpet, 27

Printed in the United States
By Bookmasters